"THE CADDO NATION"

Texas Archaeology and Ethnohistory Series

THOMAS R. HESTER, EDITOR

"THE CADDO NATION"

ARCHAEOLOGICAL

AND ETHNOHISTORIC

PERSPECTIVES

---

by Timothy K. Perttula

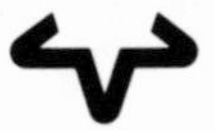

UNIVERSITY OF TEXAS PRESS, AUSTIN

Printed in the United States of America

First edition, 1992

Requests for permission to reproduce material from this work should be sent to Permissions, University of Texas Press, Box 7819, Austin, TX 78713-7819.

♾The paper used in this publication meets the minimum requirements of American National Standard for Information Sciences—Permanence of Paper for Printed Library Materials, ANSI Z39.48-1984.

LIBRARY OF CONGRESS CATALOGING-IN-PUBLICATION DATA

Perttula, Timothy K.

"The Caddo nation" : archaeological and ethnohistoric perspectives / by Timothy K. Perttula. — 1st ed.

p. cm. — (Texas archaeology and ethnohistory series)

Includes bibliographical references (p.) and index.

ISBN 0-292-71150-6 (alk. paper)

1. Caddoan Indians—First contact with Europeans. 2. Caddoan Indians—History—Sources. 3. Caddoan Indians—Antiquities. 4. Ethnohistory—Southern States. 5. Epidemics—Southern States—History—Sources. 6. Southern States—Antiquities. I. Title.

II. Series.

E99.C13P47 1992

976'.01—dc20

91-46225

CIP

To Alex D. Krieger

CADDOAN ORIGIN MYTH

They came from under the ground through the mouth of a cave in a hill which they call Cha'kani'nă, "The place of crying," on a lake close to the south bank of Red River, just at its junction with the Mississippi. In those days men and animals were all brothers and all lived together under the ground. But at last they discovered the entrance to the cave leading up to the surface of the earth, and so they decided to ascend and come out. First an old man climbed up, carrying in one hand fire and a pipe and in the other a drum. After him came his wife, with corn and pumpkin seeds. Then followed the rest of the people and the animals. All intended to come out, but as soon as the wolf had climbed up he closed the hole, and shut up the rest of the people and animals under the ground, where they still remain. Those who had come out sat down and cried a long time for their friends below, hence the name of the place. Because the Caddo came out of the ground they call it ină, "mother," and go back to it when they die. Because they have had a pipe and the drum and the corn and pumpkins since they have been a people, they hold fast to these things and have never thrown them away.

From this place they spread out towards the west, following up the course of Red River, along which they made their principal settlements. For a long time they lived on Caddo Lake, on the boundary between Louisiana and Texas, their principal village on the lake being called Sha'chidĭ'ni, "Timber hill."

—J. MOONEY
The Ghost-Dance Religion, and the Sioux Outbreak of 1890

Contents

Illustrations

Tables

Preface

Contact between Europeans and native Americans in the New World has over the last five hundred years forever changed the cultural and social character of both peoples. This interaction, which continues today in a multiplicity of ways, has left in its wake unprecedented and catastrophic native American population losses and dispossession of traditional homelands. The ideas, people, and products from Europe and the United States that have been thereby introduced have altered in many ways the traditional nature of native American lifeways. At the same time, this contact has called attention to the rich cultural heritage of native Americans, to the strength of their spirituality and beliefs, and to the tenacity with which they have held to their traditional homelands and way of life in the face of unwavering and unrelenting cultural contact.

I examine here through archaeological, historical, ethnographic, and archival means the nature of contact and interaction between the Caddoan Indian peoples of Texas, Louisiana, Oklahoma, and Arkansas and Europeans—especially the Spanish and French—and the Euro-Americans. The Caddoan Indian peoples lived in the region for over a thousand years before they had any contact with Europeans; the culmination of over three hundred years of contact was expulsion from their homelands and forced removal to Indian Territory in 1859.

The emphasis in this study on the archaeological, ethnohistorical, and archival records dealing with the effects of European contact on native Caddoan peoples can be summarized in the form of the two following questions, which are derived from the classic study by Edward Spicer (1962) entitled *Cycles of Conquest:* What are the principal ways in which Caddoan groups responded to European contact? What happened to their traditional cultures as a result of the manifold effects of contact? As such, these questions focus on the record of Caddoan cultural change initiated by European explorers and settlers in the region since ca. 1540 and the de Soto–Moscoso *entrada*.

The focus of much current archaeological and ethnohistorical research in the United States is on the systemic relationship between the archaeological and ethnographical records (i.e., the records gathered by anthropologists, traders, missionaries, explorers, and others about native American groups), and this study of the Caddo nation is solidly in that tradition. While both the archaeological and ethnohistorical perspectives hold considerable promise for elucidating the processes of native American cultural change and acculturation, it is only in concert that a broader understanding can be reached of what Bruce Trigger (1985) calls "Native history." Concern with the Caddoan peoples of Texas, Louisiana, Oklahoma, and Arkansas brings to the forefront again that Caddoan Indian peoples played a significant role in the Euro-American settlement of the area in the eighteenth and nineteenth centuries and in the European and American political arena of those times.

The detailed examination of the Caddoan archaeological record is of singular importance for the Protohistoric period (1520–1685) because processes of indirect, sporadic, and intermittent contact, and any initial changes in Caddoan lifeways brought about by European contact, are difficult to document thoroughly or explicitly from an ethnohistorical and ethnographic perspective. Profound demographic, social, and political changes could have occurred prior to the onset of face-to-face European contact with Caddoan groups because of the introduction and widespread diffusion of diseases and European material goods without European knowledge (Dobyns 1983; Ramenofsky 1990). Thus, even limited contact by Caddoan peoples with Europeans, or their products, could affect native American cultures in very fundamental ways, and only the study of the archaeological record can provide information about them.

At the same time, there is much of interest in the ethnographic, archival, and historical records for studying culture contact between Caddoan peoples and Europeans. These data provide specific details of change and traditional lifeways in a number of dimensions, particularly in such facets as political organization, language assimilation, settlement and community structure, religious persistence, and economic systems that can only be indirectly and poorly comprehended in the archaeological record. With the integration of such diverse sets of information—the archaeological, ethnographic, archival, and historical—we can explore the long-term effects and consequences of European contact on Caddoan peoples, discuss the processes and causes responsible for cultural change among Caddoan Indian groups between ca. 1540 and 1859, and lay the groundwork for a coherent history of the relationship between Caddoan peoples and Europeans.

The major conclusions of this study of Caddoan and European contact can be summarized as follows: First, severe population loss among many Caddoan peoples, beginning in the sixteenth century, occurred as a consequence of acute epidemic diseases introduced by the Europeans. The introduction and diffusion of these diseases occurred well before any substantial ethnographic descriptions of the Caddoan peoples were recorded. Second, these population losses, which continued episodically from ca. 1540 to 1890 and totaled an estimated 94 percent, were apparently accompanied by reductions in social and political complexity as well as changes in Caddoan settlement density and organization. These population losses are not uniform temporally or spatially and may have been heavier along the major rivers (such as the Red River), where Caddoan population densities at first contact were at their highest levels. Third, regional abandonments because of depopulation and mobility (following the introduction and adoption of the horse by Caddoan peoples in the late seventeenth century) are thought to be related to the development of Caddoan confederacies—The Kadohadacho, the Hasinai, and the Natchitoches—and to the coalescence over time of formerly separate Caddoan ethnic and tribal entities. Fourth, these confederacies, particularly the Hasinai confederacy in East Texas, maintained an active trade relationship with the French and Spanish through the Contact period, as is clearly demonstrated in both the archaeological and historical records. They also participated strongly in the fur trade developed by the French. Fifth, these confederacies were the preeminent native American political entity in that part of the Spanish Borderlands West until about 1800, when waves of immigrant Indians and Euro-Americans from east of the Mississippi River began to move into Louisiana and Spanish Texas. And, sixth, Caddoan communities that existed in small dispersed groups and formal settlements along the minor streams, tributaries, and hinterland areas do not appear to have been depopulated as severely as were large Caddoan riverine communities on the Red River (such as the Kadohadacho and related groups). Consequently, it is mainly the small dispersed Caddoan groups who made up the Hasinai confederacy, who were subsequently described ethnographically by Europeans and Euro-Americans, and who are the best known from historic times. Many of the Caddoan groups described in the late seventeenth and early eighteenth centuries by Europeans ceased to exist by the late eighteenth century.

Acknowledgments

This study is a product of my doctoral dissertation completed in 1989 at the University of Washington in Seattle. It has been my great privilege over the last seventeen years to have received advice, assistance, and research and moral support from a wonderful group of people across the country while I was pursuing a research interest in Caddoan archaeology and ethnohistory. First initiated by my undergraduate mentor at Ohio State University, Dr. William S. Dancey, this interest was later fostered by Dr. Alex D. Krieger (truly the father of Caddoan archaeology) and guided by Dr. Robert C. Dunnell, chairman of my graduate committee at the University of Washington. I also wish to acknowledge the support of the rest of my dissertation committee—Dr. Donald K. Grayson, Dr. James B. Watson, Dr. Julie Stein, and Dr. Stephen C. Porter—during the course of my research and dissertation efforts.

Working in the Caddoan Area has given me the opportunity to share in many diverse and wide-ranging discussions concerning the archaeology of the states of Missouri, Oklahoma, Arkansas, Louisiana, and Texas and also to interact with persons directly involved in research in this area. This interaction has been, and will remain, a great benefit to my own continuing research in Caddoan archaeology and ethnohistory.

I am especially indebted to Dr. Dee Ann Story (surely the mother of Caddoan archaeology), Dr. James E. Bruseth, Jeff Richner, Dr. Mark Lynott, Dr. C. Reid Ferring, Paul McGuff, Dr. Kathleen Gilmore, Elton Prewitt, Janice Guy, Bob D. Skiles, Nancy Kenmotsu, Duane Peter, Bonnie Yates, Daniel McGregor, and Dr. S. Alan Skinner for their support and encouragement in pursuing East Texas archaeology. Lee Johnson, through some well-placed and pointed comments, has caused me to take another look at issues and inferences with a more critical eye. Special thanks are extended to Jeff Richner for giving me the opportunity in 1975 to participate in the Tennessee Colony Lake project on the Trinity River, my first, albeit indirect, introduction to one brand of Caddoan archaeology.

Drs. Ann Early, Gayle Fritz, George Sabo III, H. F. "Pete" Gregory, David Kelley, Dan Rogers, Don Wyckoff, Jerry Galm, Burt Purrington, Robert L.

Brooks, Susan Vehik, James A. Brown, W. Ray Wood, and James E. Price contributed more than they know to my understanding of the Caddoan and Mississippian archaeological records in Arkansas, Louisiana, Oklahoma, and Missouri. Don Wyckoff and Ann Early deserve additional heartfelt thanks for helping me when I came to work in the Ouachita Mountains on the McGee Creek Project in 1982, and they have been most gracious ever since in sharing ideas and information with me. Pete Gregory sent me an impassioned and eloquent letter in 1981 (which I still read from time to time) that probably did more than anything else to redefine my consideration of the strengths of the Caddoan peoples during the Contact era and brought me a bit out of the academic cloud, but not as far, perhaps, as Pete urged.

My fellow graduate students were a considerable source of support and encouragement during the long period of research and writing. I want to extend thanks to Drs. G. Tom Jones, Ann Ramenofsky, Patrice Teltser, and Sarah Campbell. Ann was especially helpful specifically because of her expertise in archaeology, ethnohistory, and contact demography in the Lower Mississippi Valley and generally because of her well-reasoned considerations of the archaeology of European contact. Our collaborative efforts during graduate school were an important part of the groundwork for the research efforts and ideas presented here.

Theresa May, executive editor at the University of Texas Press, guided this fledging author through the publication process, and her positive attitude was a considerable comfort during manuscript revision and final editing. Dr. Thomas Hester, general editor of the Texas Archaeology and Ethnohistory Series, provided critical support during the initial stages when the manuscript was under consideration.

A host of avocational archaeologists and landowners out there have aided me (and many other archaeologists) in the quest to better understand the archaeology of the Caddoan peoples. Without their interest, cooperation, and goodwill, research on Caddoan archaeological problems would be well-nigh impossible.

Special thanks go to my parents and my wife, Cecile, for their understanding and support. Cecile, along with Kathy Roemer, did most of the typing and figure layout and unravelled the complexities of various computer programs. I hope that this book is in some measure a recompense for that support.

Finally, I reserve a special acknowledgment to the Caddoan peoples of past, present, and future. May you prosper and continue to inspire. *Hoke-ehunnohsah!*

PART 1

Contact and Theoretical Issues

1 / Introduction

The Texas [Hasinai Caddo] are lively by nature, clear-sighted, sociable, proud and high minded . . . of great heart, and very quick in military activities. With their friends they keep unchangeable peace, and with their enemies they never, or very seldom, make peace.

—*Fray Juan Agustín de Morfi, ca. 1780*

The first known European explorers of the Caddoan Area in the Spanish Borderlands West were the two hundred or so ragged and exhausted members of the de Soto–Moscoso *entrada* in 1542. In their search for treasure and great wealth, the members of the Spanish de Soto *entrada* hoped to discover native civilizations to exploit in La Florida similar to those encountered earlier in the sixteenth century by Spanish conquistadores in Mexico and Peru (Quinn 1979, 2:93–96). That no such native American civilizations were discovered in these wanderings does not lessen the overall importance of the de Soto *entrada* and its various chronicles for the archaeologist and ethnographer concerned with understanding the nature of aboriginal lifeways in the southeastern United States (Hudson et al. 1985; Hudson, DePratter, and Smith 1989).

The de Soto chronicles introduce us to the Caddoan peoples, one of many aboriginal societies described as living west of the Mississippi Valley in the general direction of New Spain. The various Caddoan societies described therein were noted to share basic similarities in material culture, behavior, and custom, but they spoke a language different from other aboriginal groups previously encountered by the Spanish (Swanton 1939). Indeed, the Spanish were unable to find a translator among the native American retinue accompanying the *entrada*. The chronicles describe these people as successful maize agriculturists as well as bison hunters and provide an initial glimpse of these aboriginal Caddoan populations who "were still in the full state of their indigenous developments" (Brain 1985a, xlvii).

We now know, 450 years later, that these peoples were southern Caddoan-speaking groups.[1] They were apparently living at the time on and between the Arkansas and Red River valleys and south into deep East Texas, now within the states of Texas, Oklahoma, Louisiana, Arkansas, and Missouri. The de Soto *entrada* provides an introduction to a native American people who had a significant role in defining the nature of the European and

American settlement of the area in the eighteenth and nineteenth centuries. The examination of the cultural contact and interaction process from an archaeological and ethnohistorical perspective is the focus of this study (see also Perttula 1989a, 1991).

It was more than one hundred years after the de Soto *entrada* that these southern Caddoan-speaking peoples again became known to Europeans through information derived from southern Plains nomadic groups who came to the Santa Fe trade fairs. Tantalizing rumors of a populous nation of Indians, soon to be known as the "Kingdom of the Tejas" (Bolton 1912), reached Spanish administrators in the Santa Fe area. Messages carried from the Tejas to the Spanish by the Jumano (a nomadic group who lived mainly in West Texas) suggested that they desired not only to initiate commerce with the Spanish but, according to the interpretations of the missionaries, desired also to be introduced to the Catholic faith. More than thirty years of propaganda efforts by the missionaries to capitalize on these desires were for nought until the political climate was right. Not until the Spanish became concerned that the French colonization of the Lower Mississippi Valley would interfere with their ambitious plans for the "Kingdom of the Tejas" and the colony of New Spain did they take action. This political and religious interplay between the Spanish and French that began in the late seventeenth century in the Spanish Borderlands West was a contributing factor to why the Caddoan peoples, located on the borders of these two political rivals, played such a pivotal role in shaping the colonization of the Red and Arkansas rivers first by the Spanish and French and then later by the Americans. Their importance is well attested to in the archival and ethnohistorical records of the colonial powers and American state (Flores 1984; Usner 1987; Winfrey and Day 1966).

The scholarly interest in the southern Caddoan-speaking peoples by ethnographers and archaeologists first began as part of a more general concern with the origins and character of the aboriginal inhabitants encountered during European and Euro-American settlement of the eastern United States and the Great Plains. The study of native American groups was an intellectual curiosity and was frequently motivated by paternalistic feelings expressed by the U.S. government, missionaries, teachers, traders, and scientists of the day for the native American groups whose history and culture was so poorly known. Nevertheless, from these efforts, particularly those of historian Herbert Eugene Bolton (1915, 1987), John R. Swanton (1942), and James Mooney (1896) of the Bureau of Ethnology in the Smithsonian Institution and George A. Dorsey (1905a, 1905b) of the Carnegie Institution, a corpus of historical and ethnographic information was compiled that was (and still is) of considerable interest to those studying the Caddoan peoples.

As I will discuss in greater detail, archaeological investigations of the material remains thought to have been left by these peoples proceeded at the same time but without an overall view and clear appreciation of the historical and developmental relationships between the Caddoan archaeological record and the ethnographically described Caddoan peoples. In large measure because of refinements in dating archaeological materials, more intensive regional investigations, and a better understanding of temporal and spatial variability in Caddoan culture within the Caddoan Area (Story 1990; Jeter et al. 1989), our perceptions of the Caddoan people have been substantially and rapidly changing.

Of late, scientific studies of the Caddoan peoples have come to emphasize cultural change over time and the meaning of cultural variations that are particular to the aboriginal populations living in the region (e.g., Schambach 1982; Jeter et al. 1989; Story 1990; Perttula 1989a). As noted, the systematic study of Caddoan archaeology and ethnography has a long and rich tradition beginning in the second half of the nineteenth century. Recent promising developments in archaeology, ethnohistory, physical anthropology, and linguistics continue the productive inquiry into the development of these Caddoan peoples and their ways of life. The studies by Chafe (1983), Gregory (1983, 1986), Phillips and Brown (1984), Rose (1984), Story (1985a), Fritz (1986b, 1989), Bruseth (1987), Sabo et al. (1988), Rogers et al. (1989), Jeter et al. (1989), and Story et al. (1990) are examples of significant recent research efforts that have illuminated many aspects of Caddoan prehistory and history. Future studies will undoubtedly contribute even further to our understanding of the cultural heritage of the Caddoan peoples.

This study attempts to examine Caddoan lifeways during a very significant period in North American history by focusing on the record of Caddoan cultural change preserved in the archaeological and ethnographic records from ca. 1520 to 1800. My primary concern is elucidating how these aboriginal Caddoan groups were affected by European contact and, likewise, how these Caddoan groups affected European societies in the Spanish Borderlands West. The emphasis on both archaeological and ethnohistorical records and on the dual nature of contact recognizes the unique but complementary promise of both disciplines for this investigation.

Examination of the relationships between the archaeological record of the Caddoan Area and ethnographically known Caddoan societies certainly exemplifies how ecological and evolutionary processes can shape the character of a native American population over the long term and, furthermore, provides the additional opportunity, through the pursuit of native American history (Trigger 1980, 1985; Axtell 1988), to address how Caddoan societies changed and/or maintained traditional cultural lifeways as a consequence of European contact and interaction over the last 450 years.

The Caddoan Area offers the further possibility of drawing upon the archaeological and ethnographic records to study aboriginal cultural change in great detail. To understand the nature of change in native American history among the Caddoan peoples during at least portions of the time under consideration foremost requires diachronic data primarily obtained from the study of the archaeological record. Certain ethnohistorical and archival records (population estimates, group movements, descriptions of significant rituals and ceremonies) are also appropriate sources of information about diachronic processes of cultural change in the Caddoan Area. These data together chronicle a specific record of change, a record that has great meaning to those who are interested in the history of the Caddoan peoples specifically and of native Americans generally.

THE CADDOAN AREA

The relationship between the Caddoan tribes or groups recorded ethnographically over the last several centuries and the geographic region containing archaeological remains presumed to represent their prehistoric ancestors has specific temporal and spatial connotations. As an ethnohistorical and ethnographic construct, the term *Caddo* had little meaning before the middle of the nineteenth century, that is, before the Caddoan peoples were removed to Indian Territory. Prior to that time the Caddo (i.e., the Kadohadacho proper) were only one of at least twenty-five distinct social entities known in the ethnographic records of the Caddoan Area (see Bolton 1987 and Swanton 1942). These were groups who had primarily lived in close contact with the Spanish and French ca. 1685–1803 and became known to chroniclers of the times.

The term *Caddo* derives from the French abbreviation of *Kadohadacho*, a word meaning "real chief" in the Kadohadacho dialect (Newkumet and Meredith 1988). However, depending upon the context, the term means several different things in anthropological and archaeological usage (Story 1978). For instance, *Caddo* or *Caddoan* can refer to a native American linguistic family or a subdivision of related dialects within that family; be a collective term for up to twenty-five related tribes or bands, three possible confederacies, or specific Prehistoric and Historic period archaeological assemblages; or mean the geographic region containing these archaeological assemblages (Trubowitz 1984, 4).

Because of the overall thrust of this study, the consideration of *Caddo* or *Caddoan* from an archaeological perspective is a necessity. What is meant by the use of the term *Caddoan Area?* Basically, archaeological areas are coherent spatial and temporal entities within which the archaeological record is similar among its various regions and different from that of other broad geographic areas that have other cultural traditions (Willey and Phillips 1958, 18–21). Behind this relatively simplistic definition then, the Caddoan Area as an archaeological concept is thus recognizable primarily on the basis of a set of longstanding and distinctive cultural, social, and political elements that have temporal, spatial, and geographic connotations. While total unanimity in definition of a complex archaeological phenomenon such as the Caddoan Area may never be reached, some basic characteristics have been outlined by Prewitt (1974, 76), namely, that the Caddo had "a large population represented by many small settlements scattered within particular resource areas; a reliance upon horticulture as one of the primary means of subsistence; differentiated and undifferentiated mound/habitation sites with structurally differentiated mound classes (producing an apparently hierarchic division of places on the landscape); differential treatment of the dead reflective of a system of ranking; indications of long-term cooperation in disposal of the dead by groups represented by some of the archaeological units."

In general, these basic characteristics of settlement, subsistence, sociopolitical organization, and mortuary treatments for the Caddoan Archaeological Area over the last one thousand years, from ca. A.D. 750 to 1750, are very similar, if not identical, to what constitutes Mississippi period cultural traditions defined in eastern North American archaeology (Griffin 1967, 1985; Muller 1978; Smith 1986, 1990; Steponaitis 1986). However, in spite of these broad similarities, the evolutionary development of the prehistoric and early historic Caddoan tradition, Caddoan archaeologists argue, took place relatively independently of Mississippi period developments in the eastern North American region (Smith 1990).

The combination of the cultural criteria outlined above, in conjunction with the specific distribution of the Trans-Mississippi South biome as defined by Schambach (1970), provides perhaps the most precise and useful geographic delineation of the Caddoan Area irrespective of its spatial extent at any one particular point in time. The area is approximately 200,000 square kilometers and centers on the Red and Arkansas rivers in portions of the states of Texas, Arkansas, Louisiana, Oklahoma, and Missouri (Fig. 1). It is characterized by an ecological or biotic community of hardwoods, pines, and interspersed prairies that is distinct from the tall-grass prairies to the north, west, and south and distinct from the floodplain environments of the Lower Mississippi Valley embayment and the Mississippian and Plaquemine peoples who lived there (Phillips 1970; Williams and Brain 1983; Schambach 1991).

The Caddoan Archaeological Area has recently been divided into three subareas, the Northern Caddoan, Western Caddoan, and Central Caddoan. Archaeological developments within each of these subareas seems to repre-

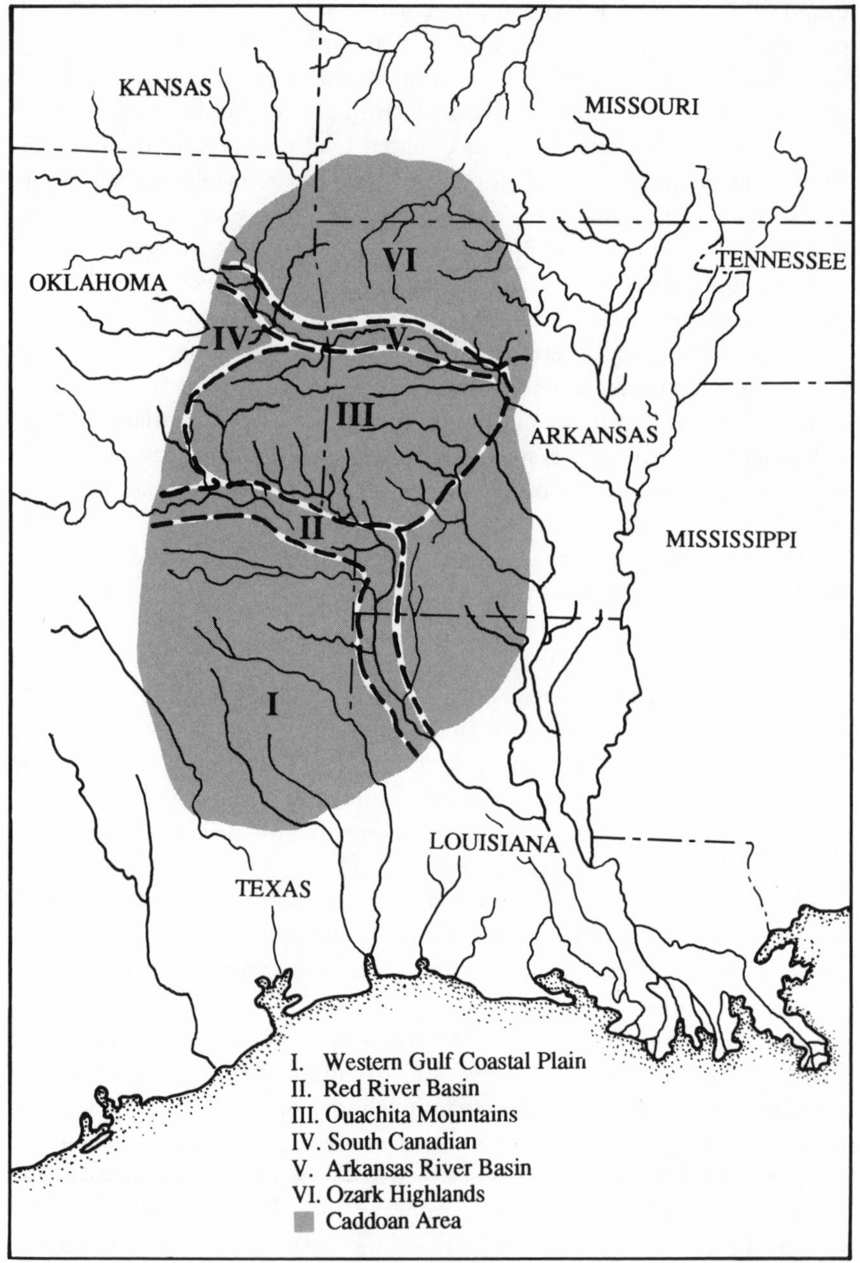

FIG. 1. The Caddoan Area: I, western Gulf Coastal Plain; II, Red River basin; III, Ouachita Mountains; IV, South Canadian; V, Arkansas River basin; VI, Ozark highlands.

sent the in situ formation of separate and complex Caddoan cultural traditions (Schambach 1983): (*a*) the Arkansas, or Northern Caddoan, subarea of northeast Oklahoma, northwest Arkansas, and southwest Missouri, including the Arkansas Valley lowlands (region V in Fig. 1), the South Canadian basin (region IV), and the western Ozark Highlands (region VI) (Brown, Bell, and Wyckoff 1978)[2]; (*b*) the western Caddoan subarea of East Texas and South-central Oklahoma, including the western Gulf Coastal Plain outside the Red River Valley (region I), and the Ouachita Mountains (region III) (Story 1981, 1990; Wyckoff and Baugh 1980); and (*c*) the central Caddoan subarea in the Red and Ouachita river valleys in Southwest Arkansas, Northwest Louisiana, and Southeast Oklahoma (region II) (Schambach 1983; Williams and Early 1990). Within each of these Caddoan subareas there were probably significant intraareal and diachronic differences in the character of individual cultures and groups (Story 1990). Many of these regional cultural differences, as well as the larger set of broad overall similarities, will be discussed in more detail as we examine the effects of cultural contact between Europeans and Caddoan peoples from subarea to subarea.

This study is divided into three sections. Part 1, which contains this introduction and chapters 2 and 3, deals primarily with theoretical and methodological issues concerning the Protohistoric and Historic archaeological records of the Caddoan Area and reviews the documentary materials pertaining to the patterns of cultural contact between the Caddoan peoples and Europeans.

Part 2, which contains chapters 4, 5, and 6, is concerned with providing an assessment of the Caddoan contact period archaeological record from areal, regional, and thematic perspectives. Emphasis is given to discerning systemic differences at particular points and intervals in time (1520, 1520–1685, and 1685–1800) in such things as mortuary variability, the construction and use of mound structures and other community facilities, regional settlement density, and the occurrence and adoption of European trade goods among Caddoan peoples that highlight contrastive changes between Caddoan riverine town communities and rural communities in gauging the effects of contact with Europeans.

Finally, in Part 3 (chapter 7), I present a summary of the specific and general findings presented in this study and conclude with remarks about the limitations and future prospects of research on the Caddoan Historic archaeological and ethnohistorical records. Major issues important in future studies of the 1520–1860 period in the Caddoan Area are (*a*) further ethnohistoric research dealing with the still poorly tapped French, Spanish, and American archival and documentary records, (*b*) the archaeology of the fur trade, (*c*) the archaeology of the removal and post-Removal period

(1840 to the present), and (*d*) analyses of the paleodemographic and bioarchaeological records necessary to directly evaluate the effects and consequences of demographic change and stress postulated in this study. This study should encourage renewed consideration of the archaeology, ethnography, and history of an important southeastern native American population occupying the Trans-Mississippi South.

2 / European Contact with the Caddo Nation: An Overview

The next day a woman, who governed this nation [*the Kadohadacho*], *came to visit me with the principal persons of the village. . . . We went together to their temple, and after the priests had invoked their God for a quarter of an hour they conducted me to the cabin of their chief. Before entering they washed my face with water, which is a ceremony among them. . . .*

The Cadadoquis [*Kadohadacho*] *are united with two other villages called Natchitoches and Nasoui* [*Nasoni*] *situated on the Red River. All the villages of this tribe speak the same language. Their cabins are covered with straw, and they are not united in villages, but their huts are distant one from the other. Their fields are beautiful. They fish and hunt. There is plenty of game, but few cattle. . . . I never found that they did any work, except making very fine bows, which they make a traffic with distant nations. The Cadadoquis possess about thirty horses, which they call* cavali [caballo, *a horse in Spanish*]. *The men and women are tattooed in the face and all over the body.* —*Henri de Tonti, 30 March 1690*

In discussing the nature of the historic period and the interaction of Caddoan peoples and Europeans between ca. 1520 and 1850, this chapter explores not only what Caddoan groups were like in the centuries after contact, but how and why the archaeological record takes the form it does. Here I assess the magnitude and consequences of European contact and the resulting transformations in historic Caddoan lifeways and systematically consider them from an archaeological perspective.

In this study, my discussions of European contact with Caddoan peoples can be divided into two periods. The first, the Protohistoric period, corresponds to the time of indirect and intermittent direct contact between European and Caddoan peoples and is comparable to the latter portion of the Late Caddoan period recently defined by Story (1900, 334). The second and subsequent period is one of direct, sustained, and continuous contact between both populations. This is also the period when immigrant Indian groups first moved into the area from east of the Mississippi River, then certain Caddoan Indian groups were moved out of their homelands into Texas, and finally all aboriginal populations were pushed out of Texas into Indian Territory. With the exception of the Alabama and Coushatta (Koasati) Indians in Southeast Texas and Southwest Louisiana, all aboriginal groups in this region left for Indian Territory or Mexico by 1859 (Prucha 1984, 354–366; Tanner 1974; Kniffen, Gregory, and Stokes 1987).

Although processes of indirect and intermittent direct contact are difficult to thoroughly document or explicate from either an ethnohistorical or archaeological perspective, it is clear that an archaeological focus on the Protohistoric period is of singular importance in the study of "initial changes brought about by European contact" (Trigger 1985, 118). In general, episodes of indirect and intermittent direct contact between Caddoan peoples and Europeans are characteristic of ca. 1520–1685.

Direct, sustained contact, the province of the historian and archivist as well as the archaeologist and ethnohistorian, was first initiated by French and Spanish exploration parties in the Caddoan Area. Settlement and colonization of selected, key sections of the region followed shortly thereafter for purposes of military, economic, religious, and political advantage. Then finally came wholesale settlement of the area in the early nineteenth century by immigrant Anglo-Americans and displaced Southeastern aboriginal groups from the expanding frontier of the United States. Although speaking of the colonial French and English efforts east of the Mississippi River, in a very appropriate sense, Axtell (1985, 3–6) depicts this period of contact as primarily one of cultural conversion and diplomacy, a "contest of cultures." This later phase of European-Caddoan interaction has lasted more than three hundred years, from 1685 to today.

As we shall see, the available ethnographic data about the Caddoan peoples mainly pertain to the first two centuries of this time period (Newkumet and Meredith 1988; Swanton 1942). The story of Caddoan life after the Civil War—during the periods of more intensive assimilation efforts, the destruction of Indian community self-government and reservation lands following the adoption of the General Allotment Act of 1887, and the implementation of the Indian Reorganization Act of 1934 and the Oklahoma Indian Welfare Act of 1936 (see U.S. Congress, Senate 1989; Debo 1942; Newkumet and Meredith 1988, 51–57, 71)—cannot be told here. It is an important story and one that deserves to be told with close attention to detail through historical studies and the words, thoughts, and actions of the Caddo peoples who lived then or were told about those times.

THE ARCHAEOLOGICAL AND ETHNOGRAPHIC CONTEXT

Before we delve into the study of contact and interaction between Europeans and Caddoan peoples in the Trans-Mississippi South, it is important to briefly review current understanding of the archaeology and ethnography of these native American groups. Until about two thousand years ago, relatively mobile hunters and gatherers who utilized naturally occurring plant and animal resources lived in the Caddoan Area. Generally speaking, after this time, some of these hunters and gatherers began to settle down within recognizable territories (Story 1985a, 44), to build structures and small communities that served as places of residence for several seasons (if not year-round), to manufacture ceramics to cook and store foodstuffs, and to develop a horticultural life-style based on the cultivation of tropical cultigens and certain native plants. The roots of the southern Caddoan-speaking peoples can be traced to these Early Ceramic or Fourche Maline cultures (Jeter et al. 1989, 196; Story 1990; Schambach 1982).

By around A.D. 800, substantial evidence in the archaeological record indicates development of a distinctive cultural tradition that has come to be referred to as Caddoan (see chapter 3 for further discussions). Archaeologists have relied strongly on the distinctive ceramics made in this area to separate the Caddoan tradition from the prehistoric cultures in the Southern Plains or the Lower Mississippi Valley, but the ceramics are only one small aspect of a much broader picture we can use to portray the prehistoric character of these Caddoan peoples. The actual processes involved in the appearance and development of the prehistoric Caddoan cultural tradition are still a matter of some debate, but generally speaking the most important factors appear to be: (*a*) the development of more complex social and political systems of authority, ritual, and ceremony; (*b*) the rise, elaboration, and maintenance of social ranking and status within the Caddoan communities and larger social and political spheres; and (*c*) the intensification of maize agriculture and a reliance on tropical cultigens over time in local economic systems (see Story 1990, 325; Perttula 1990).

During prehistoric times the Caddoan peoples lived in dispersed communities of grass- and cane-covered structures, which frequently were associated with grass-covered arbors and ramadas. These communities were composed of isolated homesteads and/or farmsteads, small hamlets, a few larger villages or "towns," and the civic-ceremonial centers. These centers were marked by the construction of earthen mounds that were used as temples, as burial mounds, and as ceremonial fire mounds (Jeter et al. 1989, 201). The civic-ceremonial centers appear to have "served a local population which [was] dispersed in small social and economic groups around the center" (Schambach and Early 1983, SW107).

The Caddoan communities were dispersed throughout the major and minor stream valleys of the Trans-Mississippi South. Although the archaeological evidence is incomplete, it appears that the largest communities and the more important civic-ceremonial centers were present primarily along the major streams—the Red, Arkansas, Little, and Ouachita rivers. None of these communities and ceremonial centers had fortifications of wooden palisades, unlike the heavily populated fortified towns of agricultural peoples in the Mississippi River Valley.

The civic and ceremonial mound centers used by the Caddoan peoples in prehistoric and historic times are a reflection of the complex sociopolitical and religious systems that evolved in the area beginning about A.D. 800. As noted, these centers probably represented "the social and economic focal point of local polities" (Rogers n.d., 5). Many of the earthen mounds were used as caps or platforms for special structures used for civic and/or religious functions. According to Story (1990, 341), these mounds probably represent "places where religious practitioners could perform sacred rites, where ritual paraphernalia could be kept, and around which members of the society could periodically congregate to reaffirm what was important and right."

The civic and ceremonial centers frequently had special mortuary roles to fulfill in prehistoric Caddoan polities. The social and political elite were typically buried in some of the earthen mounds, and they were accompanied by many elaborately made grave goods, including "ornaments of marine shells and copper; delicate, long stem (*sic*) clay pipes; stone effigy pipes; large quartz crystals; minerals including galena, bauxite, and glauconite; expertly chipped arrow points placed in quivers; exceptionally large and well made bifaces or knifes; and ceremonial (spatulate-shaped) celts" (Story 1990, 339). Many grave goods were manufactured of nonlocal materials and had to have been obtained through long-distance trade networks (Vehik 1990).

During prehistoric times Caddoan peoples developed a successful horticultural economy based on such tropical cultigens as maize, beans, and squash as well as such native cultigens as maygrass, amaranth, chenopods, and sunflowers (Fritz 1986b; Perttula 1990). Stable carbon isotope ratios of Caddoan skeletal remains clearly indicate that by ca. 1100 to 1300 most of the Caddoan groups were consuming large amounts of maize (Burnett 1990b, Table 11-24), and maize was quite likely the most important food source for Caddoan peoples after that time. Wild plant foods, including annuals, fruits, roots, seeds, and nuts, were gathered along with a wide variety of small to large game animals.

The game animals supplied items of clothing, tools, and equipment as well as necessary food. Deer (particularly the white-tailed deer), rabbits, raccoon, fish, turkey, squirrel, and turtles were some of the more important sources of meat to the Caddoan diet. Bison and bear were commonly exploited for their meat and furs, particularly so in the Arkansas River Basin of eastern Oklahoma and in the western portions of the Ozark Highland (Sabo et al. 1988).

The Caddoan peoples in prehistoric times made beautiful artistic as well as functional ceramic wares from the locally abundant clays. The fine wares, the elaborately decorated and slipped bowls and bottles of many forms and shapes commonly included as grave goods, must be considered some of the finest aboriginal ceramics manufactured in North America (Holmes 1903). Also an integral part of the ceramic technology were the large utility ware jars and plain vessels employed by the Caddoan peoples for cooking, serving, and storing. These vessels often attained impressive sizes, sometimes being several feet in height and diameter, particularly after the development of maize agriculture in the area.

The Caddoan peoples had a sophisticated technology based on the use of stone, bone, wood, shell, and other media for the manufacture of tools, clothing, basketry, ornaments, and other items. Because of preservation conditions, much of the archaeological evidence for Caddoan technology is unfortunately limited to the more durable items of stone and bone. Readers who are interested in the broader range of artifacts manufactured by such groups as the Caddo should examine the books by Kniffen, Gregory, and Stokes (1987) and Newkumet and Meredith (1988). They provide much useful information on the aboriginal manufacture of clothing, adornments, basketry, and wood items by the Indians of Louisiana, including the Caddoan peoples, and the Hasinai Caddo in Oklahoma.

The stone technology was based on the manufacture of the arrowhead for the bow and arrow; the groundstone celt and chipped ax for removing trees and brush and turning over the soil; and a wide variety of small hand-held stone tools for such tasks as scraping hides, cutting bone and wood, and piercing leather. Locally available lithic raw materials were usually employed for the manufacture of these tools, but nonlocal lithic raw materials (and finished tools made of these materials) were also obtained in trade (Brown 1983; Perttula 1990). Bone was made into tools such as awls, beamers, scoops, digging implements, and hoes and was also fashioned into ornaments, beads, and whistles. Mussel shells were altered to form small but surprisingly durable digging implements and hoes, and locally available gastropods were made into beads worn around the neck or on the ears. Although rare, marine shell from the Texas and Florida Gulf Coast that had been obtained by the Caddoan peoples through trade was used in the production of shell pendants, gorgets, beads, and cups. These items were usually included as grave goods with the social and political elite.

The development and maintenance of long-distance east-west and north-south trade networks were notable features of the prehistoric Caddoan cultural tradition. Traded were such items as bison hides and salt; such raw materials as copper, stone, and marine shell; and such finished objects as pottery vessels and large ceremonial bifaces (Brown 1983; Creel 1991a; Early 1990; Vehik 1988, 1990). Many of the more important trade items, particularly the marine shell and copper objects, were obtained from areas more than three hundred miles away from the Caddoan Area. Although much of the archaeological evidence for the Caddoan long-distance trade and exchange networks occurs in contexts predating 1400, which may indicate a decline in the importance of long-distance trade after that time, in 1542 when Moscoso visited Caddoan groups in East Texas he noted evidence of cotton and turquoise. The cotton must have come from the southwestern United States, and analysis of some of the turquoise indicates the Albuquerque, New Mexico, area as the source (Brown 1983).

In historic times the Caddoan nation comprised at least twenty-five separate groups, bands, or tribes. These were organized into loosely affiliated kin-based groups referred to by European observers as the Hasinai, Kadohadacho, and Natchitoches confederacies. The Hasinai groups lived in the Neches and Angelina River valleys in East Texas, the Kadohadacho groups on the Red River in the Great Bend area, and the Natchitoches groups on the Red River in the vicinity of the French post of Natchitoches established in 1714.

The Caddoan peoples are matrilineal, tracing descent through the maternal line rather than through the paternal. This carries over into the kinship terms used by the Caddo: the father and father's brothers are called by the same term as the mother and the mother's sisters. The Caddoan peoples also recognized and ranked clans named after such animals as the eagle, panther, beaver, raccoon, bear, crow, wolf, and bison, and marriage typically occurred between people of different clans rather than between people of the same clans (Rogers n.d., 9).

Religious and political authority in Caddoan society in historic times was vested in a hierarchy of positions within and between the various affiliated communities and bands (see Wyckoff and Baugh 1980; Swanton 1942). The key positions were the *xinesi* (pronounced SEE-neeh-tsi) (Newkumet and Meredith 1988, 56), the spiritual leader; the *caddi* (pronounced CAH-de), or village headman; and the *canahas* (pronounced cah-NA-ha), subordinate headmen or village elders (Wyckoff and Baugh 1980, 234–235; Newkumet and Meredith 1988, 56–57).

The xinesi was apparently both a political and religious leader, and the position was inherited. The power of the xinesi was not absolute. Although the other leaders owed their allegiance to him, his power depended partly on the influence he wielded in the decision-making process of the Caddoan-affiliated communities under that allegiance. The roles of the xinesi included "maintaining the temple containing the sacred perpetual fire; acting as a religious leader for 2 or more of the formally allied villages; mediating between the deities and the people, especially the nominal decision makers for each village; and leading and participating in certain special rites (i.e., first fruits, harvest, and naming ceremonies)" (Wyckoff and Baugh 1980, 234).

The caddi was the principal headman, chief, or governor of a Caddoan community. This was also an hereditary leadership position (Newkumet and Meredith 1988, 56). While the caddi was primarily responsible for making the important political decisions for the community, he was assisted by the canahas in various governing duties, including sponsoring important ceremonies, conducting councils for war expeditions, and conducting the calumet (or peace pipe) ceremony with visitors to the village.

War leaders and warriors (the *amayxoya*) were also important members in the Caddoan sociopolitical structure. The warriors who had achieved victories in war were called *amayxoya,* and the war chief was elected by the general populace from among that rank. During a war expedition, the war chief was recognized to have complete authority over the course of the war and its Caddoan participants.

In religious matters, the Caddoan peoples looked to the xinesi and the other priests for mediation with the *Caddi Ayo,* or Ah-ah-ha'-yo, the supreme god. The xinesi was the head priest, and he communicated with the gods and "heavenly children" to pass on their wishes to the Caddoan peoples. Using the important themes of fire, corn, pipes, and drums in the forecasting, early spring planting, first fruits, and after-harvest ceremonies (Sabo 1987, 29), the xinesi linked and imbued everyday life with the supernatural powers and the supreme god and was thought to have further aided communication with them on behalf of the Caddoan peoples. According to Rogers (n.d., 14), "every aspect of Caddo life was inseparably linked through ritual to the supernatural powers which could aid or as easily do harm, if proper actions were not taken to placate and give homage where due. The most important ceremonies reflected themes of great concern to the Caddos, including hunting, warfare, and especially the fruits of cultivation. Corn was the most important crop and was at the center of major ceremonies."

The dispersed settlement pattern described above for the prehistoric Caddoan peoples continued into historic times. The scattered farmsteads, hamlets, and affiliated villages were distributed wherever there were good arable lands and ready sources of water, especially dependable springs and flowing creeks. Public buildings, the fire temple, and the compounds of the xinesi and the caddi, were kept distinct from the typical settlements of the community, and these buildings and special residences were constructed under the direction of the caddi. Earthen mounds were no longer constructed and used by Caddoan peoples after ca. 1700.

The annual cycle of the Caddoan peoples was based on the importance of farming, hunting, fishing, and collecting of wild plants. Certainly the cultivation of crops, especially corn, was of primary significance to the Caddo. They cultivated two varieties of corn, an early or "little corn," planted in April and harvested in July, and a "flour corn," planted in June and harvested in September as the harvest of the Great Corn (Kniffen, Gregory, and Stokes 1987, Fig. 23).

Corn was processed and eaten in a variety of ways and was augmented by the cultivation of squash, beans, pumpkins, and other cultigens. European crops, such as the watermelon, were introduced and adopted by the Caddoan peoples as well (Blake 1981). Wild plants and animals were gathered when they were available. Wild plant foods were plentiful May through November, and game animals, like deer and turkey, were hunted in the fall months. The deer was considered the primary game animal, but after the introduction of the horse, many of the Caddoan groups began to participate in communal bison hunts during the winter months on the prairies to the west.

Although the Caddoan peoples did not have fortified villages and did not congregate in nucleated communities for protection, they did engage in war with certain enemies. The Choctaw, Chickasaw, Osage, Wichita, and Tonkawa Indians were traditional enemies of the Caddoan peoples in historic times (Newkumet and Meredith 1988, 73). In most cases, warfare amounted to little more than organized raids to capture or scalp one or a few individuals, though the Caddoan and Wichita groups were frequently captured by the Choctaw, Chickasaw, and Osage and sold to the French and English colonists and traders. However, on occasion, great victories were achieved by the Caddoan peoples when large numbers of the enemy were either killed or captured and many trophy heads and scalps were gathered to be displayed in the xinesi's compound. According to Newkumet and Meredith (1988, 73–74), the Caddo recall these historical relationships "with good humor. Hasinai singers have removed from the turkey dance sequence some songs recalling military victories over the Choctaw and the Osage. This was done so that no one would be embarrassed when Choctaw and Osage members attended Caddo dances."

FIRST ENCOUNTERS, 1520 – 1685

The earliest explorations by Europeans of the general area or margins of it (Milanich and Milbreath 1989a, 1989b) began shortly after Spain's Indies commerce was formally organized in 1503 by the creation of the Casa de Contratación (Arnold and Weddle 1978, 63). As part of the regulation and encouragement of New World trade, explorations of the Gulf Coast were carried out from Florida to Tampico throughout the early sixteenth century. In fact, Pineda in 1519 successfully explored and mapped what is now known as the Texas coastline (Weddle 1985). While no documentary evidence exists for direct European contact with Caddoan peoples through these initial forays, Europeans were already conducting slave raiding and native resettlement projects along the Texas coast by 1550 (Bolton 1912).

Shortly after this, Álvar Núñez Cabeza de Vaca and companions, shipwrecked survivors of the Narváez Florida expedition, traveled and traded along the Texas coast from 1528 to 1534 (Bandelier 1904). While Swanton (1942, 29) does not believe that Cabeza de Vaca actually encountered any Caddoan peoples during his wanderings, his dealings in the exchange of native American goods, including marine products, stone, and wood, between coastal and inland groups, suggest that he might have traveled in the region. In *The Florida of the Inca* Garcilaso de la Vega (1951, 482) noted that, during the 1542 Moscoso exploration in what is thought to be East Texas,

> throughout the province of Guancane [in East Texas] many wooden crosses had been placed on top of the houses. . . . The explanation for this circumstance . . . was that the people here had received news of the benefits and marvels Alvar Núñez Cabeza de Vaca and Andrés Dorantes and their companions had performed . . . within the provinces of Florida. . . . And even though it is true that Alvar Núñez and his companions did not come to this particular province or to a number of others which lie between it and the lands where they traveled, still the fame of the deeds performed by God through these men eventually, by passing from hand to hand and from land to land, reached the province of Guancane.

In any event, direct contact between Cabeza de Vaca and Caddoan peoples in East Texas cannot be established by historical documentation. Nevertheless, the possibility exists that if it did take place, the typhoid and measles carried by the Narváez party could have been transmitted to native American groups living elsewhere along the Texas Coast and then inland to Caddoan groups through aboriginal trade and other contact (Dobyns 1983, 261). Thus, the Narváez and Cabeza de Vaca exploration is an important benchmark for the initiation of contact between European groups and native Americans in the Spanish Borderlands West (Hester 1989b, 199).

In 1542, the de Soto *entrada,* led by Luis de Moscoso following the death of de Soto along the Mississippi River near present-day Memphis, passed into the Caddoan Area, spending several months among Caddoan groups who lived between the Ouachita and Trinity rivers (Swanton 1939; Young and Hoffman in press). At this point the *entrada* of de Soto, and what was left of his six hundred men, was already three years old, and had taken them on a circuitous route through the southeastern United States and then to the Mississippi River in May 1541 (Hudson 1990).

Within what is now recognized as the Caddoan Archaeological Area, Moscoso described the provinces of Naguatex, Nondacao, and Guasco, for example, as groups that had dense populations in scattered settlements and abundant food reserves of maize (Swanton 1939, 258–280). My examination of the route of Moscoso (see Perttula 1989a, 88–99), utilizing known locations of such aboriginal trails as the Caddo (Strickland 1942) and Hasinai (Wedel 1978) traces, the initial routes of the Camino Reales (Corbin 1991), Caddoan language names (Chafe 1983, in press), accounts of the expedition, and archaeological data (Thurmond 1990a, 1990b; Schambach 1989), suggests that his route passed through settlements of aboriginal Caddoan groups known archaeologically as the Late Mid-Ouachita (or Social Hill), Belcher, Texarkana, Titus, and Frankston phases (Fig. 2).[1] These archaeological phases will be discussed further in the next chapter, but the important point here is that the identification of these phases allows us to discuss the social and cultural character of Caddoan populations living at this time in greater detail than would otherwise be possible (Thurmond 1985; Johnson 1987).

This proposed route of Moscoso differs in some respects from that outlined by Swanton (1939) and more recently by Hudson (1985, 1986, 1990) and associates (Hudson, DePratter, and Smith 1989). Other proposed routes of Moscoso in East Texas (Castaneda 1936; Williams 1942; Woldert 1942) are less in accordance with archaeological, ethnographic, and geographical data because they range farther north and west in Texas than seems warranted. They are not discussed here.

There are four accounts available from the expedition, but only three pertain to the Caddoan Area because the last part of the Ranjel narrative is missing. The accounts of Fidalgo of Elvas and Luis Hernández de Biedma are firsthand reports from members of the *entrada* written in 1554 and 1557, contain descriptive and statistical information, and generally corroborate each other (Brain, Toth, and Rodriquez-Buckingham 1974, 239–243). The Garcilaso de la Vega account was written from the reminiscences of several participants fifty years after the *entrada* and was only published in 1605 (the Varner and Varner edition in 1951). As a historical document, therefore, it is generally acknowledged to be of secondary value because of apparent fabrications in the text and its lack of correspondence in detail with the other narratives.

The classic reconstruction of the de Soto route of exploration by Swanton (1939) has been the subject of several subsequent studies (Brain 1985a, 1985b; Hudson et al. 1984, 1985, 1989; Hudson 1986, 1987a, 1990; Milanich 1987b; Schambach 1989; Kenmotsu, Bruseth, and Corbin 1992). This discussion is limited to those segments of the route following the *entrada*'s crossing of the Mississippi River and the movement of the de Soto expedition into the Arkansas River basin of central Arkansas.

After crossing the Mississippi River near present-day Commerce Landing, Mississippi (Morse and Morse 1983, Fig. 13-2), not far south of present-

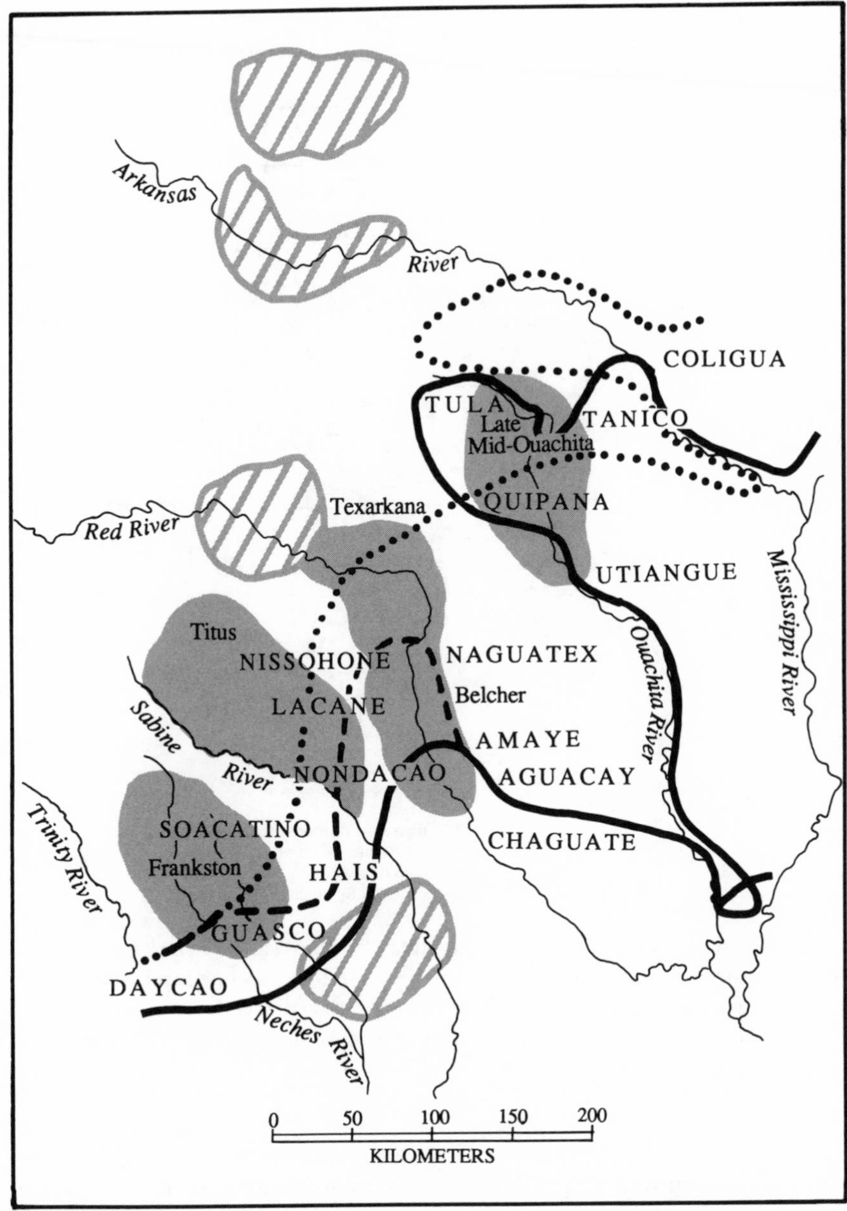

FIG. 2. Proposed de Soto–Moscoso routes and the Caddoan Area. The suggested locations of aboriginal provinces are shown relative to the distribution of the Frankston, Titus, Belcher, Texarkana, and late Mid-Ouachita phases, ca. 1540: *solid dots,* de Soto route (Hudson 1986); *dotted line,* de Soto route (Perttula, this volume); *solid line,* de Soto route (Swanton 1939); *screened cells,* archaeological phases; *striped cells,* other Caddoan phases.

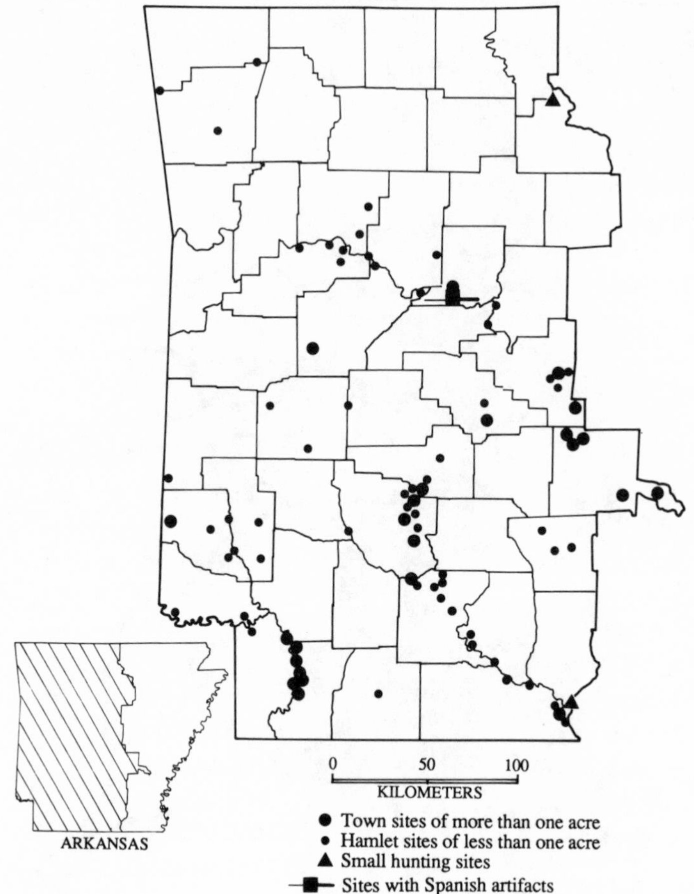

FIG. 3. Protohistoric sites in Caddoan area of Arkansas: *large circles,* town sites of more than one acre; *small circles,* hamlet sites of less than one acre; *triangles,* small hunting sites; *large squares,* sites with Spanish artifacts (from the Arkansas Archeological Survey, Automated Management of Archeological Site Data in Arkansas data base).

day Memphis in June 1541, the de Soto expedition spent several months in the Mississippi Alluvial Valley of eastern Arkansas among large populations of Mississippian peoples in the provinces of Pacaha, Cosqui, and Aquixo. There are a few sites in this region with sixteenth-century Spanish artifacts (Fig. 3). Then they moved in a north and westerly direction toward the Ozarks and the Arkansas River in their hopeful search for gold and passage to the South Seas, coming first to the Coligua province on the White River in east-central Arkansas (Hudson 1990). Hudson and Morse (in press) identify the Coligua province archaeologically as the Mississippi period Greenbrier phase along the western lowland and Ozark escarpment. From Coligua, they encountered other provinces and towns between the White and Arkansas rivers, finally setting out from Tanico toward the south and "the best populated land thereabout" (Elvas in Robertson 1933, 194), where they might be able to travel through without mishap or "in which he [de Soto] could winter the people." Tanico is usually placed in the vicinity of Hot Springs because of the well-known and large warm springs there (Brain 1985b, xl, liv), but warm springs and salines are common in many of the drainages of the Ouachita Mountains as well. Hudson (1990) places the Tanico in the Carden Bottom area of the Arkansas River in west-central Arkansas (see Fig. 3). A sixteenth-century Clarksville copper bell has been recovered from one of the Carden Bottom sites (Brain 1975b). In any event, the Spaniards next encountered people of the province of Tula.

The language and customs of the Tula were not like those of other groups previously encountered by the Spanish. They offered fierce resistance to the Spaniards, used large spears, practiced head deformation, and had facial tattooing (Swanton 1942, 30–31). After the Spanish subdued the Tula, the *cacique,* or tribal leader, of the Tula province brought bison hides as a gift, explaining that "nearby to the north were many cattle. The Christians did not see them nor enter their land, for the land was poorly settled where they were, and had little maize" (Elvas in Robertson 1933, 199). From the description of this location, the Tula appear to be referring to the area of the northern Ouachita Mountains in the Petit Jean and Fourche la Fave valleys or to the region further north in the Arkansas River basin in the general vicinity of Fort Smith (Hudson, DePratter, and Smith 1989, 89).

There is some question whether the Tula were Caddoan people (Swanton 1942; Early 1982b). Resemblances in customs (i.e., head deformations and facial tattooing) between the Tula and groups later encountered by the *entrada* that are certainly now known to be Caddoan appear to support such an ethnic relationship. However, there is no definite archaeological evidence to denote the presence of sixteenth-century Caddoan archaeological sites in either the eastern Ouachita Mountains (Early 1982b, 46), the Ozark Highland, or the Arkansas River basin in western Arkansas (see Fig. 3).

Deciding not to stay in Tula for the winter, de Soto continued to search for a province that could support and provision the expedition through the winter. Based on information gathered from Indians captured in the Caddoan province of Quipana, south or southeast of Tula, the two closest provinces were Utiangue or Autiamgue (Hudson 1990, 121) downstream on the Arkansas River and Guahate (Naguatex) to the south by overland routes. Both were within a week's journey of Tula and Quipana. He chose to winter at Utiangue, alternatively in the vicinity of Camden on the lower Ouachita

River (Dickinson 1980; Swanton 1939, 258), or south of Little Rock on the Arkansas River (Hudson 1990; Schambach 1989, 13).

The identification of Guahate with the province of Naguatex on the Red River later visited by the *entrada* in June 1542 appears to correspond well with the information available on directions and distances provided in the Elvas and Biedma chronicles (Strickland 1942, 112–114). The trail between Quipana and Guahate, an eight-day journey, presumably followed the Caddo Trace described in 1713 in more detail by Joutel (1906) that ran from the Ouachita River to the Red River, and from the Ouachita River to the lower Arkansas and the Quapaw people living there. An eight-day journey from Quipana to Naguatex, a twenty-three league trip (Pichardo in Hackett 1931–1946, vol. 3) based on the distance of a six-day trip between Quipana and Utiangue, places the Naguatex crossing of Red River in the Long Prairie area near where Lewisville, Arkansas, is now (see Fig. 2).

Swanton had located the Moscoso crossing of the Red River just above Shreveport, Louisiana, based on old ferry crossings and the presence of a group of mounds (the Mounds Plantation site reported by Webb and McKinney [1975]) located above the city (Swanton 1939, 275). However, at the time of the *entrada,* the Caddoan utilization of Mounds Plantation was quite minimal (Webb and McKinney 1975, 122) and certainly could not represent the major Caddoan riverine community described by the Elvas chronicles (Robertson 1933, 244). Unfortunately, Biedma does not mention the Naguatex province after describing the journey of the *entrada* to Aguacay province east of Amaye province, which Schambach (1989, 19) locates north of Texarkana in the vicinity of Ogden, Arkansas (see Fig. 2). Placing the crossing approximately eighty kilometers north of Shreveport puts the Naguatex province squarely in the Great Bend locality of the Red River, one of the foremost sociopolitical centers of Caddoan life ca. 1540. The largest surviving Caddo Mound, the Battle Mound, was the premier Late Caddoan period civic-ceremonial center in the entire Caddoan Area, and it was here during the Belcher phase that Caddoan culture reached its precontact peak in population and sociopolitical complexity (Schambach 1983, 1989, 20). The Battle Mound and associated sites are located on Long and Chicaninna prairies, specifically on the left (descending) bank of the Red River. There is a large cluster of Protohistoric period Caddoan sites in this area of southwest Arkansas (see Fig. 3).

In light of the fact that the Late Caddoan period settlements of the Red River Great Bend region appear to cluster into two localities, the Amaye province Texarkana phase cluster limited to the Upper Great Bend and the Naguatex province Belcher phase cluster in two localities downstream (see chapter 3), Strickland's (1942, 119–120) discussion of the etymology of *Naguatex* is particularly pertinent. According to Strickland, *Naguatex* is a transliteration of Caddoan cognates *nawi* and *tash* (*techas*) meaning "friends down there" (Strickland 1942, 120). Conceivably then, the Naguatex, or Nawitash, refers to the fact that they were downstream friends of the Texarkana phase groups in the upper Great Bend of the Red River.

The death of de Soto on the Mississippi River at the province of Guachoya in the spring of 1542 "freed the survivors from continuing upon the original objectives of the expedition. There was only one thought shared by all: to escape from the whole dreadful adventure. Under the leadership of Luis de Moscoso, they officially decided it was hopeless to seek the sea . . . in fact, the cavaliers were clearly reluctant to take to boats . . . and instead determined to march west in the direction of New Spain" (Brain 1985b, xlv).

Moscoso's expedition to the Caddoan Area in 1542 came by way of the Lower Mississippi Valley and the Tensas Basin, passing through the Caddoan provinces of Chaguate and Aguacay where the Indians made salt (Swanton 1939, 273). These provinces may be in the Saline Bayou and Bayou Dorcheat basins east of the Red River, but Hudson (1990) and Schambach (1989) place them in the Ouachita and Little Missouri drainages in southwest Arkansas where productive salines are known (Early 1990) and clusters of Protohistoric Caddoan period sites are apparent (see Fig. 3). Out of the salt-producing areas, the next indications of Caddoan peoples were in the province of Amaye about thirty kilometers east of the Red River (Swanton 1939, 274). The Amaye, Naguatex, and Hacanac, or Lacane, peoples together attacked the Spaniards prior to their reaching the Red River but were not able to stop them from crossing the Red River the next day into the Naguatex settlements. It was abandoned, but they saw evidence of much available food on hand. Swanton (1942, 32) noted that the province of Naguatex "is represented as the most fertile and populous of all the provinces through which the army passed during this expedition, and though they plundered its granaries in July on their way west, when they returned in October these were refilled."

When leaving Naguatex Moscoso's native guides, who were obtained after the Spanish burned several villages and seized captives (Elvas in Robertson 1933, 246), advised him to turn away from the Red River and proceed southwest (see Fig. 2). Whether this was a way to discourage further exploration of the Red River or was an isolated plan of action by the guides, they eventually brought the Moscoco *entrada* into East Texas. Even this was with reluctance, however, for according to Elvas (in Robertson 1933, 247), "the guides, who were guiding the governor, if they had to go toward the west, guided them toward the east, and sometimes they went through dense forests, wandering off the road. The governor ordered them hanged from a tree and an Indian woman, who had been captured at Nissohone, guided him, and he went back to look for the road. Two days later, he reached another wretched land, called Lacane."

From the narrative by Elvas it is clear that a definite aboriginal trail existed from the Red River southwest into East Texas that the Caddo guides either did or did not try to follow in their attempts to delude the Spanish. This can only be the Hasinai Trace (Wedel 1978, 3), known as Trammell's Trace in the nineteenth century (Williams 1979), that crossed a series of tributaries of the Red River between the Sulphur and Sabine rivers before running to the Caddoan settlements in the Neches and Angelina river valleys (Kenmotsu, Bruseth, and Corbin 1992). The provinces of Nissohone and Lacane would, therefore, appear to have been located on tributary streams of the Red River, probably on the Sulphur River and Big Cypress Bayou, respectively (Thurmond 1990b; Schambach 1989, Fig. 2; Kenmotsu, Bruseth, and Corbin 1992).

Except for the provinces of Nondacao, thought to be on the Sabine River, and Guasco on the Neches River, intervening groups, if mentioned, are generally characterized by the de Soto chronicles as having relatively small populations. Neither the area nor the settlements appeared to be notably fertile or infertile, and neither contained abundant reserves of maize. This description certainly includes the Nissohone, Lacane, and Hais (or Aays) provinces as well as others. As Biedma (Bourne 1904, 181) put it when referring to the Soacatino, "It was among some close forests and was scant of food."

In the province of Guasco in the Neches/Angelina River basin of East Texas (see Fig. 2) the Spanish noted that there was plenty of corn as well as turquoise and shawls of cotton that had been brought from the direction of the sunset (the southwest) (Bourne 1904, 181). From there Moscoso continued west some six to ten days to a river named Daycao, beyond which lived another group of Indians who did not cultivate the soil, nor did they speak a language intelligible to the East Texas Caddoan groups. The river Daycao may be the Trinity, Navasota, Brazos, or Colorado rivers in north-central or Central Texas (Hudson 1990, 122; Kenmotsu, Bruseth, and Corbin 1992). The area west of Guasco was apparently not permanently occupied by Caddoan peoples but was sometimes used by them to hunt deer (Elvas in Robertson 1933, 252).[2] After finding little to commend the area to the Spaniards—"The land was so poor they did not find half an alquire of maize" (Elvas in Robertson 1933, 252–253)—they returned to Guasco. From there they returned by the same route through the Caddoan Area until they reached the Ouachita River. Then they crossed over to the Mississippi River and settled in Aminoya on the Mississippi River. That winter they built a number of boats, and in the summer of 1543 they started down the Mississippi River. They reached Panuco on the Mexican Gulf Coast about two months later (Hudson 1990, 100–101; Swanton 1939, 280).

It may never be possible to reconstruct the route of the de Soto *entrada* across the Caddoan Area. Unlike the Mississippi Valley and interior Southeast (Brain 1975b, 1985a; Ewen 1988; Hudson, Smith, and DePratter 1984; Mitchem 1989; Mitchem and McEwan 1988; Morse and Morse 1983), where there is some consensus that sixteenth-century *entrada* artifacts have been identified in archaeological sites, artifacts pertaining conclusively to the de Soto expedition have not been located in the entire Caddoan Area (Dickinson 1987; Schambach and Early 1983, SW115). However, one intriguing possibility for early Spanish contact–related goods are the chalice-like vessels found at three mid–sixteenth-century Titus phase sites in the Cypress Creek drainage of East Texas (see Thurmond 1990b; Turner 1978, 98; and this book's appendix).

Turner (1978, 100) suggests that the ceramic "chalices" found at the Titus phase sites were copies of stemmed wine glasses, stemmed cups, or stemmed goblets in the possession of individuals in the de Soto *entrada.* Deagan (1987, 127–155 and Figs. 6.2a–b, 6.33a–b, 6.37b, 6.42, and 6.45) illustrates sixteenth-century Hispanic bottles, goblets, decanters, vases, and *almorratxa* that have a form similar to that of the stemmed vessels recovered in the Titus phase sites. These Titus phase sites are in the general vicinity of the province of Lacane (Hudson 1990; Perttula 1989a; Thurmond 1990a, Fig. 35) visited by Moscoso.

Swanton (1939, 348 and map 9) equates the Lacane with the ethnographically recorded Nacao, a poorly known Caddoan group loosely affiliated with the Hasinai confederacy. The Nondacao and Nissohone of the chronicles are probably the Nadaco (or Anadarko) and Nasoni groups of the eighteenth-century ethnographic records. Later population remnants of these groups apparently lived in the same approximate areas of the Sabine and Sulphur rivers as they did in 1542 when they were described by the de Soto–Moscoso chroniclers. If this reconstruction of the Moscoco *entrada* is reasonable, both the Nondacao and Lacane groups may have been among those Caddoan groups living on the Sabine River and Cypress Creek drainages in the mid–sixteenth century who produced the chalicelike vessels from a Spanish model (Perttula et al. 1986, 184; Thurmond 1990a, 233).

While there was no direct observation of the transmission of epidemic diseases during the de Soto *entrada,* it is probable that Caddoan groups were being affected by infectious diseases through this first phase of contact (Ramenofsky 1982, 255–259, 1986). Smallpox, some form of tuberculosis (Clark et al. 1987), and certain disease zoonoses (such as typhus, plague, and malaria) could all have been introduced to the New World by de Soto and the *entrada*. It is important to note that while the effects of the de Soto *entrada* were probably not particularly significant in the sense of European goods and products being made available and introduced to the Caddo peoples, the ultimate biological effects of the *entrada* are manifold and cannot be so easily overlooked. This is because in "virgin soil" conditions such as North America, the introduction of an exotic virus such as smallpox can result in upward of 100 percent mortality (Ramenofsky 1987b; Upham 1986; Crosby 1986). We will return to this topic in subsequent chapters, where the archaeological and bioarchaeological evidence for contact with Europeans will be reviewed in greater detail.

Following the Moscoso *entrada,* there is no recorded European contact directly with Caddoan peoples until the Hernando Martín and Diego del Castillo expedition to the Jumanos in 1650 (Bolton 1920, 314). The settlement of Santa Fe by the Spaniards in 1600 and then the seventeenth-century exploration of the plains to the east (Vehik 1986; Quinn 1979, vol. 5) by the Spaniards, among whom were traders and missionaries, increased intersettlement contact between Plains groups and those of other areas (Spielmann 1989) who were involved in what Baugh calls the "Southern Plains macroeconomy" (Baugh and Swenson 1980; Baugh 1982).

As previously noted, the Spanish first heard about the "Great Kingdom of the Tejas" in the mid–seventeenth century from Jumano middlemen who ranged from the Rio Grande to East Texas carrying goods back and forth to aboriginal trading fairs held in the southern plains (Bolton 1912). The Hernando Martín–Diego del Castillo expedition in 1650 and the Mendoza-López expedition in 1683 both reached the western boundaries of East Texas Caddoan country, the latter receiving "ambassadors" from the Tejas or Hasinai Caddo. There is no documented evidence, however, that any goods of European manufacture were traded or given to these Caddoan groups during these expeditions, though it is likely that East Texas Caddoan peoples had already acquired some goods indirectly from the Spanish settlements in New Mexico or Coahuila (Bolton 1987, 135; Swagerty 1989).

The Jumano Juan Sabeata (Kelley 1955) described the Tejas as "a settled people [who] . . . raised grain in such abundance that they even fed it to their horses" (Bolton 1920, 314). Sabeata also mentioned that two Tejas messengers told him "that into this eastern region Spaniards are entering by water in wooden houses, and that they barter and exchange with the said nations of the Texas" (Pichardo, pt. 1, para. 156, in Hackett 1931–1946, vol. 1).

With this and later news of La Salle's expedition along the Texas coast (Weddle 1973), Spanish efforts became concentrated on not only finding La Salle, but in reaching and converting the country of the Tejas before the French did (Bolton 1912). This ushered in sustained direct contact between

TABLE 1. Documented Expeditions: Possible Direct and Indirect European Contact in the Caddoan Area, 1519–1683

1519	Pineda's exploration of the Texas Gulf Coast
1528–1534	Alvar Núñez Cabeza de Vaca expedition
1542	de Soto–Moscoso expedition
1650	Hernando Martín and Diego del Castillo expedition
1683	Mendoza-López expedition

Caddoan groups and Europeans that continues to this day, begun by Spanish missionaries and French traders after ca. 1685 (Swanton 1942).

The basic import of the de Soto–Moscoso expedition in 1542 is that these Spanish explorers documented and described aspects of Caddoan settlement, subsistence strategies, aboriginal routes of travel and trade, and social organization that in broad scope are consistent with and reflected in the archaeological record of the Caddoan Area (Story 1990; Jeter et al. 1989). Other documented Spanish travels during the Protohistoric period (Table 1) are very widely separated in time and space and provide no direct information about the Caddoan peoples except their general location, since no direct contact was made with them. Descriptions by Juan Sabeata of the Jumano and the earlier observations of the Moscoso expedition chroniclers indicate Caddoan peoples living in the western subarea of the Caddoan Area were in regular contact with aboriginal peoples living in the southern plains and the Southwest. Through them they obtained aboriginal products such as ceramics, lithic raw materials, and bison hides, and Spanish products without the direct participation of the Spanish. These important Spanish products included horses, horse gear (for instance, bridles and saddle gear), ornaments, and clothing (Griffith 1954; Swagerty 1989).

Between 1520 and 1685, various Europeans actually lived in the Caddoan Area less than a half a year in total. It is virtually certain that most Caddoan peoples during that time never saw a European. This is not to suggest that the Caddoan groups did not know about the Europeans or were not aware of their movements, only that there was no sustained contact between them until Spain and France committed themselves to colonization in the late seventeenth century. As a consequence, artifactual evidence of this phase of European contact in the Caddoan Area will be minimal, for as Krieger (in Davis 1961, 120) pointed out some years ago, "In any one site, something like twenty beads and two bits of iron may be all that can be found to represent perhaps a century of contact; and this being true, there must be scores of sites actually occupied during the same 'historic period' from which the archaeologist cannot recover a single European object."

MORE ENDURING EUROPEAN CONTACT, 1685 – 1800

The second phase of European contact in the Caddoan historic period began with the renewed exploration of the Mississippi Valley following the establishment of the Illinois colony by the French in the 1670s. Initially explored in 1673 by Marquette and Joliette to the mouth of the Arkansas River (Delangez 1946), the Mississippi River in 1682 was fully explored to its mouth by La Salle. This was followed three years later by another expedition directed by La Salle that was intended to colonize the area and link the Gulf Coast with the growing French colonies of Illinois and Canada (Margry 1877–1886). For unknown reasons, this expedition missed the mouth of the Mississippi River and came to shore on the Texas Gulf Coast at Matagorda Bay (Cox 1922; Gilmore 1986b).

La Salle made several trips from Fort St. Louis to explore the region and try to find the Mississippi River, visiting the Hasinai (or Cenis, as the French transcribed it) in 1686 before turning back with several horses purchased from the Hasinai. Another effort was made in 1687 by most of the survivors at Fort St. Louis to reach the Mississippi River. La Salle was, however, murdered by several of the men part way through the trip, and the remaining party decided to stay on with the Hasinai to live. Several of the men, including Henri Joutel and Jean Cavelier, brother of Sieur de La Salle, eventually moved on toward the Illinois colony, passing through the Red and Ouachita River valleys with the assistance of the Kadohadacho and Cahinnio Caddoan groups living there, until they reached the Arkansas Post on the lower Arkansas River (Delangez 1938; Joutel [1713] 1906). The Arkansas Post had been established by Henri de Tonti in 1686 (Delangez 1944).

The threat of French settlement in an area the Spanish considered officially under their hegemony initiated serious Spanish efforts to settle and missionize the country east of New Mexico and the Rio Grande known to them as the "Kingdom of the Tejas" (Bolton 1912). At the same time, the French were determined to take advantage of the La Salle explorations of the Lower Mississippi River Valley to extend their claims to the region. This was followed shortly thereafter by the English colonies established along the South Atlantic Coast who wished to extend trade routes west to native American groups living on the Mississippi River and the Texas Gulf Coast (Crane 1929; Woods 1980; Coker and Watson 1986; Usner 1989).

The years between 1685 and 1714 were then a time of continual French and Spanish exploration of the Caddoan Area. European knowledge about the geography, territory, and native peoples living in the Lower Mississippi Valley and its western tributaries increased as changes in maps of the area show clearly (Jackson, Weddle, and DeVille 1990).

Information supplied by native American groups about other populations and resources in particular areas was often the impetus for further exploration and subsequent European settlement. For instance, Pierre Le Moyne d'Iberville obtained information in 1699 from the Taensa Indians (in Northeast Louisiana) about the Caddoan peoples that led to the first exploration of the Red River by St. Denis in 1700 (Cox 1906) and the establishment in 1714 of Fort St. Jean Baptiste aux Natchitos (Natchitoches). D'Iberville was told by the Taensa that he "shall come to a river on the left side that is named Tas[s]encougoula [Red River], in which he [the Taensa mapmaker] shows two branches: on the west one are eight villages, which he calls Yatache' [Yatasi], Nachthytos [Natchitoches], Yezito, Natao, Cachaymoua, Cadodaquio [Kadohadacho], Nataho, Natsytos. The fifth and sixth of these villages M. Cavelier visited on his way back overland from the Senys [Hasinai] to the Acansa. From the Senys to the Cadodaquio they found to be a distance of 53 leagues" (McWilliams 1981, 71–72).

The European political relationships, trade and religious objectives, and the larger spheres of influence controlled by the Spanish, French, and British in the developing world economy all played a part in determining the degree and kind of involvement they had in the Caddoan Area between ca. 1685 and 1800 (see Braudel 1984, 21–85, 387–429; Wallerstein 1974, 1980; and Wolf 1982, 129–231, for discussions of world economies). Trade contacts, rumors of settlement, and exploration by one government were responded to in kind by the others as part of the unstable process of colonization (Table 2). The nature and character of sustained European contact in this second phase has been so comprehensively discussed (e.g., Bolton 1915, 1987; Giraud 1957, 1963, 1974a, 1974b; Cox 1909; Fieldhouse 1966; Galloway 1982; Gibson 1989; John 1975, 1985; Surrey 1916; Swagerty 1984; Usner 1987; Wade 1989) that a detailed summary is not necessary. The following considerations thus concern only the critical parameters of Spanish, French, English, and American contact as manifest in the Caddoan Area.

Spanish objectives in the Caddoan Area, the province of Texas, were basically designed to achieve political and religious goals involving the Caddoans. Their purpose was to "convert him, to civilize him, and to exploit him"(Bolton 1917, 45). In other words, the Spanish colonial policy aimed to combine the political ends of the state in holding and expanding the frontier colonies (Fig. 4) with the religious purpose inherent in Spanish civilization (Dobyns 1980; Fairbanks 1985; Gibson 1989). To do this, a system of missions and presidios (forts to protect the missionaries and converts) was established in what is now East Texas and western Louisiana between 1691 and 1721 (Habig 1984).[3] The actual timing of mission settlement and abandonment in the province of Texas closely followed political motivations of

TABLE 2. Major Documented Expeditions and Events: Direct European and North American Contact with the Caddoan Peoples, 1685–1810

	FRENCH
1685–1687	La Salle expedition, establishment of Fort de St. Louis on Matagorda Bay, Texas, and travels to the Hasinai, Kadohadacho, and Cahinnio
1690	Henri de Tonti travels to Kadohadacho and Hasinai in search of La Salle
1700, 1705	Exploration of Red River by Louis Juchereau de St. Denis
1714	Establishment of Fort St. Jean Baptiste aux Natchitos (Natchitoches) on Red River by St. Denis
1719	Exploration of Red River and Canadian River by La Harpe and Du Rivage; establishment of French trading post among the Kadohadacho
1721	Establishment of French trading post among the Wichita on the Arkansas River in Northeast Oklahoma by La Harpe
1740	Mallet party of voyagers reach Santa Fe, then descend Canadian and Arkansas rivers
1741	Fabry de la Bruyère expedition to New Mexico via the Arkansas and Canadian rivers, returning by way of the Kadohadacho
1750	French traders from Natchitoches living among the Wichita on Arkansas River
	SPANISH
1690	Alonzo de León and Fray Massanet travel to the Hasinai to establish the first two Spanish missions
1691	Don Domingo Terán de los Ríos exploration of Hasinai and Kadohadacho country
1693	Spanish missions withdrawn
1716–1717	Reestablishment of Spanish missions in East Texas and Northwest Louisiana by Domingo Ramón. A presidio was established at Nuestra Señora de los Dolores de los Tejas among the Hasinai

the Spanish government in response to French exploration (Corbin 1989, 269–270). As Bolton (1917, 50) pointed out many years ago:

> The missionaries of the northern frontier had long had their eye on the "Kingdom of Texas" as a promising field of labor, and had even appealed to the government for aid in cultivating it. But in vain, till La Salle planted a French colony at Matagorda Bay. Then the royal treasury was opened, and funds were provided for missions in Eastern Texas. The French danger passed for the moment, and the missions were withdrawn. Then for another decade Father Hidalgo appealed

TABLE 2. (*Continued*)

	SPANISH (*Continued*)
1721	Presidio at Nuestra Señora de Pilar de los Adaes established by Aguayo expedition
1731	Los Adaes becomes the capital of the Province of Texas. All but two Spanish missions (Los Adaes and Concepción) abandoned in East Texas and Northwest Louisiana
1767	Louisiana ceded to Spain by France; Spain bans Indian slavery
1772	All Spanish missions abandoned in provinces of Texas and Louisiana
1774	Settlement of Nuestra Señora del Pilar de Bucareli made by Spanish Adaesanos on Trinity River at the El Camino de Real crossing
1772, 1778 1779	Expeditions by de Mézières, lieutenant-governor of Natchitoches, as ambassador to the Hasinai, Kadohadacho, and Wichita tribes
1779	Settlement at Nacogdoches established by Spanish Adaesanos from Bucareli
1788	Exploration of north-central and northeast Texas by Vial and Fragoso enroute from Santa Fe to Natchitoches
1790	Territorial disputes between Spain, France, and the United States. Spanish open boundary of Texas province to Anglo-Americans and native Americans living east of the Mississippi River
	UNITED STATES
1803	Sale of Louisiana to the United States is completed
1804	Exploration of the Ouachita River by Hunter and Dunbar by orders of President Jefferson
1806	Exploration of the Red River by Freeman and Custis by orders of President Jefferson
1809–1810	Exploration by Anthony Glass of the Red River, Sulphur River, and the Wichita tribes at Spanish fort

> in vain for funds and permission to re-establish the missions. But when St. Denis, agent of the French government of Louisiana, intruded himself into Coahuila, the Spanish government at once gave liberal support for the refounding of the missions, to aid in restraining the French.

The missions were dependent, therefore, upon the frontier political situation for government support as well as upon their presumed success in converting the Caddoan peoples in the vicinity to Christianity. They were set up in such a way that it was necessary to try to induce the Caddoan

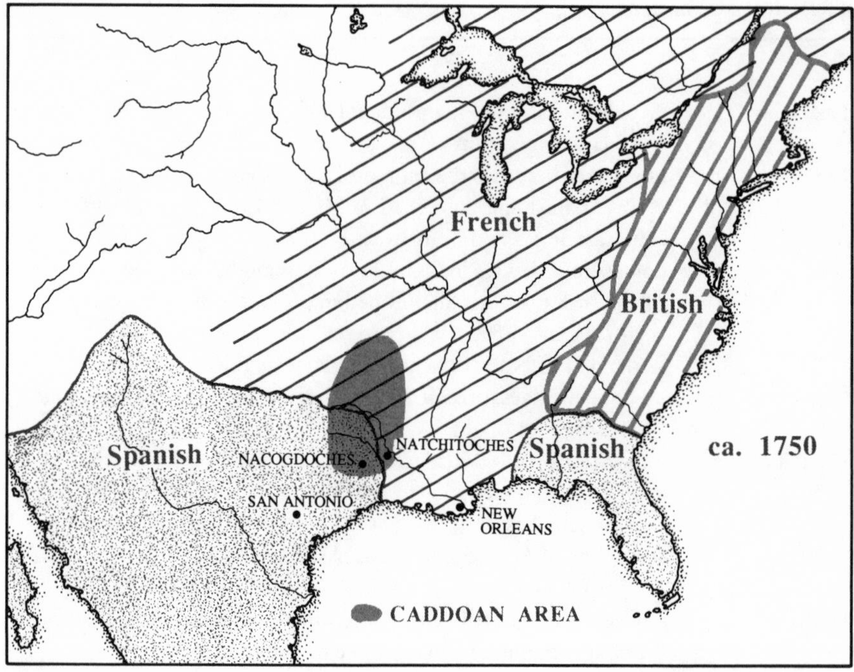

FIG. 4. The Caddoan Area and territories under the control of the Spanish, French, and British, ca. 1750.

peoples to settle in proximity to the Spanish missions; to have them participate in the religious, social, and economic activities devised by the missionaries (Espinosa 1716); and to try to create a supporting peasantry and feudal system (Hudson 1981, 167–168). The primary inducement was the message of Christianity, rather than physical force, and it was not dependent upon the extensive use of giving European goods as gifts and presents to the different Caddoan groups as the French so successfully did.

Periodic inspection reports of the missions in East Texas (Buckley 1911; Kress and Hatcher 1932; Murphy 1937) lamented not only their lack of success in converting the Hasinai Caddo (except at death), but also the poor economic and military situation at these settlements, which were so far from Spanish supply centers on the Rio Grande and in Coahuila. Each inspection led to the recommendation that the Caddo missions should be abandoned, and when the political setting was stable, these recommendations were followed.

Therefore, the Spanish missions in the Caddoan Area lasted only a short time among the Hasinai and East Texas tribes (1690–1693 and 1716–1772). Because of French trade encroachments, the Caddoan peoples were

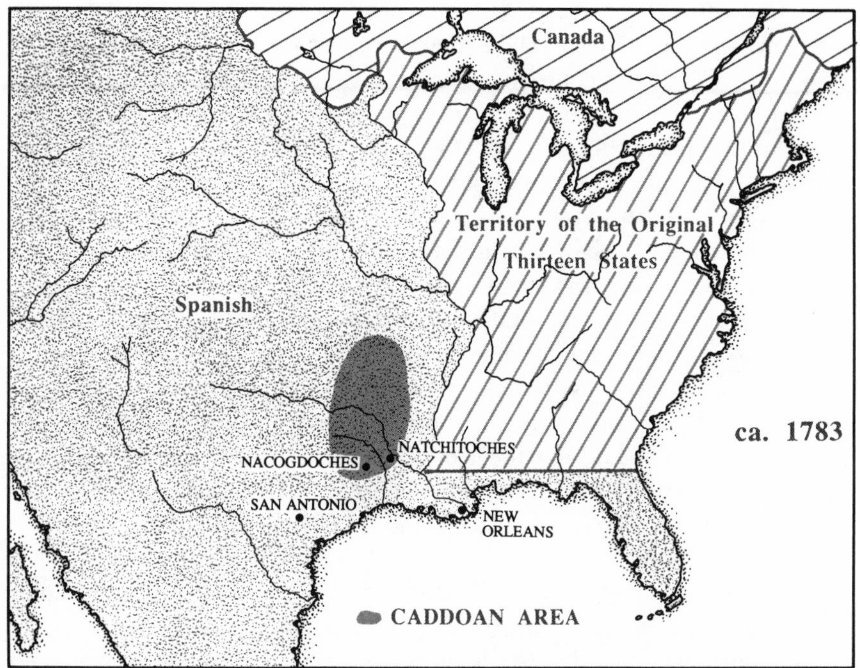

FIG. 5. Spanish Territory and the territory of the original thirteen states of the United States of America, 1783.

able to acquire trade goods and supplies they found useful for their own purposes without developing any material dependence upon the Spanish, who were not in a position to foster trade relationships with them. The religious message of the Spanish missionaries was equally inefficient, linked as it was soon to be with the episodic epidemics occurring among the Caddoan peoples after ca. 1687 and the Caddoan belief that the Spanish were the cause of those epidemics (Ewers 1973; Leutenegger 1979). The missions were established in close proximity to large numbers of Caddoan settlements in East Texas, and thus even their failure to induce the Hasinai to settle at the mission compounds in large numbers probably did not offset the spread of diseases from the Spanish to the nearby Hasinai and from there to elsewhere in the Caddoan Area.

Changes in Spanish Indian policy toward the Hasinai Caddo began when French Louisiana in 1767 became part of the Provincias Internas of Nueva España (Fig. 5), and the missions were abandoned in East Texas (Berry 1917; Holmes 1975; Kinnaird 1949). At that time, attempted means of Indian control became based more firmly on the system of distributing annual gifts to the friendly tribes and supplying them with regularly licensed traders with access to desired goods, as the French had tried to do under their administration in Louisiana. The earlier policy of narrowly restricting trade among the Caddoan peoples in an attempt to force their dependence upon missions for supplies had failed for the simple lack of supplies, causing the Caddoan groups to "illegally" deal with the nearby French, who were able to provide contraband goods in quantity. After 1767, expenses in the provinces by the Spanish government expressly included this "friendship to the Indian population." These gifts amounted to between only 2 and 5 percent of the budget between 1766 and 1776 but steadily increased to between 10 and 40 percent of the total budget after 1776 (Archivo General de Indios, Legajos 597) as a result of increased Spanish ventures in mediating English and American incursions along its borders (Bolton 1914, 1:79).

Other attempts to offset English influence in the Mississippi Valley and Louisiana led to the development of a Spanish Louisiana policy (*a*) to induce Choctaw, Chickasaw, Alabama, Coushatta, Delaware, Shawnee, and Cherokee tribes to settle in Louisiana and (*b*) to issue land grants to Anglo-Americans who swore allegiance to the Spanish Crown (Din 1973; Kinnaird and Kinnaird 1980). By 1790 these "immigrant" Indians and Anglo-American settlers began moving into Louisiana and Texas (Hatcher 1921), quickly outnumbering the Caddoan inhabitants of the area. This created further conflict between different aboriginal groups competing for fur resources (Strickland 1937) that was to continue and intensify under Mexican and American administrations in Texas. White (1983, 92–93) provides a useful discussion of 1790s Choctaw hunting strategies west of the Mississippi River and the intensification of warfare with the Osage and Kadohadacho that continued into the first quarter of the nineteenth century as a result of their resettlement in Louisiana.

French objectives in the Louisiana colony were firmly based on developing a mercantilistic trade policy whereby New World goods were produced at a lower cost and/or higher profit than they could be in France and were then sent to France for sale (Eccles 1973). In addition to the fur trade, wood, cotton, rice, and indigo were major goods produced in French Louisiana in the eighteenth century (Surrey 1916). While goods other than furs were produced mainly with slave laborers (including Apachean Indians supplied to the French colonists by the Wichita and Hasinai [Gregory 1973, 261–266]), the eighteenth-century fur trade clearly involved both the Indian and French populations (Usner 1981, 1985).

At least for the French, involvement in the fur trade was particularly strong in the first half of the eighteenth century, prior to the stabilization of the French Louisiana economy around other exportable goods (Surrey 1916). To pursue their policies, they tried to develop and foster regular and dependable relationships with Indian groups by which to acquire necessary products from them without disrupting local alliances and interactions (Wade 1989). That the French-Indian or Indian-Indian alliances were meant to create an economic setting conducive to French profits did not always mean that the status quo was maintained from year to year. How these relationships worked out depended on information received from the traders and coureurs de bois operating in the hinterlands and on Indian efforts to manipulate current trade networks to their own benefit.

Groups such as the Osage and Wichita, who consistently tried to maintain a favorable middleman role with the French and other Indian groups, thereby recovering more trade goods for themselves, were not always considered friendly by the French (and later the Spanish) because of their efforts to control and restrict trade for their own benefit (John 1975; Bailey 1973). Goods were then restricted, and the French would try, usually unsuccessfully, to replace them as middlemen by financing direct trading ventures to other interested aboriginal parties who had theretofore dealt with the more powerful Wichita and Osage middlemen.

For all intents and purposes, the French colonial policy can be described as monopolistic but accommodative. The French wished to exclusively control the economic exchange and trade with the Indians but were willing to accommodate short-term relationships with some of these Indian groups that were not as profitable as the long-term ones. This accommodation arose not only from the logistical difficulties of carrying out trade ventures in virtually unknown regions of their territory with poor means of supply, but also from their having to rely initially on the aboriginal community for critical food items that they could not produce themselves in adequate quantities (Usner, in press). This requirement was never overcome completely during the French control of the Louisiana colony (Clark 1970). In its accommodation, it approached a symbiosis because of the mutual relationship between the native Americans and the French colonists. For Indian products to have sufficient value to increase production, goods of "interest" to the Indian had to be offered in return; in the long run, one was not feasible without the other.

Annually supplying goods or presents to the Indians in return for products (at a set, negotiated price) desired by the French for export was a cornerstone of French colonial commercial policy in Louisiana (Usner 1987, 171–172). Regulation of market prices in the fur business by merchants and traders was based not only on the understanding of commercial profit as overseen by the French government, but was also an accommodation "to Indian insistence that trade be contained within the political sphere of relations" (Usner 1987, 175). Indian "clients" repeatedly bargained for more favorable exchange rates, using differences in the quality and expense of French versus English merchandise as a bargaining tool with the French and

Spanish Louisiana colonial governments. New Orleans was the entrepôt of the French colonial economy, serviced by Indian clients throughout the Mississippi Valley and its western tributaries.

The Caddoan tribes were only one of the French colonial economy's clients, and based on the amount of annual goods distributed, they were a subsidiary group when compared with the Arkansas or Quapaw, Tunica, and Mobilean tribes closer to New Orleans. Because of this, the Tunica were apparently able to exploit their position as middlemen dealers with the Caddoan peoples and French in the horse and salt trades (Brain 1979, 1989; Usner 1987, 187) by controlling the movement of goods on the Red River below Natchitoches.

The British played a late, albeit marginal, role in the Spanish Borderlands West inasmuch as their trade activities were concentrated mainly to the east of the Mississippi River (Woods 1980). By the time of the cession of French Louisiana to Spanish control in 1767 (see Fig. 5), the British trade network extended from the Atlantic Coast to the Mississippi River, and efforts were under way to penetrate Louisiana and the Gulf Coast of the Texas province (Stevens 1916). British objectives were comparable to those of the French in that they were designed to take advantage of all opportunities to garner a profit in the Indian trade (see Hudson 1981, 168; Nash 1972; White 1983). Throughout the 1770s and 1780s, English traders were reported to have been living among the East Texas Caddoan tribes, even at Natchitoches, and Indian groups were also going to the British suppliers and trading houses to purchase goods directly from them (Bolton 1914, vol. 1). Because they were relatively inexpensive, British manufactured goods continued to be purchased by the Spanish and then the Americans as part of the maintenance of the annual gifts policy (Purser 1964; Whitaker 1928).

CONTACT OF THE CADDOAN PEOPLES WITH PEOPLE OF THE UNITED STATES AND THE REPUBLIC OF TEXAS

From the 1790s international considerations, especially the containment of the United States east of the Mississippi River (see Fig. 5), dominated Spain's concerns in its Texas and Louisiana colonies. Any explorations of the Louisiana-Texas frontier by the United States were considered by Spain as threats to her territorial integrity (Flores 1985, 3). Along the boundary between Spain and the United States the allegiance of the various Indian nations (such as the Caddo, Wichita, and Comanche) of the Provincias Internas was perceived by the Spanish government as a critical factor in controlling the frontier, thus stalling U.S. expansionist policies in the Southwest. By 1790 Americans from east of the Mississippi River, including the Natchez District and West Florida, had begun to conduct trading ventures in horses and guns with the Texas Indians (Kinnaird 1932). Spain responded by abolishing any trade ties with the post at Natchitoches in favor of a more strictly controlled overland exchange of goods through supporting the trading house of William Barr, Edward Murphy, and Samuel Davenport in Nacogdoches (Flores 1985, 11). East Texas Caddoan peoples had frequented Nacogdoches as a place of trade since 1779, when it became the Spanish distribution center for annuities and presents (John 1975).

The 1790s were a period of growth in the American fur trade, and another major growth period in the industry was recorded from 1800 to 1808 (Clayton 1967). According to annual reports of the secretary of the treasury, beaver was the primary fur resource in the trade 1790–1820. As previously noted, the Kadohadacho and Hasinai participated in the trade from the outset, and their respective contributions to the fur trade were considered important parts of the Spanish and Louisiana economies (see Magnaghi 1978; Ewers 1969, 47–48; Flores 1984; Peake 1954, 17–18). According to Flores (1984, 274), "In 1812 Dehahuit of the Caddos entered a special request with Thomas Linnard at the Natchitoches factory to order 20 beaver traps for them, since 'The Beaver trade would be beneficial [to them] as Beaver abound in and about their country.'"

Following its purchase of the Louisiana Territory in 1803 the United States moved rapidly to explore the boundaries and character of this newly acquired territory (Fig. 6). It was considered important for the federal government to also establish commercial and political relationships with resident aboriginal groups, among them certain Caddoan tribes.

Accordingly, in 1805 Natchitoches became the site of a U.S. factory system (Prucha 1962). Dr. John Sibley was appointed as the acting Indian agent. The Kadohadacho, Petit Caddo, and the Yatasi frequented the government trading house, exchanging "furs from the bear, the deer, the beaver, the otter, and other animals . . . for carbines, merchandise, tobacco and firewater, of which they are very fond" (Padilla [1820] 1919, 47). Juan Antonio Padilla goes on to note that the Kadohadacho "are faithful in keeping their contracts; for the merchants of Natchitoches advance them munitions, trifles, and liquors at a good rate of exchange for furs."

The Freeman and Custis expedition of 1806 on the Red River, sponsored by the Jefferson administration (see Table 2), followed specific guidelines on intercourse with the Indians that were the product of standing U.S. policy for over a decade (see Turner 1977, 66–67; Prucha 1984, 89–114). In a letter to Thomas Freeman written in 1804, President Jefferson outlined his instructions for establishing Indian relations (quoted in Flores 1984, 322–323):

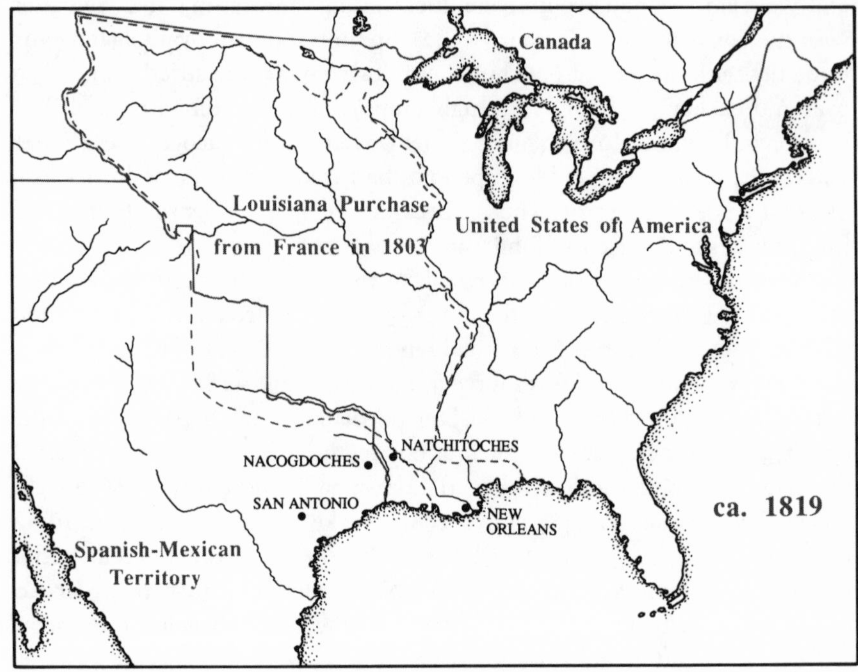

FIG. 6. The United States of America and Spanish-Mexican Territory in 1819. Note the overlap between the 1803 Louisiana Purchase and Spanish-Mexican Territory in Texas.

> Court an intercourse with the natives as intensively as you can . . . our first wish will be to be neighborly, friendly and useful to them and especially to carry on commerce with them on terms more reasonable and advantageous for them than any other Nation ever did: Confer with them on the points most convenient as mutual frontiers for them and us say that we have sent you to enquire into the nature of the Country and the Nations inhabiting it to know their wants and the supplies they will wish to dispose of and that after you shall have returned with the necessary information we shall take measures with their consent for setting trading houses among them at suitable places that in the mean time the same traders who reside among them or visit them and who are now become our citizens will continue to supply them as usual and that they will find us in all things just and faithful friends and patrons.

Freeman presented this message from the United States to the Kadohadacho chief Dehahuit at the Alabama-Coushatta village on the Red River in Northwest Louisiana in July 1806. Dehahuit was the son of the "Great Peacemaker" Tinhiouen, a Spanish medal chief who had mediated between the Spanish and Wichita-Taovayas on several occasions in forming treaties of peace (Bolton 1914, 2:141, 1915, 121–122) many years earlier. The Kadohadacho chief replied to Freeman in prophetic words, here paraphrased (Flores 1984, 163):

> That being well treated by the French while under their Government he loved them, that under the Spanish Government he was well treated and he loved them, that now it had pleased the French (for what reason he knew not) to give them up to the Americans, he loves them and hopes they will love and treat him as well as the French and Spanish did and that he doubts not that will be the case as two years have now elapsed since he came under their Government and has not yet had any cause for complaints. He added that he was sensible the Supreme Being had made a difference between us and his people, that he had been pleased to endow us with more sense and that he had also seen proper to grant us means which they were entirely destitute of; he therefore would look to them for protection and comfort, to be his father, brothers and friends.

Following the abandonment of the Freeman and Custis expedition on the Red River in Northeast Texas because of Spanish interference, which was related to questions concerning the actual boundary between Spanish Texas and the Louisiana territory, the United States initiated a border "war" with Spain. The end result was the 1806 Neutral Ground Agreement specifying that the Arroyo Hondo, rather than the Sabine River to the west, was the eastern boundary of Spanish Texas. Consequently, possession of the Red River was unresolved, as was the territorial allegiance of the Kadohadacho (Flores 1984, 287) since the neutral zone to all intents and purposes partitioned the Kadohadacho territory (now around Caddo Lake) between Spanish Texas and the United States. Dehahuit commented on this partition by noting that "the other day when I saw the Spaniards on one side of me, and your people on the other, I was embarrassed—I did not know on which foot to tread" (Flores 1984, 163).

In an effort to restrict the activities of American traders among the Indian groups in Texas, Spanish officials formulated a new policy whereby those Indian groups who dealt with the traders from Natchitoches (organized by Dr. John Sibley) were to be punished by being deprived of Spanish trade from Nacogdoches (Flores 1985, 23). A Spanish trading post at Bayou Pierre was also established in 1808 by Marcel Soto, but it proved uncompetitive with the American trade from the Natchitoches agency (Flores 1984, 307). Well-financed trading ventures from Natchitoches continued in Texas, with horses, mules, furs, and other products being exchanged by the Texas Indians in return for guns, lead, and powder from American traders such as Anthony Glass of Natchez (Flores 1985).

While these American trading ventures continued, actual settlement of the Red River, its tributaries, and the neutral ground between Louisiana and Texas began in earnest (Strickland 1937; Haggard 1945). By 1818 about three thousand settlers from the Midwest and upper South had squatted illegally in Caddo country along the south side of the Red River from the Great Bend to the Kiamichi River (see Lottinville 1980, 170–172). Although occasional settlers along the Red River were removed by American soldiers sent from Fort Smith or Natchitoches, Anglo-American settlements and populations increased up to and beyond the time of the Texas Revolution in 1836 (American State Papers 1832–1834; Strickland 1937, 64–238). Flores (1984, 308) notes that "after the Adams-Onis Treaty of 1819 made the Red River the international boundary, and particularly after Mexico finally threw off the yoke of Spanish imperial rule two years later, Anglo-Americans quickly poured into Northeast Texas."

This settlement expansion was also accompanied by another influx of aboriginal groups from east of the Mississippi River and from the Arkansas River, including Choctaw, Cherokee, Delaware, Kickapoo, Quapaw, Shawnee, Delaware, and Koasati groups (Anderson 1990; Everett 1990; Ewers 1969; Kniffen, Gregory, and Stokes 1987; Williams 1964).[4] These groups exchanged skins, corn, pumpkins, and beans at the trading house at Nacogdoches (Swanton 1942, 88), as well as with the American government traders at the new agency house at the mouth of the Sulphur River. In 1828, more than 40,000 deer skins, 1,500 bear skins, 1,200 otter skins, and 600 beaver skins were brought by native Americans to trade in Nacogdoches (Ewers 1969, 47). As the frontier moved west, Caddoan Indians in Louisiana became more isolated in the Anglo-American community and were under continual pressure from these settlers and from the immigrant Indians (Swanton 1942, 88; Williams 1964, 557). Magnaghi (1978, 170) noted that by 1817 "few Indians traded at Natchitoches any longer because of hostile reactions from white settlers and because they could get higher prices for their furs at Alexandria, Opelousas, and Spanish Nacogdoches."

In Texas the situation was much the same, though settlement pressures from Anglo-Americans did not impinge on Caddoan lands until after 1830 (see Strickland 1937, 318–355). Stephen F. Austin, impresario, viewed the aboriginal populations of Texas as a hindrance to the security of settlement (Barker 1925), and in general "early Texans excluded Indians . . . from their future Texas" (Doughty 1987, 31).

Following the death of the Caddo chief Dehahuit in 1833, American pressure in Louisiana on the new Caddo chiefs led to the ceding of their homelands within the limits of the United States on 1 July 1835 (Swanton 1942, 89–92). For $80,000 the Caddo relinquished their lands and agreed to move at their own expense within one year of the treaty date; they moved to Texas just prior to the establishment of the Republic of Texas in 1836 (Fig. 7). The term *Caddo Nation* came to be associated with the Cherokee as well as with the Hasinai, Anadarko, and other related tribes in East

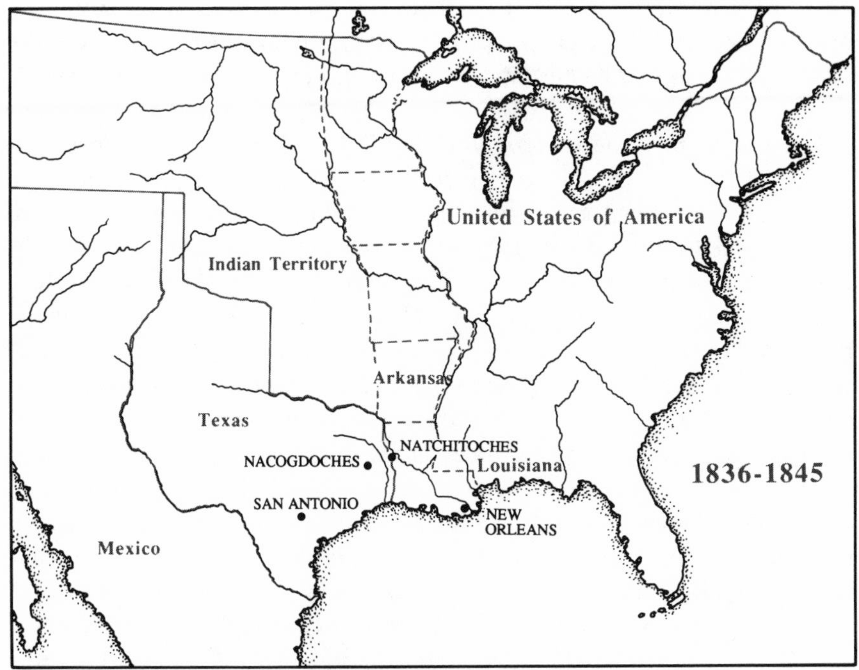

FIG. 7. The United States of America, the Republic of Texas, and Mexico, 1836–1845.

Texas, and the Indians became subject to repressive measures of successive Republic of Texas administrations (see Neighbours 1973, 1975) because of the suggestion that they had instigated or perpetrated depredations, which began in 1837, along the East Texas frontier (Strickland 1937, 320; Swanton 1942, 95). These purported depredations or threats of warfare were frequently linked with Mexican plots to recover Texas from the Republic of Texas (Strickland 1937, 326–328, 332).

By the early 1840s, the Caddo Nation was composed of remnants of the Kadohadacho, Hasinai, and other once-independent Caddoan tribes. By this time, they had essentially been pushed out of East Texas, along with the other Indian groups who had signed the Treaty of Peace and Friendship with the Republic of Texas in 1843 at the conclusion of concerted Anglo-American hostilities (Swanton 1942, 97; Strickland 1937, 355). In 1846 the Kadohadacho, Hasinai, and Anadarko lived together in a village of about 150 houses on the Brazos River near the present community of Waco, Texas. Shortly thereafter they moved near the Clear Fork of the Brazos to maintain their distance from the Anglo-American frontier communities in that part of the Republic. From 1846 until 1854, when the U.S. government and the

Texas legislature saw to it that the Texas Indian Reservation was founded on the Brazos River (Neighbours 1957, 1973), Anglo-American and Caddo relations were overtly hostile (see Prucha 1984, 1:354–366; Swanton 1942, 98–102).

Previous to this, the Caddo, Wichita, Tawakoni, and other tribes had requested that the special agent for the Indians in Texas, Jesse Stem, tell the U.S. government "that their relations with the Government should be established on a more certain and permanent basis; that a permanent boundary should be fixed, so that they might have a country where they could be secure from encroachments of the white settlements, and where they could build up their villages and cultivate their corn fields without the constant fear of being driven further back, and compelled to abandon their homes, the fruit of their labor, and the graves of their kindred" (Reports of the Commissioner of Indian Affairs 1851, 260–261, quoted in Swanton 1942, 100).

The Texas Indian Reservation lasted only till 1859, however, because of the same frictions between white settlers, Indian agents, and the tribal members that had characterized the Indian situation in Texas since 1836 (see Neighbors 1973; Swanton 1942, 108–109). Accordingly, in August 1859 the "Caddo Nation," about 1,050 people in number, were removed to the Indian Territory and the Wichita agency in western Oklahoma.

3 / Archaeology and the Contact Era: Theory and Methodology

The angel of death seems to have preceded rather than followed the white man, and testimony is practically unanimous that the aborigines decreased steadily and in many instances rapidly from the time of their first appearance. —*John Swanton, 1911*

An understanding of the theoretical and methodological issues important to the overall study of the Caddoan Historic archaeological record may begin with an overview of archaeological research in the Caddoan Area since ca. 1900. My emphasis in providing that overview is on a critical analysis of past archaeological research at sites with Protohistoric and Historic Caddoan period occupations. Of special interest are investigations concerned with shaping concepts of the nature of the Caddoan archaeological record in the Contact era. Present approaches and models dealing with Historic period cultural change in the Caddoan Area are also imporant. To provide the research framework for the detailed examination of contact and interaction between Caddoan and European peoples, I also review theoretical and methodological issues involved in the study of the Caddoan historic archaeological record. Issues I address include assumptions of systemic continuity and the objective use of the ethnographic record (Dunnell 1991), the implications of European acute diseases for any trends in Caddoan population decline or growth, definitions of contact as used herein, the temporal framework of contact, population estimations, and regional settlement parameters. Finally, to examine the changing character of Caddoan lifeways between ca. 1520 and 1800, I present a series of research expectations and research problems.

I summarize the history of archaelogical research in the Caddoan Area (see also Guy 1988, 1990; Jeter et al. 1989; Sabo et al. 1988) to provide the framework for more specific discussions of the Protohistoric (1520–1685) and Early Historic(1685–1800+) periods that follow in Part 2 of this study (chapters 4 through 6). My focus is on research relating to Caddoan archaeological sites occupied during those two time periods and to models developed to better understand and explain the character of the Contact era archaeological record.

EARLY INVESTIGATIONS AND THE DEVELOPMENT OF ARCHAEOLOGICAL CONCEPTS

Early nineteenth-century European and Anglo-American speculations about the Mound Builders and their origins (Gibson 1985a, 29–34) were the precursors to modern archaeological Caddoan Area research. Questions about the origins of the American Indians, especially incongruities between European expectations about the kinds of aboriginal societies that were capable of building mounds and the observed nature of native American societies in the eighteenth and nineteenth centuries, led to the development of several competing theories that proposed to explain the relationship between aboriginal Americans and the construction and function of earthen mounds (Willey and Sabloff 1974, 30). These ranged from speculations that the mounds were built by Aztecs or by other "vanished" peoples (Scandinavians, Hindus, or Israelites) to the more realistic suggestions that the earthworks were indeed of native North American Indian origin (Haven 1856; Silverberg 1968; Trigger 1986b).

Some of the first observers and travelers in the area, most notably H. M. Brackenridge (1814), Peter Custis (Flores 1984), and Amos Stoddard (1812), described mounds and abandoned Indian villages along the Red and Ouachita rivers in the states of Louisiana, Arkansas, and Texas. These descriptions were in the naturalist tradition typical of the time (Gibson 1985a). The writers were not specifically "interested in collecting archaeological information. Rather they attempted to record data about, and make observations on, everything they saw in their travels" (Willey and Sabloff 1974, 29). Neither Brackenridge nor Stoddard believed, however, that the mounds they saw were built by native North Americans.

The next phase of archaeological activity in the Caddoan Area focused on the description and recovery of artifacts from newly discovered mounds and/or cemeteries. The earliest published descriptions of this work were by T. P. Hotchkiss of Shreveport, who reported finding an Indian grave and artifacts in the Wallace Lake area near Shreveport in Caddo Parish (Neuman 1984). As Story notes (1978, 57–58), this period of nascent archaeological research was dominated by the collection of specimens for museums and private ownership. Consequently, little useful information was gathered on the actual provenience or association of specific artifactual remains, and much of the less striking material was either overlooked or discarded during the excavations.

From a current perspective little substantive information on Caddoan peoples or their prehistory was gained by this type of work prior to the 1890s. Even the investigations by Edward Palmer in Texas and Arkansas

1879–1880 (McVaugh 1956; Jeter 1990) and by the Division of Mound Exploration of the Bureau of Ethnology, founded in 1881, had a negligible impact on the basic understanding of the region's archaeology (Smith 1982, 51). Field operations of the Division of Mound Exploration were carried out in the Trans-Mississippi South 1882 to 1884 and 1889 to 1890 (Smith 1982, 1985), but this work constituted only an incidental part of the Thomas (1894) and Holmes (1903) monographs on the archaeology of the eastern United States. As a result of the incidental nature of the Division of Mound Exploration work in the Caddoan Area, the region as a whole was not incorporated into major archaeological syntheses of the eastern United States until after the 1930s (Ford 1936; Ford and Willey 1941).

INITIAL TYPOLOGICAL AND CHRONOLOGICAL ORGANIZATION, 1900 – 1940

The second major period of Caddoan Area archaeological research began in the first decade of the twentieth century with the initial efforts of Clarence B. Moore of the Philadelphia Academy of Science (Moore 1908, 1909, 1912, 1913). Moore concentrated on exploring mounds along the Red and Ouachita rivers (Fig. 8), recording sites, conducting excavations, and publishing selected results of his work in lavish and well-illustrated monographs. Moore's importance comes from the fact that he was the ground breaker in investigating the archaeological record of an area that had not yet been recognized as distinctive in terms of such elements as mound construction, mortuary practices, and ceramic styles. Moreover, he is often the only primary source on many Caddoan mound groups that have been subsequently destroyed by meanderings of the Red River (Schambach 1983, 11).

Moore excavated several hundred Indian burials at the Glendora and Keno sites on the Ouachita River in north-central Louisiana, including many that had European trade items as grave goods, and he also conducted investigations at Protohistoric period sites throughout the Ouachita and Bartholomew drainages in south-central Arkansas and north-central Louisiana (Belmont 1985; Jones 1985; Kidder 1986, 1987, 1988). He also excavated a number of cemeteries in the Great Bend area of the Red River in Southwest Arkansas that apparently represent Belcher and Chakanina phase components of the Caddoan post-1520 archaeological record (see below and Schambach 1983; Trubowitz 1984).

Archaeological research activities throughout the Caddoan Area began in earnest shortly after Moore's explorations. M. R. Harrington followed up Peabody and Moorehead's 1903 excavations in Southwest Missouri at

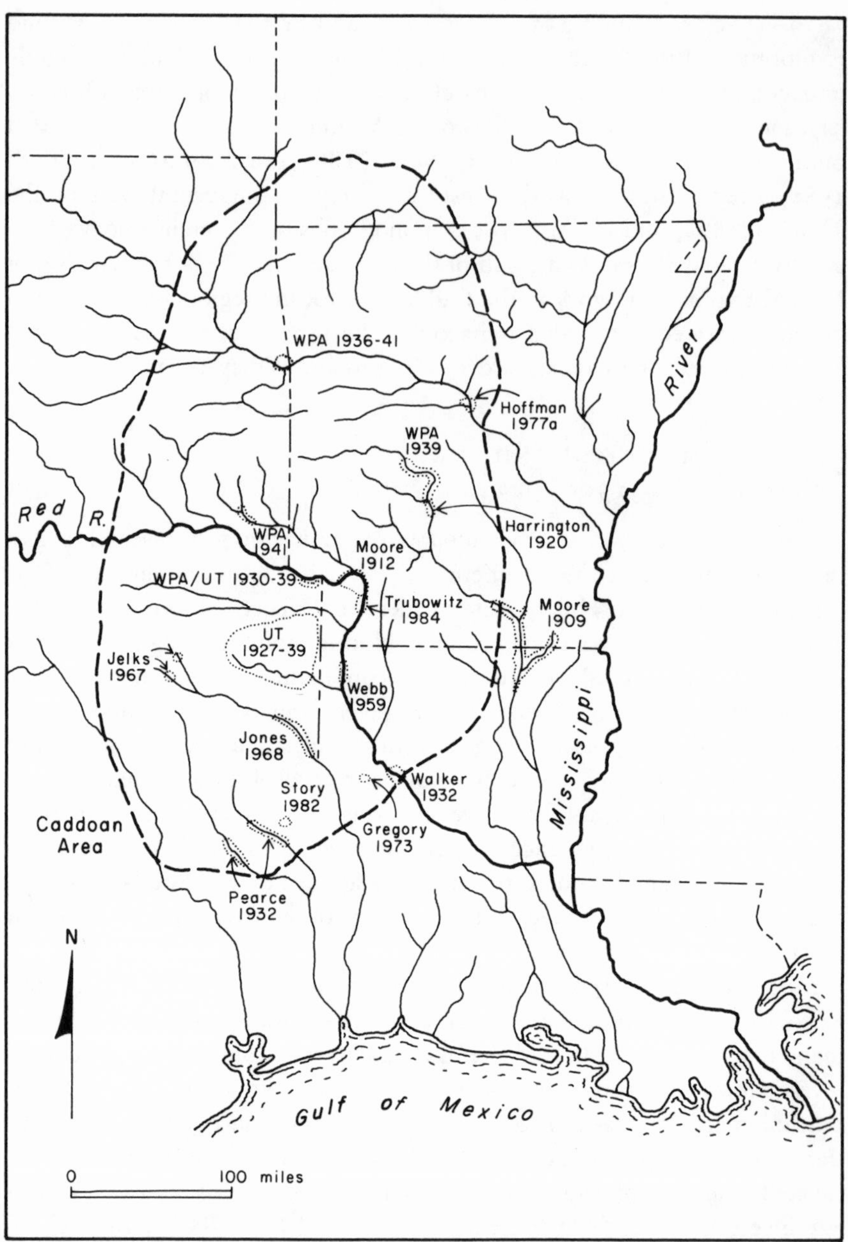

FIG. 8. Significant archaeological research activities relevant to 1520–1800.

Jacob's Cavern, McDonald County, by beginning explorations of rock shelters along the Grand River in eastern Oklahoma during the autumn of 1914 (Harrington 1960; Peabody and Moorehead 1904). Extensive excavations of rock shelters in Southwest Missouri and Northwest Arkansas were then initiated by the Museum of the American Indian in 1922 (Harrington 1960, 6). Joseph Thoburn began excavations at the Spiro Site in Oklahoma in 1916 (Albert 1984, 46), and Harrington was commissioned in 1917 by the Heye Foundation to continue Moore's work in Southwest Arkansas. J. E. Pearce of the University of Texas started explorations of East Texas Caddoan sites in 1919, but little work was accomplished until the 1930s on sites apparently dating to periods of European contact (Barnard 1939; Davis 1979, 165; Pearce 1919).

Probably the most important result of the archaeological research conducted up to 1930 in the Caddoan Area was the association of archaeological remains from Southwest Arkansas to a known Caddoan ethnographic group, the Kadohadacho (Harrington 1920). This association led to the use of ethnographic and ethnohistorical records in helping interpret the Caddoan Area archaeological record. At the same time, and probably inspired by the "culture area" approach of Holmes (1914) and Wissler (1914), the Red River area and Northeast Texas were compared in a fledgling manner with the archaeological record of the eastern United States (Pearce 1932a, 1932b, 1932c; Walker 1932). The Caddoan Area as an organized entity in an archaeological and taxonomic sense, therefore, extends back only about sixty years.

The association of historic European trade goods with what was recognized as distinctively Caddoan pottery helped considerably to consolidate and extend the association between Caddoan ethnic groups and peoples to the prehistoric archaeological sites that had been uncovered in the area. As Walker (1932, 43) observed:

> A year ago last summer [1931] an Indian burial ground was accidentally discovered near Natchitoches [Louisiana], which yielded elaborately engraved and incised, highly polished pottery associated with European trade objects. . . . Its significance lies in the fact that we have been able to identify this site as the probable one occupied by the Natchitoches Indian village visited by Henri de Tonti in 1690. . . . This pottery is possibly one variant of a more general Caddoan ceramic type which we may expect to find in adjacent parts of Texas and Arkansas, but it gives us what we hope will be the key to the major archaeological problem in Northwestern Louisiana, the temporal and areal extent of Caddoan culture.

Pearce (1932c, 53) also remarked upon an association of European goods with aboriginal burial sites in East Texas (see also Jackson n.d.a, 1932). These associations seemed to confirm the identification of the archaeological remains as belonging to another Caddoan ethnographic group, that of the Hasinai tribe (Bolton 1908, 1987).

Further discoveries in Arkansas, Texas, and Louisiana at that time exemplified the archaeological approach that was used in establishing possible ethnic and cultural links between postcontact tribal histories (after ca. 1520) and precontact archaeological cultures (Dickinson 1941; Dickinson and Dellinger 1940; Walker 1936). This approach has become known as the direct historical approach (Dixon 1913; Steward 1942). By 1940, only in Oklahoma and Missouri were direct associations of this kind between European goods and Caddoan archaeological remains still lacking; the situation in these two states has not changed much in this respect since that time (Sabo 1986; Sabo et al. 1988; Rohrbaugh 1984).

The application of the direct historical approach drew upon considerable historic and archival research (e.g., Bolton 1914, 1915; Hackett 1931–1946; Griffith 1954; Margry 1877–1886; Parsons 1941; Sibley 1933; Swanton 1911, 1942) that could be used to locate and characterize particular Caddoan tribal entities described in the ethnographic and historic records. Once these locations were established, the archaeologist attempted to pinpoint specific archaeological sites in those places that were temporally relevant to known historic events (e.g., Walker 1935, 1936; Johnson and Jelks 1958; Jelks 1970; Jones 1968).

Of course, the association between a historic description and the archaeological record was initially dependent upon the recovery of European trade goods together with aboriginally manufactured cultural materials such as pottery and stone tools. When this was accomplished, the archaeological and ethnic association established through the direct historical approach was then extended to other archaeological locations in the region having apparently similar cultural materials but wholly lacking European goods (Hodges 1957). This extensional argument was the basis for the earliest attempts at Caddoan space-time systematics (Sayles 1935), but it was unsuccessful with the Caddoan sites clearly predating the introduction of European materials because of the imprecise and limited chronological framework for Caddoan archaeology and prehistory that existed at that time.

CULTURE HISTORY

The change in the archaeological discipline from a concern with culture's geographic variations to an awareness of temporal variation—what is termed *culture history*—began in the Caddoan Area after 1930 as more localized, long-term archaeological programs funded by state educational institutions and private foundations were developed (Story 1978, 58). James A. Ford

(1936, 6) had noted "that no true treatment of materials in an area can ignore temporal relationships" and had demonstrated methods in the Lower Mississippi Valley of constructing chronologies (i.e., ceramic stylistic seriations) that were apparently applicable to archaeological materials in the Caddoan Area. Nevertheless, chronological relationships within the area were unrefined until at least a decade after the construction of the Lower Mississippi Valley regional culture history.

In Arkansas, Samuel Dellinger continued and systematized archaeological research initiated by Mark R. Harrington (1924, 1960) at dry bluff shelters in the Ozarks (see Fritz 1986b). New research was initiated in the state with Works Project Administration (WPA) funding in the late 1930s (Lyon 1982; H. Davis 1983, 14). Beginning in 1927 with Laura Spelman Rockefeller Foundation funding, field parties from the University of Texas worked annually to 1936 throughout East Texas (particularly in the Big Cypress Creek basin [see Fig. 8]), concentrating on the excavation of late Caddoan period (ca. 1400 and later) cemeteries, but occasionally trenching trash middens and mounds (Barnard 1939; Thurmond 1990a). Jackson (1934, 1935) and Pearce (1932a) had concluded that the diversity in material culture in pipes and ceramic and shell artifacts found in East Texas Caddoan sites supported the notion of a "considerable tendency towards unity within the river valleys and towards noticeable diversity as one goes from one valley to another" (Pearce 1932c, 53).

E. B. Sayles (1935) in *An Archaeological Survey of Texas* defined the Red River and Hasinai phases using differences in the types of artifacts collected under the direction of Pearce and Jackson, particularly the elaborately decorated ceramic vessels recovered from cemeteries. The Red River phase was presumed to be the precursor to the phase of the historic Kadohadacho and related Red River Caddoan groups, while the Hasinai phase was thought to be related to the Hasinai confederacy in the Neches-Angelina drainages (Sayles 1935, 84–85 and Table 7).

The collection emphases of and techniques utilized by Pearce and Jackson were unfortunately poorly suited to the development of a systematically applicable spatial-temporal framework in the Texas part of the Caddoan Area. Systematic selection biases in sites of certain types (i.e., a preference for cemeteries and burial mounds) chosen for excavation in combination with an atemporal perspective meant that the Sayles system was ineffective as a cultural-historical device and a poor means of interpreting accumulating data in a temporal fashion. Sayles's framework was never seriously employed in the Caddoan Area work and was forgotten when a more robust typological and chronological scheme was developed in the 1940s by Alex D. Krieger (1944, 1946) and Clarence H. Webb (1945, 1959).

During the 1930s WPA projects were conducted at many of the known major Caddoan mound and habitation sites, only a few of which contained materials of Protohistoric or Early Historic period affiliation. These projects include unpublished records of excavations at the Adair mound site in Southwest Arkansas (Early 1985, 1988), work at the McCurtain phase McDonald and Clement sites in Southeast Oklahoma (Bell and Baerreis 1951; Wyckoff and Fisher 1985), and the extensive 1938–1939 excavations at the Hatchel and Mitchell sites on the Red River in Bowie County, Texas (see Davis 1970; Wedel 1978; Creel 1982c, 1991b). Projects directed by Dickinson and Lemley (Dickinson 1936; Dickinson and Lemley 1939; Lemley 1936) were completed in Southwest Arkansas. In Texas and Oklahoma, projects were directed by H. Perry Newell, William Beatty, William Duffen, David Baerreis, and Phillip Newkumet. Public works projects in the Caddoan Area were not conducted in Louisiana (Ford 1951; Lyon 1982).

Although still concerned with the "augmentation of the corpus of reliable data and analysis and comprehension on a broad basis" (Spaulding 1983, 25), archaeologists working in the Caddoan Area during this era began to appreciate the spatial and temporal complexity of what had been subsumed under the general term *Caddo* and started to question how these archaeological manifestations related to those in other areas of the eastern United States, the Southwest, and Mesoamerica (Krieger 1947; Webb and Dodd 1939, 1941). As a result, no longer was the consideration of cultural variation in the area kept separate from ongoing investigations of chronological interrelationships in Caddoan Area archaeology.

The foremost concern of WPA archaeologists in the eastern United States was the spatial-temporal organization of the region's prehistory (Willey and Sabloff 1974, 121). By 1936 Ford had established a number of Lower Mississippi River and Lower Red River Valley ceramic complexes, or "horizons," based upon surface collections and excavations in Louisiana and Mississippi (Ford 1936). One of the complexes, a Caddoan ceramic complex, was placed on the same temporal level as the Tunica and Natchez complexes—as a historic entity on Ford's Horizon III.

In the late 1930s in Texas, Krieger began to supervise the WPA laboratory in Austin. Using information on Caddoan archaeological sites with stratigraphic information from the Neches (e.g., Newell and Krieger 1949) and Red River Valleys (e.g., Webb and Dodd 1941), Krieger produced the first systematic syntheses of the culture history in the Caddoan Area. This culture history sequence was based on the Midwestern Taxonomic System (MTS) (McKern 1939).

The MTS created classificatory units through the development of trait comparisons at varying levels of similarity. The most basic level is the *com-*

ponent, which McKern (1939, 30) defined as "the manifestation of any given focus at a specific site." These components, the building blocks of the MTS, are recognized by developing and comparing lists of linked and diagnostic traits, including stylistic, technological, and functional traits (Dunnell 1971, 177). The higher level groupings of *focus, aspect, phase,* and *pattern* are then developed by successively comparing these formal traits to create higher levels of abstraction (i.e., an agricultural pattern versus a hunting-gathering pattern). As the groupings proceed to higher levels, the relative similarity between classificatory units decreases commensurately (Dunnell 1971, Fig. 21). Thus, foci (which are composed of a number of components that share a great number of traits) are more similar to each other in formal terms than are aspects, which are composed of a number of foci, and so on up the taxonomic ladder.

Krieger (1944, 1946) defined two major time periods, the early Gibson Aspect and the later Fulton Aspect, along with thirteen foci. The Alto and Glendora foci, two of the thirteen foci, were known from only a few widely separated sites and hence lacked a true spatial distribution (Fig. 9).

According to Krieger, the Gibson Aspect (including the Alto focus) was dated 1100–1450, the Fulton Aspect 1450–1650, and the historic Caddo occupation (the Glendora focus) subsequent to that (Krieger 1946). The differences between Krieger (1946) and present-day chronological schemes are not great (see Thurmond 1985; Schambach 1983; Wyckoff and Fisher 1985; Neuman 1984), with the exception that Krieger was inclined to place the Gibson Aspect earlier than the Mississippi period in the southeastern United States since he had aligned it with the Troyville and Coles Creek periods of the Lower Mississippi Valley (Ford and Willey 1941). At that time, these temporal estimates were not based on methods of absolute dating, and the chronologies (and chronological relationships) tended to be foreshortened.

The most relevant and comparative cultural sequences for Krieger's work in the Caddoan Area were in the southwestern United States and the lower Mississippi River Valley. He commented that "the generally recognized Puebloan time scale . . . provides the basis for extending datings eastward (from the Rio Grande to the Mississippi). Puebloan trade sherds, stratigraphic data, and documentary materials are used to determine the age of these cultures" (Krieger 1946, Fig. 18). The alignment of the Caddoan Area's culture history with these sequences, particularly that of the lower Mississippi River Valley defined by Ford and Willey (1941), was a primary impetus in the organization and expansion of Caddoan archaeological research, regardless of whether the focus was on Prehistoric, Protohistoric, or Early Historic period manifestations in the regional archaeological record.

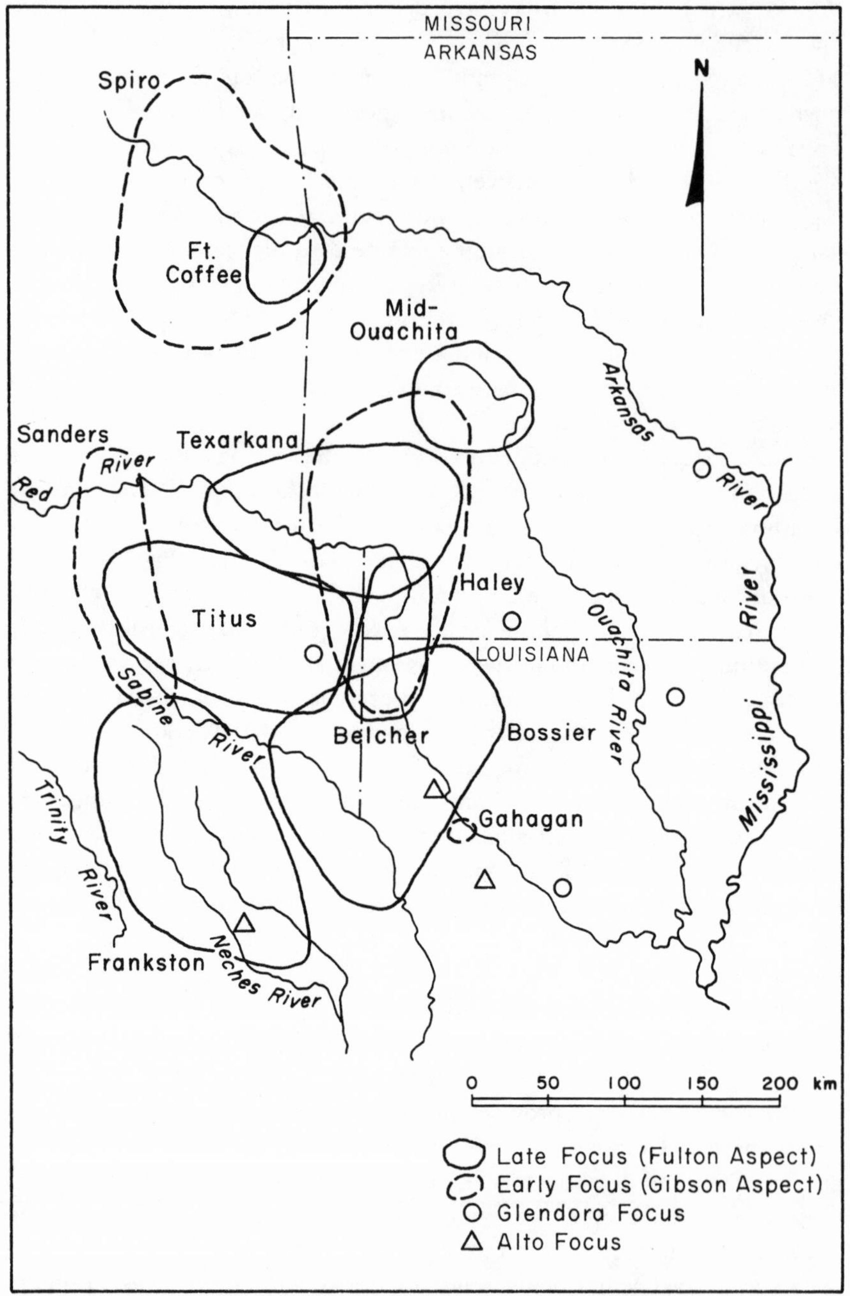

FIG. 9. Distribution of Gibson and Fulton aspect foci defined by Krieger (1946). The triangles and circles represent individual components of the Alto and Glendora foci. Neither focus had a realistic spatial distribution when it was initially defined.

While Krieger concentrated his efforts in synthesizing Caddoan archaeology and its Texas expression (Suhm, Krieger, and Jelks 1954), local Caddoan sequences were also developed in eastern Oklahoma (Bell and Baerreis 1951; Orr 1952) and on the Red River in Louisiana (Webb 1959).

The cultural-taxonomic classifications defined by Krieger (1946) for the Caddoan Area were applied in specific cases with not much realistic appreciation of the cultural context or variability inherent in the units themselves. That is, contextual biases in unit formulation, whether they were of Prehistoric or Historic period affiliation, were not explicitly recognized for a class of entities (i.e., components) or the problems in association were ignored in lieu of typological and trait descriptions. Interpretations of the archaeological record were instead seemingly governed by the unstated assumption that the entire range of Caddoan cultural variability within any defined focus should be represented at every site or component of the period. Where it did not, the archaeological record was often partitioned into foci that manifestly separated functionally specific components of the same temporal period (see Johnson 1987, 2; Perttula et al. 1986, 41–43).

This problem in cultural classifications is potentially acute with Caddoan Historic period components because European trade goods are sparse in Caddoan sites predating 1730, and they are concentrated in cemetery contexts. Associated habitation sites may be overlooked because of the gross nature of chronological associations that currently exist in the Caddoan Area archaeological record (see Story [1990] and my Part 2, chapters 4 and 5). For example, at the Deshazo site, whose Historic Caddoan Allen phase occupation "began in the latter half of the 17th century and lasted until the early part of the 18th century" (Story n.d., 517), extensive excavations in the habitation area produced only a handful of European trade goods. In the associated cemetery for adult interments, however, a number of the burials contained many glass beads, gun parts, hawkbells, metal knives, and other trade goods. The burials of the children were placed in subfloor pits beneath the structures, and they were not associated with European trade goods. Archaeologists used ceramic seriations (Fields 1981) and archaeomagnetic samples from the habitation area to effectively link the two functionally different parts of the Historic Caddoan Allen phase component.

The poor control of temporal variation within components, especially between functionally distinct aspects of a single (and probably contemporaneous) settlement meant that European goods by necessity had to be recovered in both occupational and mortuary contexts before the total assemblage character of a Protohistoric or Early Historic period component, or groups of components, could be accurately ascertained (see Trubowitz 1984, 40). As an illustration, consider the Kinsloe focus, a Historic Caddoan period focus on the Sabine River in East Texas (see chapters 4 and 5).

This focus was defined by Jones (1968) on the basis of aboriginal cultural materials and European trade goods recovered from burial proveniences at seven sites. No excavations were conducted, however, in associated habitation contexts to aid the broader characterization of the focus. This precluded relating mortuary data to a larger conceptualization, namely, that the Kinsloe focus represents some of the eighteenth-century settlements made by Nadaco Caddo groups. Limited excavations at one of the Kinsloe focus habitation sites by Clark and Ivey (1974), however, produced evidence that (*a*) the occupation probably dated to the first quarter of the nineteenth century, which was compatible with historical and archival information, and (*b*) while thought to be undiagnostic, aboriginal materials at the site could be stylistically and technologically discriminated from Caddoan assemblages in the locality known to be of either late Prehistoric or Protohistoric age (Clark and Ivey 1974; Webb et al. 1969).

In many ways, the investigation of the culture history of the Caddoan Area laid the framework and the basic building blocks that must be understood to meaningfully grasp the Prehistoric and Historic periods' archaeological record of the Caddoan peoples. Conceptually, these investigations concentrated on temporal variation within the Caddoan Prehistoric and Historic archaeological sequence, linked taxonomic units with other archaeological traditions and cultures through comparison of distinctive cultural traits such as ceramics and mound building, and attempted to establish the geographic parameters of these cultural and taxonomic entities. After the construction of local and regional sequences of taxonomic entities, the cultural and behavioral meaning of the entities could be (at least hypothetically) considered further.

Through the archaeological identification of components and the definition of a plethora of foci, phases, complexes, and other culture history constructs, the archaeological record of the Caddoan Area is fairly well comprehended. Nevertheless, this pursuit of culture history, first erected and systematized by Krieger (1944, 1946) and Webb (1959), has had far-reaching consequences in terms of our ability to address broader and more significant research problems and questions by employing the area's impressive archaeological record. In the main, the issues of taxonomy and chronology continue to dominate the archaeological investigations being conducted in the Caddoan Area. However, since the late 1960s (see below) the consideration of culture history has been rightly tempered with a more realistic appreciation of (*a*) the social and cultural complexity and variability that characterizes the Caddoan peoples' past, the end product being a diverse archaeological record, and (*b*) the natural processes (such as bioturbation and pedoturbation), which have altered and formed the archaeological record available for scrutiny and study.

DIVERSE PARADIGMS AND APPROACHES, 1960S TO THE PRESENT

The 1960s ushered in a new boom in the level of archaeological activity in the Caddoan Area as a result of federally sponsored reservoir salvage projects. Forced to work in areas where little or no archaeological work had been done, Caddoan archaeologists started to question the twenty-year-old temporal-spatial systematics in detail and began to perceive the Caddoan archaeological record in different terms. Edward Jelks (1961, 74), for instance, in discussing excavations at Texarkana Reservoir in the lower Sulphur River in Northeast Texas, noted that "differences in quantitative representation of pottery types . . . [at sites of the Texarkana focus] emphasize a general observation that a focus [as that classificatory unit has been applied in the Caddoan Area] is not necessarily a closely integrated complex of traits found with little or no variation from site to site."

Dissatisfaction with the classification scheme, coupled with a general interest in temporal-spatial systematics, continued through the early 1970s. The introduction of the phase scheme (Willey and Phillips 1958; Phillips 1970) and the type-variety system (Schambach and Miller 1984) into studies of the Caddoan Area from those of the Lower Mississippi Valley resulted in the recognition of new cultural units that were not always intended to be comparable to previously defined units (e.g., Williams 1964, 560–561).

The concept of phase has been described by Willey and Phillips (1958, 22) as "an archaeological unit possessing traits sufficiently characteristic to distinguish it from all other units similarly conceived, whether of the same or other cultures or civilizations, spatially limited to the order of magnitude of a locality or region and chronologically limited to a relatively brief interval of time." Thus, a phase has a "formal content," a "distribution in geographical space," and a "duration in time."

The basic building blocks of the phase are components, as in the previous discussion of the MTS, and the integration of such cultural-historical units as components and phases is attempted through the development of local and regional temporal sequences. Broader integrative units include the *horizon* (a broad and rapidly spread constellation of contemporaneous cultural traits and assemblages), the *tradition* (a temporally persistent constellation of systems of related nature), and *periods* (broad chronological units) (Willey and Phillips 1958, 33, 37, 69).

As Story and Davis (1983, 11) pointed out when discussing the shift from the use of foci to the use of phases in the Caddoan Area, "when cultural units were first defined as a focus, then subsequently as a phase . . . in many, but not all cases, the terminological change has been accompanied by a substantive change in definition. The terms *complex* and *manifestation* have been used in the literature when recognition of the cultural unit is based on limited data and the definition is provisional."

This substantive redefinition did not radically depart from the Krieger scheme per se because it was still based on the long-held assumptions of change and continuity embedded in phases or foci that grounded the earlier temporal-spatial systematics (Hoffman 1971; Wyckoff 1974). As an illustration, when the larger regional framework of the Gibson and Fulton aspects was replaced, it was replaced only by a Pan-Caddoan Caddo I–V period scheme (Davis 1970). The use of periods in this context is totally compatible with the definitions of *period* proposed by Krieger (1953, 247) some years earlier. Periods were chronological units defined to give a temporal character to formal content-based *stages,* which Krieger (1953) conceived of as "dominating patterns of economic existence," such as Paleo-Indian, food-gathering, food-producing, and urban life stages. Stages have never been fully employed in the Caddoan Area as a classificatory and interpretive framework, though the actual use of the Caddo I–V period scheme sometimes verges toward stages.

Each period in this scheme (Table 3) is assumed to represent a supra-cohesive temporal unit entirely applicable across the entire Caddoan Area. Changes from period to period in culture content (e.g., ceramic and lithic tool assemblages, construction of mounds, use of cemeteries, settlement character) follow uniformly by definition from one regional and/or local cultural sequence to the other. This is implied in the unspecified basic assumptions of any areal/regional chronological framework: (*a*) that change occurs on the order of the "areal" rather than at the regional scale, (*b*) change is synchronous and episodic, and (*c*) change is comparable from one regional cultural sequence to another.

As an ordering device, the Caddo I–V period framework is useful to the extent that it demands a consideration of the building of regional chronologies and is therefore a warrant to relate contemporaneous regional manifestations in a consistent manner. Yet its utility is in large measure misleading because of the characterizations of change it unwittingly fosters about the Caddoan archaeological record (Story 1981, 1990). Actual applications of the Caddo I–V periodization rely on the gross character of the periods, as primarily recognized for the Red River (the Great Bend and Northwest Louisiana sequences), though what is detected in the archaeological record may be ignored or misrepresented in attempts to bring each regional developmental sequence into conformance with the overall areal framework.

A reaction to the inadequate understanding of change expressed in the Gibson-Fulton scheme has been to develop and refine classificatory and cultural taxonomic schemes at a smaller scale, such as the region or locality

TABLE 3. Regional Cultural Sequences in the Caddoan Area

Time (A.D.)	Arkansas Basin[a]	Great Bend[b]	Little River[c]	Northwest Louisiana[d]	Middle Red[e]	Ouachita River[f]	Southern Ouachita Mtns.[g]	Cypress Creek[h]	Upper Sabine[i]	Neches[j]	Western Ozarks[k]
Caddo 1800									Norteno/		
V		Chakanina		Little				Hunt	Kinsloe	Allen	
1700				River/							
				Lawton		Deceiper					Neosho
Caddo 1600		Belcher/		Belcher	McCurtain	Social Hill		Titus			
									Forest		
IV	Fort	Texarkana								Frankston	
									Hill		
1500	Coffee		Saratoga								
								Whelan			
				Bossier			Mtn.				
		Belcher/									
Caddo 1400						Mid-	Fork/				
		Texarkana	Mineral								
III					Sanders	Ouachita	Buckville				
			Springs								
1300								Period			
	Spiro	Haley									
								II			Loftin
			Graves'	Haley							
Caddo 1200											
			Chapel								
II									Pecan	Alto	
1100							Hochatown		Grove		
Caddo 1000			Miller's			Pre-Mid		Period			
	Harlan	Lost		Alto							
I			Crossing			Ouachita		I			
		Prairie			Apple						
900											

[a]Bell 1984; Brown 1984a; Rohrbaugh 1984.
[b]Schambach 1983.
[c]Hoffman 1983.
[d]Hoffman 1970; Webb 1983.
[e]Krieger 1946; Rohrbaugh 1973; Wyckoff 1974.
[f]Schambach and Early 1983.
[g]Wyckoff 1974; Early 1983.
[h]Thurmond 1981.
[i]Bruseth and Perttula 1981; Jelks 1967; Jones 1968.
[j]Story and Creel 1982.
[k]Perttula 1984; Sabo et al. 1982.

proposed by Willey and Phillips (1958) (see Table 3 and Fig. 10). In some of the more detailed and better understood local Caddoan sequences—the Great Bend (Schambach 1983; Trubowitz 1984) and the Neches (Story and Creel 1982; Story n.d.) localities—descriptions of cultural classificatory units have been formulated that can be readily understood to refer to large-scale trends in adaptation that are independent of stylistic considerations. That is, the cultural classificatory units are imbued with a sense of "culture," with past lifeways and with good solid information on how Caddoan peoples once lived. Archaeological research elsewhere in the Caddoan Area may yet come to emulate these broader conceptualizations of Prehistoric and Historic period cultural change, and this will occur when each region's archaeological record is structured and synthesized beyond only the basic temporal-spatial analyses (Thurmond 1985; Johnson 1987).

The first important change in the description of the Historic period archaeological record since the early 1970s concerns refining the regional Caddoan chronology. This has been based on a combination of ceramic seriations and recognition of stylistic horizons (Schambach and Miller 1984; Fields 1981), albeit with an incomplete and regionally biased sample of radiocarbon, archaeomagnetic, and thermoluminescence dates (Wolfman 1984, 260–261; Story 1990). Of Protohistoric and Early Historic period Caddoan sites, only the Cedar Grove site has a sufficiently large sample (N = 21) of absolute dates from several contexts to begin discussing occupation date ranges and temporal spans in specific calendrical terms, though, unfortunately, precise concordance between the radiocarbon and thermoluminescence dates at the site was poor (Wolfman 1984, 261). Other post-1520 Caddoan sites have typically less than two or three absolute dates (Story 1990, 325–338).

This limited sample clearly is not adequate to establish reasonable temporal estimates for occupations, particularly when there are multiple serial occupations at the sites. Archaeomagnetic dating is in its infancy in the Caddoan Area (Wolfman 1982), and thermoluminescence dating of ceramics has yet to be meaningfully applied across the area (Perttula, Turbeville, and Skiles 1987). Given the usually limited suitable organic material at Caddoan sites, secular variation in C14 in the last four hundred years, but the abundance of ceramics at all sites, it would appear that thermoluminescence dating and selected accelerator radiocarbon dating efforts (Browman 1981) offer better opportunities in the long run for the resolution of Caddoan chronological problems in the Contact era.

Another important change that has recently taken place in Caddoan archaeology concerns developing methods to designate historic cultural entities such as foci, phases, and clusters (Story and Creel 1982, 30–34) to best relate them to "classifications used in processual studies, such as settle-

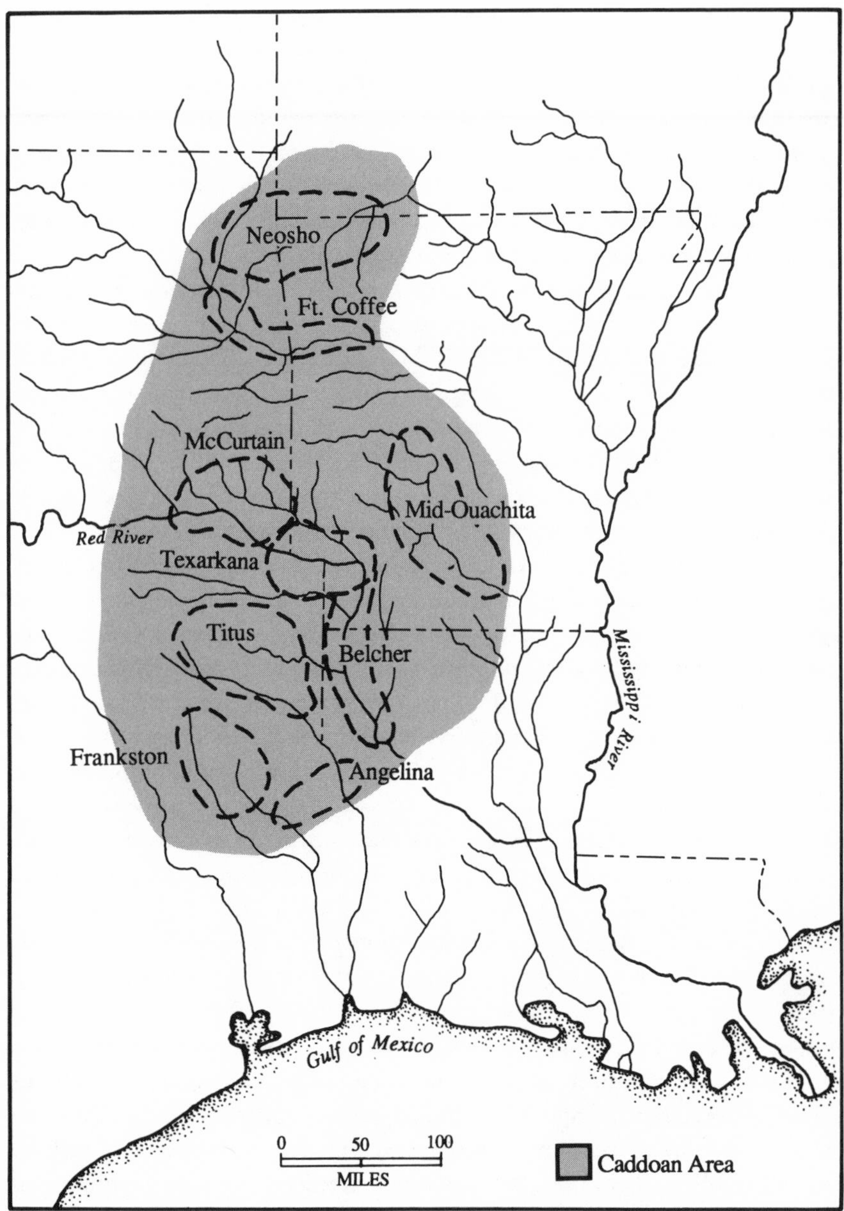

FIG. 10. Distribution of Caddoan phases at initial contact with Europeans, ca. 1520.

ment pattern types, levels of socio-political organization, and exchange networks" (Story and Creel 1982, 29). Almost without exception, archaeological models dealing with these issues of Caddoan sociocultural reconstruction and systemic cultural behavior are based explicitly on ethnographic analogies derived from studies of documentary and archival sources concerning the Caddoan peoples in Northeast Texas, known historically as the Hasinai confederacy (see Woodall 1969; Gilmore 1983; Story and Creel 1982; Thurmond 1985; Wyckoff and Baugh 1980).

Models of social groupings, social structure, and settlement patterns based on historical documents are used as guidelines for interpreting the empirical content of the archaeological record. These documents essentially provide the means whereby reconstructions of past behavioral patterns are to be tested with the archaeological record (Dunnell 1986, 40) and the ethnographic present is extended into the past (Trigger 1983, 440).

The goals of culture history and cultural reconstruction in twentieth-century American archaeology and anthropology are products of a consensus in the discipline that have set certain precedents in how processes of European contact and aboriginal cultural change are to be considered (see Dunnell 1986, 35). This is particularly the case in the reliance upon ethnographic descriptions by archaeologists to build inferences and extend analogies about the past (Trigger 1986b). As was said many years ago, if archaeology afforded a means to extend existing knowledge of living groups into the past, then "it is only through the known that we can comprehend the unknown, only from the study of the present that we can understand the past; and archaeological investigations therefore must be largely barren if pursued in isolation and independent of ethnology" (Dixon 1913, 565). The interest expressed by Dixon was not so much in documenting the effects of European contact on native American groups per se, but was rather to study native American systems free of European influences (Swanton and Dixon 1914). Since these native American cultures free of European influences only existed in the prehistoric archaeological record and interpretation relied upon ethnographic models, anthropologists constructed an ethnographic record, as a composite empirical generalization composed of time-transgressive data, direct observations, interviews, and analysis of disparate traits, that allowed the past to be reconstructed through the technique of the *ethnographic present,* which was placed just prior to European contact (Kroeber 1939).

All of this information had to be carefully evaluated because it had passed "through a cultural screen by which the recorded native behavior has been filtered" (Story 1978, 52). The result is usually an ahistorical, synchronic description that is first used as a description of a systemic and functioning whole and then secondarily employed as explanatory analogs to reconstruct the past. As a consequence, trait continuities in the ethnographic record become synonomous with systemic cultural continuities through time. Inasmuch as ethnographic analogs are dependent upon the assumption of systemic cultural continuity for them to have meaning, the relevance of proposed continuities as analogic sources are thus also subject to questions of appropriateness (Trigger 1981a).

If using the ethnographic present as a source for interpretive analogs is called into question, then so must the ethnographic descriptions that make up the ethnographic present. It is not unusual that traditional descriptions of the ethnographic present are often compiled from tribal groups that were approaching demographic collapse and/or extinction, and thus they are doubtful interpretive analogs for specifying precontact and postcontact systemic cultural relationships (Trigger 1981a, 12–13; Wilson and Rogers 1992; Dunnell 1991).

Steward (1954, 296) has noted that "even limited contacts with Europeans . . . may affect Indian society in a very fundamental sense." However, the duration or intensity of that interaction between different cultural systems is only one aspect of the broader process of episodic contacts between Europeans and native Americans. For example, the impact of European epidemics could have had enormous consequences for shaping the nature of European contact with native Americans and could have substantially altered aboriginal societies prior to the actual onset of direct, face-to-face, and sustained European contact. Because the effects of European contact were under way well before the compilation of the earliest written records, unless archaeologists have overestimated the impact of disease pathogens, they are confronted with a "traumatic historic rupture in the evolution of culture in North America . . . like an archaeological Grand Canyon, more easily looked across than spanned or jumped" (Mason 1976, 335).

Therefore, relying upon the ethnographic record alone to study the contact process usually underestimates the extent to which European contact affected or changed over the long term the character of aboriginal societies. Trigger (1983, 440) notes that "an increasing number of ethnologists and ethnohistorians are beginning to recognize that only archaeological data can provide a true base line for measuring changes brought about by a European presence in North America." The focus upon traits and particular cultural practices described by living informants, rather than on the assessment of the systemic context of these traits, precludes describing systemic discontinuity or defining the significant processes responsible for the persistence, alterations, and changes in cultural behavior that ultimately shaped the native American ethnic groups of the ethnographic record.

An effective utilization of ethnographic analogies, based on a fictive "ethnographic present" and the direct historical approach, is something that archaeologists should only consider exploring once they "have detailed the changes in material culture that occurred during the protohistoric and early historic periods. This alone produces sufficient continuity in the archaeological record to permit archaeological and ethnohistorical data to be compared in detail for the early historical period, and the resulting understanding of the archaeological record to be used as a basis for interpreting earlier periods" (Trigger 1983, 440).

There have recently been a number of very interesting studies of the Caddoan Historic archaeological and ethnohistorical records. These studies, by Gregory (1973, 184–294, 1980, 358–360), Trubowitz (1984, 1987), Gilmore (1986a, 33–37), and Sabo (1987, 1989, in press) do not primarily concern themselves with verifying and correlating the ethnographic content of Historic Caddoan archaeological and cultural entities. Rather, they are more concerned with relating particular regional models of cultural systems, typically dealing with economic strategies, trade, and interaction with Europeans, to expectations derived from ethnohistorical research and general considerations of the Caddoan archaeological record. Sabo (1987), however, has mined the primary historical and archival documents to try to understand how the Caddoans strived to adjust their world view at contact to accommodate the European explorers and how the cultural categories and cognitive structures of the Caddoan peoples were transformed to lessen the impact of that contact. All of these studies have illuminated the Caddoan Historic archaeological and ethnohistorical records and have brought us closer to a more complete understanding of the Caddoan peoples during the Contact era.

Trubowitz's (1984, 1987) Contact era model for the Great Bend region of the Red River is a case study that deals with such factors as (*a*) the type and accessibility of European goods and ideas, (*b*) population size, (*c*) social structure, and (*d*) native health conditions to try to explain changes in the Caddoan Contact era archaeological record. The model was devised to help explain the lack of evidence for direct European contact at sites, such as Cedar Grove, which seemingly date to the first quarter of the eighteenth century (Trubowitz 1984, 270), though there is some question about the terminal date of the Caddoan occupation at them (Story 1984, 278–279). The Great Bend Contact era model presumes to address diachronic questions of Caddoan contact and interaction with Europeans, but because of the nature of the archaeological record in the region the end product essentially depicts the contact process in a synchronic manner.

Differences in the amount of European trade goods at Caddoan sites in the Great Bend area are hypothesized to be the result of a redistribution system that limited the accessibility of European goods only to high-status groups and individuals within Kadohadacho society. The existence of a redistribution system and a ranked social structure in the archaeological record of the Great Bend region at that time is not based so much on empirical grounds as it is on suggested patterns of cultural behavior derived from limited documentary accounts (e.g., Hatcher 1932, 33–35) and from accounts of mortuary data scattered throughout the Caddoan Area (e.g., Gregory 1973). Means to assess the behavioral reconstructions independent of the means by which they were made have not been offered. Trubowitz (1984, 40) also assumes that because face-to-face contact between the Kadohadacho and Europeans did not take place until late in the Contact era (after 1690), the introduction of epidemic diseases would have had little effect on population reduction or social structure until after ca. 1730 in the Great Bend area. This position fails to take into account the diffusion potential of directly transmitted viruses and zoonoses spread through intermediate vectors independent of direct human contact (see Ramenofsky 1986, 1987a, and 1987b). It also overlooks that even though only a limited number of epidemics may have occurred in the Great Bend before 1730, a reduction in their effects is not implicit.

Gilmore's investigation of the archaeology of the Roseborough Lake site, the probable location of the 1730s–1770s French post St. Louis de Cadohadacho, was concerned with discerning the structure of economic and social interaction between the French soldiers and traders at the post and the Nassonite Caddo living near the fort (Gilmore 1986a). Because of the known intermarriage of the Frenchmen with Caddoan women at the post, certain processes of French-Indian acculturation and hypotheses about the mestizo character of the population there were examined utilizing specific aspects of the archaeological record (e.g., the abundance of native-made pottery and the presence as well as coassociation of native dwellings and European-style dwellings). The pattern of acculturation appears to reflect the integration of native women into the households of the French post community (Gilmore 1986a, 39) and is probably reflected as well in continuities in subsistence strategies (see Yates 1986, 124) that denote French solutions to subsistence problems quite similar to those described for the earliest Spanish colonists of Florida (Reitz and Scarry 1985, 92–99).

Other aspects of the *mestizaje* process, including changes in social status, sex roles, and ideological and technological factors (see Deagan 1983, 263–271), in the French and Caddoan Indian populations are still poorly understood because of the limited investigations of the internal structure of the community itself. Without the systematic consideration of how spatial and social variability within the site, or in the French and Indian communities, is expressed in the archaeological record, the significance of acculturative and adaptive processes in this contact and frontier society will not be understood in a meaningful manner.

Gregory's perspective concerning the Caddoan Contact era archaeological record is a holistic one in the sense that transformations in Caddoan society are viewed within a context that considers social, economic, religious, ecological, and acculturative factors in a systemic way (Gregory 1973, 1980, 1986). Changes or differences in the Historic Caddoan archaeological record are not interpreted with reference solely to Historic Caddoan ethnic or linguistic differences (Gregory 1973, 291), but are primarily conceptualized to be the result of a European-Indian symbiosis developing out of a long-standing prehistoric Caddoan pattern of economic interaction that was then extended to include European groups.

Such Historic period innovations in economic strategies as the participation in the hide and horse trades or large-scale population movements are therefore interpreted by Gregory (1973, 293–294) as functional responses to changing trade networks, Osage encroachments, and the Caddoan acquisition of commodities desired by the European community. In many ways Gregory presented an elegant model of Caddoan lifeways in the Historic period, first, because the model highlighted the dynamic interplay between two different cultural systems and, second, because it also changed the emphasis of study for the Caddoan Historic period away from an ethnocentric model of European dominance and Indian subordination (Gregory 1981, 127) to a more realistic consideration of European-Indian interaction that can be used to understand how Caddoan cultures changed after European contact. That is, the Caddoan peoples played a large role in determining and shaping the effects of contact between themselves and Europeans based in large measure on their perceptions of who the Europeans were.

A critical failing of Gregory's approach, however, is the lack of consideration given to the impact of European-introduced diseases on Caddoan peoples in terms of population decline and cultural discontinuity. As discussed below, factors of disease introduction and diffusion must be taken into consideration to arrive at a more comprehensive understanding of Caddoan culture change and systemic continuities in the Caddoan Historic archaeological and ethnohistorical records (Perttula 1989a, 1991).

Sabo (1987) has closely examined Spanish and French eighteenth-century accounts of the Caddoan peoples to try to determine how their conceptions of the world (and their culture) were changed as a result of contacts and interactions with Europeans. The examination is from "the native point of view" (Sabo 1987, 25), in so far as possible, and utilizes accounts of Caddoan ceremonialism to reconstruct those key cultural categories and symbols employed by the Caddoan peoples at contact that illustrate significant structural relationships within their society. These most important categories identified by Sabo (1987, 34) for the Caddoan peoples include "a social order reproduced from cosmology, a notion of power corresponding to the hierarchical position ascribed to various beings (human and supernatural), and a concept of sacredness pervading many cultural institutions and formal practices."

From these perceptions and cultural categories, Sabo (1987, 1989) employs the ethnohistorical record quite successfully to illustrate in various respects how Caddoan societies were transformed or, conversely, how cultural conceptions were maintained as a consequence of European contact. Changes in economic concerns, a deemphasis on sacred rituals and religious bases of authority, and an overall secularization of status and political positions were some of the shifts whose symbolic representation in Caddoan ritual can be identified in the ethnohistorical records. He also discusses how the Caddoan world view was expanded to incorporate the Europeans, initially as sacred beings, then as secular individuals concerned with political and economic questions, and finally as people who must be kept separated from the maintenance of such traditional and sacred Caddoan affairs as the decisions on who wields political and religious authority (Sabo 1988). Newkumet and Meredith (1988) also address these questions. The incorporation of the Europeans into the Caddoan world is thought to have been effective, at least for a time, as a means to "maintain cultural viability in the context of a world no longer controllable by traditional notions of order and balance" (Sabo 1987, 44–45).

Many of the conclusions offered by Sabo (1987) have archaeological implications that may be of utility in understanding the character of the Protohistoric and Historic Caddoan archaeological record; for example, the increasing secularization of Caddoan society and the deemphasis on matters of sacred ritual. These implications will be discussed below and explored further in Part 2.

There have been many changes and innovations in archaeological method and theory since the 1960s in North America (see Meltzer, Fowler, and Sabloff 1986, 8–17). These changes have been associated with substantial (if fluctuating) levels of federal and state support for archaeological research. However, the impact of the last twenty years of change in archaeology has not been fully felt in Caddoan archaeology, for better or worse.

Basically, the period since the 1960s has been one of filling in gaps in the regional Caddoan archaeological record (Hoffman 1971; Story 1981; Gregory 1980; Wyckoff 1980). It has also been one of launching investigations in new archaeological and geographical situations within the Caddoan Area, of devising different technical and methodological strategies to better interpret the record, rather than one of theoretical development (Meltzer 1979). Finally, it has been a period when understanding of the Caddoan archaeological record has fostered a greater appreciation of the dynamic, diverse, and variable Protohistoric and Historic periods in the Caddoan

Area (Woodall 1969; Gregory 1973; Perttula and Ramenofsky 1982; Trubowitz 1984; Gilmore 1986a).

THEORETICAL AND METHODOLOGICAL CONCERNS

Theoretical and methodological issues considered directly pertinent to and important in a study of Protohistoric and Historic period archaeological and ethnohistorical records in the Caddoan Area include the following: the recognition of contact in the archaeological record; the temporal framework of contact, depopulation, and the derivation of population estimates (Zubrow 1990); regional and local settlement parameters; and paleodemographic questions. One of the more critical concerns discussed here is the introduction and diffusion of European acute diseases at various times among the Caddoan peoples and the implications of these episodic epidemics for demographic and adaptive changes in Caddoan populations.

The interpretation of the Caddoan archaeological record in the periods following initial European contact has been consistently based on the assumption that there was a systemic cultural continuity between the Late Caddoan, the Protohistoric, and the Historic Caddoan periods. In a review of the Caddoan Historic archaeological record, Gregory (1973, 293–294) summarizes the prevalent view: "Certain patterns, established by the 1400s, were still functional in the eighteenth century. . . . This paper has attempted to remodel the eighteenth-century data in such a manner that these continuities are reflected in the interpretations and so the various Caddoan enclaves can be seen in a systemic way. . . . Consequently, the 'changes' in Caddoan culture so often attributed to European influence merely reflect the adaptability of traditional economic strategies."

Further, the presumed strength of the cultural continuity has been accepted as demonstrating a resistance to the effects of European cultures by Caddoan peoples that other native American groups did not possess (Brain 1983). For instance, Webb and Gregory (1978, 17) have stated that "contrary to many other southeastern Indian groups, the Caddoan people seem to have clung tenaciously to land and leadership even after the coercive effects of European contact. The fact that their roots extended into prehistory gave them strength and selfconfidence. They kept their faith and polity, and their traditions remain even today."

This depiction of adaptability of Caddoan peoples, coupled with the general lack of direct conflict with Europeans, has been made all the more sensible because of many of the ethnographic accounts and testimonies by Caddoan leaders throughout the eighteenth and nineteenth centuries. In 1830, for instance, Jean Louis Berlandier noted that the Caddo (referring to the Kadohadacho) "proudly recall their ancient lineage and power, and claim rights preeminent to those of all the other natives in the immense lands of Texas. General Terán [see Terán 1870] once asked their chief whether his people's lands lay in Mexico or in the United States. Once the chief had got the question straight, he answered that he was neither on Mexican nor United States territory, but on his own land which belonged to nobody but him" (Ewers 1969, 107).

Berlandier then goes on to point out, however, that the Kadohadacho in 1830 cultivated "very little land," followed the migrations of the buffalo herds, and did a "thriving trade in furs," which were exchanged in Natchitoches and other U.S. government trading houses or agencies among them (Ewers 1969, 107).

Thus, while I do not wish to deny the historical record or the picture it paints of the political relationships and alliances of the time, to rely on the testimony of then-active participants to depict the "contest of cultures" (Axtell 1985) is to negate an objective consideration of the changes to aboriginal peoples brought about by Europeans in North America (Trigger 1983, 440). Many important cultural changes took place in native American societies long before the first in-depth accounts of aboriginal peoples were recorded by European explorers and settlers. Thus, the study of the archaeology of this general period is essential to the comprehensive consideration of native history in the Contact period, as is the further integration of the ethnographic, ethnohistorical, and archaeological records as comparable or complementary data sets that are informative about the culture contact process (see Washburn 1989; Wilson and Rogers 1992).

The nature of European contact in the Caddoan Area from an aboriginal perspective has two important but related components: (*a*) the relative intensity of face-to-face contact and (*b*) the types of products associated with particular phases of face-to-face contact. The temporal and spatial character these two components manifest signify different and changing levels of European–native American interaction in the Caddoan Area (Trubowitz 1984, 30, 35; Perttula and Ramenofsky 1982). The manifestations range from the intermittent procurement of European goods by native Americans without any actual European participation or cognition and the intermittent and exploratory observation and meeting of native Americans by Europeans, to sustained year-round and generational contact of large numbers of Europeans with native Americans in combination with the regular use and exchange of European products.

Diseases introduced by the Europeans must be considered independent of direct contact because their transmission is not inherently determined by the nature or duration of face-to-face contact (see Crosby 1986, 195–216). Indeed, the effects of diseases introduced in the New World were probably most virulent during the initial phase of exposure to native Americans, rather than after repeated direct contact had been established (Crosby 1967; Dobyns 1983). Episodes of disease epidemics became more frequent as the intensity of contact increased, though it is probable that each episode had less of an effect on mortality than had previous episodes (Robinson, Kelley, and Rubertone 1985). In the Caddoan Area of Texas, there were eight known epidemic events between 1691 and 1816, or one epidemic event every 15.6 years. Population decline was a consequence of the epidemics, which came at regular intervals (every ten to twenty years) after direct contact had been established (Reff 1987b). As a result, there was usually a new group of nonimmune individuals, children and young adolescents, who were exposed to the disease. This resulted in high subadult mortality and further diminished the population growth potential of this native American group. In a real sense, therefore, the introduction of certain diseases by Europeans is a type of product. Their importance for studies of culture contact in the Caddoan Area must be determined by their character and pervasiveness in the record.

There also is abundant archaeological and ethnohistorical evidence that there were changes in native American demography and a diffusion of European goods that preceded actual European colonization and settlement in the southeastern United States (Dobyns 1983; Swanton 1939; Smith 1987; Milanich and Milbrath 1989b). Consequently, ethnographic descriptions and cultural reconstructions based on documents written primarily during the period of direct European contact and settlement cannot automatically be considered relevant to "pristine," or precontact, native American societies. There was a lag in information obtained by Europeans that was recorded after the initial intermittent and/or indirect contact of native Americans with Europeans. This lag persisted until the time when permanent European settlement and direct recording of events took place on a regular sustained basis because of face-to-face contact. European products noted to have been present among the Caddoan groups (most notably the Hasinai) in the 1680s are known to have reached them prior to sustained European settlement and trade operations (Hatcher 1927, 1932; Griffith 1954; Schilz and Worcester 1987). Bolton (1987, 135) notes that the Hasinai had obtained indirectly from the Spaniards hawkbells and shells that they wore around their necks or used as ornaments on clothing.

Other types of products introduced by the Europeans to North America included dry goods and clothing that could not be manufactured by the native Americans themselves and animals, either livestock that could not be produced or European domesticated animals that could eventually be raised without European assistance or technology. European products preceded sustained European exploration and settlement in the Caddoan Area by an unknown length of time, perhaps by as much as thirty years or more.

Direct contact between Caddoan peoples and Europeans denotes exploration and/or colonization efforts that include permanent settlement and the trade of European products. Because it is sustained, it is to a large measure dependent for its initial form upon the distinct material items brought for trade by both cultures, the Europeans' variegated motivations that dictated how interaction with aboriginal populations should occur (McEwan and Mitchem 1984; Poyo and Hinojosa 1988), and the selection and integration of those ideational and technological elements within both cultural systems through time.

RESEARCH ISSUES

In what ways did Caddoan Indian society and culture change or remain the same as a result of European contact and interaction? How is it possible to discuss, measure, and evaluate cultural change among the Caddoan peoples during these time periods using the archaeological record? One of the key issues that must be addressed in this study is the timing and magnitude of demographic change in Caddoan cultural groups caused by the introduction of European acute epidemic diseases because they affect the maintenance of sociopolitical cohesion, short- and long-term nutrition and health conditions, and the overall quality of Caddoan lifeways (Perttula 1989a; Ramenofsky 1987b; Trubowitz 1984). How do researchers address the issue of demographic change and the impact of diseases?

Henige (1986, 303–305) has thoroughly reviewed the documentary evidence used by Dobyns (1983) in *Their Number Become Thinned* in arguing that periodic epidemics or pandemics caused dramatic population declines among North American Indians before 1565 and rather convincingly refutes the value of documentary sources as the sole means of demonstrating population reduction during this early period (see also Milanich 1987a, 174). Instead, Henige (1986) proposes that "arguments of silence," in this case the native American archaeological record of the sixteenth and seventeenth centuries, be employed to demonstrate independently the timing and magnitude of such a population decline or demographic collapse and thereby corroborate and extend the historic record.

Recent archaeological and bioarchaeological research in many regions of North and South America has shown that the lifeways of most aboriginal peoples were significantly "altered by changes produced by a European presence . . . long before the first detailed accounts of those groups were recorded" (Trigger 1983, 439–440). In addition to cultural changes that must have occurred because of basic differences in social and political organization, religious beliefs, and technological parameters between Europeans' and native Americans' two autonomous cultural systems, European-introduced diseases on aboriginal populations increasingly have come to play a significant interpretive role in the study of the impact of European contact (Dobyns 1966, 1983; Milanich and Milbrath 1989a).

With the aid of written documentation, historians, demographers, and anthropologists have provided important comparative data on reductions in populations among aboriginal groups around the world as a result of European-introduced diseases. Significant research has been published on the demographic issue in South America (Hemmings 1978), Mexico and Central America (Cook and Borah 1971–1974; Crosby 1967; Borah 1964, 1976; Joralemon 1982), Australia, New Guinea, and New Zealand (Jacobs 1971, 1974; Crosby 1986). Native American cultures in Alaska (Wolfe 1982, Krech 1983) and diverse regions within the North American continent have also been studied from this perspective (Thornton 1986, 1987; Thornton and Thornton 1981; Crosby 1972, 1976, 1987; Duffy 1953; Dobyns 1984; Johansson 1982; Cronon 1983; Cook 1937, 1973, 1976; Martin 1974, 1978; Jackson 1985, 1986; Merrell 1984; Newman 1976; Ubelaker and Jantz 1986).

Only within the last ten years or so, however, have archaeologists and bioarchaeologists begun to give careful attention to the demographic issue or, moreover, to the importance in both disciplines of interpreting and understanding this record of contact cultural change in the New World in light of European-introduced diseases and their diffusion (Trigger 1985; Milanich 1987a; Ramenofsky 1987b, 1990). Important new contributions and reevaluations of the sixteenth- and seventeenth-century archaeological and bioarchaeological records include studies by Cook (1981) of South America and Walker, Lambert, and DeNiro (1989) of California as well as those of Reff (1985, 1987a, 1987b), Riley (1986), Stodder (1986), Merbs (1989), and Upham (1986, 1987) of the greater Southwest.

A number of researchers who study the Great Plains of North America have also pursued this issue (Bradtmiller 1983; Hanson 1987; Lehmer 1977; Palkovich 1981; Trimble 1985, 1986; Yelton 1985). Similar types of archaeological, bioarchaeological, and ethnohistorical studies concerning the effects of European-introduced diseases on native Americans in the northeastern United States (Bradley 1987; Brenner 1988; Crosby 1988; Robinson, Kelley, and Rubertone 1985; Snow and Lanphear 1988; Snow and Starna 1984; Spiess and Spiess 1987; Trigger 1981b), Florida and the Caribbean (Deagan 1984, 1985; Fairbanks 1985; Hahn 1986; Milanich 1987a, 1988; Mitchem et al. 1985; Mitchem and Hutchinson 1986, 1987), the Gulf Coast (Aten 1984; Davis 1984), South Texas (Miller 1988), and the southeastern United States are available for comparative purposes (Blakely 1988; Blakely and Detwiler-Blakely 1989; Brown 1982, 1985; Burnett 1990c; Milner 1980; Curren 1984; Dickens, Ward, and Davis 1987;

Dye and Brister 1986; Fish and Fish 1979; Fitzhugh 1985; Larsen 1987a, 1987b; Muller 1986; Ramenofsky 1985a, 1986; Smith 1984, 1987, 1989; Thomas 1987).

Implications and Consequences of European Acute Diseases on Caddoan Populations

Significant epidemic diseases that were introduced in the Caddoan Area included smallpox, measles, plague, diphtheria, whooping cough, trachoma, and influenza, among others (Ewers 1973). None of these diseases were present in North America before the arrival of Europeans (Crosby 1986, 197–198).

According to Ramenofsky (1982, 80) all introduced European diseases shared certain characteristics affecting exposed populations:

1. Exposure and infection for most of the diseases resulted in permanent or long-term immunity.
2. Therefore, if populations lacked familiarity to such diseases, they had no immunity and were considered virgin colonizing territories for the reproduction of the infectious agents.
3. In such populations, the infestation was acute and epidemics erupted.

The increasing mortality of adolescents and young adults from virgin soil epidemics decreased population fertility (Burnet and White 1972). This decrease was accompanied by episodic infections that killed those born between epidemics who had no previous exposure or immunity to the European-introduced diseases.

In Texas there were epidemics among such native American groups as the Comanche, Apache, Karankawa, Wichita, and Tonkawa at "least once each generation from 1731 to 1877" (Ewers 1973, 107), a time for which some documentation exists (Table 4). The cumulative effect of these recorded epidemics among the Texas Caddoan groups was a known 94 percent population reduction between 1690 and 1890 (Ewers 1973, Table 1). Taking into consideration, therefore, the possibility that the more virulent and devastating epidemics occurred between 1520 and 1690 but were not well recorded historically, the combined effect on aboriginal populations was unparalleled (Thornton 1987; Vehik 1989).

One of the more important aspects of the demographic issue that has been recently raised is disease diffusion (e.g., Dobyns 1983; Ramenofsky 1987b, 1990). Essentially, the concept of disease diffusion concerns the potential of introduced diseases to be diffused in advance of direct transmission from European settlers and explorers and how such unrecorded disease outbreaks could be transmitted and diffused beyond points of initial introduction (Ramenofsky 1990; Trimble 1988).

TABLE 4. Known Epidemics in the Caddoan Area of Texas

Date	Type of Disease
1691	Unidentified
1718	Unidentified
1731	Smallpox
1759	Measles
1777–1778	Cholera or bubonic plague
	Smallpox
1801–1802	Smallpox
1803	Measles
1816	Smallpox
1864[a]	Smallpox
1867[a]	Cholera
1892[a]	Measles, influenza, whooping cough

Source: Based on Ewers 1973.

[a]Recorded among the Caddoan peoples living in Indian Territory within the present boundaries of Oklahoma.

Dobyns (1983, 337) points out that diseases such as smallpox, measles, and bubonic plague may spread widely and rapidly on a continental level and that the initial virgin soil episodes of disease transmission were pandemic and caused the greatest mortality. He identifies major epidemics—"decisive demographic events of the first magnitude in terms of their influence on native American settlement and population" (Dobyns 1983, 337)—in 1519–1524, 1564–1570, 1613–1619, and 1633–1639 (Table 5). The diffusion of disease pathogens from Cuba and Mexico is assumed to have had a deleterious effect over a large section of North America, in these cases from Florida north to New England and perhaps into the North American Great Plains. Vehik (1989, Table 11) has identified possible epidemics on the southern plains with high mortality rates in the years 1617–1619 and 1635–1638.

Deagan (1985) and Ramenofsky (1985a, 1987b) and Ewers (1973) include only a few suspected epidemics in Florida, the lower Mississippi Valley, and Texas (see Table 5). The divergences between the authors in Table 5 point out quite clearly their different perspectives on what they believe constitutes disease contact and documentary evidence for the occurrence of epidemics at those times. Direct references to epidemic episodes typify the lists provided by Deagan, Ramenofsky, and Ewers. The others are those disease outbreaks that Dobyns (1983, 8–32) has speculated diffused from Mexico and Cuba.[1] A list compiled by Vehik (1989, Table 11) for the

TABLE 5. Known or Suspected Sixteenth- and Seventeenth-Century Epidemics in Florida and Texas

Florida (Dobyns 1983)	Florida (Deagan 1985)	Texas (Ewers 1973)
1513		
1519		
		1528
1535–38		
1545–48		
1549		
1550		
1559		
1564–1570	1570	
1585–86	1586	
	1591	
1596		
1613–17	1613	
	1617	
1649	1649	
1653		
1659	1659	
	1670	
1672	1672–74	
1675		1674–75
	1686	1686
		1691

Note: Ramenofsky (1985a, 1987b) recognizes an epidemic in the lower Mississippi Valley in 1698.

southern plains of North America includes possible epidemics in 1535, 1592–1593, 1647–1648, and 1671 that may be related to those diseases identified by Dobyns (1983) as having diffused from Mexico or eastern North America.

Ramenofsky's analyses of the diffusion potential of the different reported (or inferred) sixteenth- or seventeenth-century diseases were based on an examination of their means of transmission to estimate (*a*) the probability by which certain diseases could have diffused to North America and (*b*) what type of spatial pattern they might take (1986, 1987a). She distinguished between directly transmitted pathogens (measles, influenza, other viruses, and smallpox) and zoonoses (typhus, plague, and malaria) transmitted through an intermediate host or vector. It is not essential for the zoonotic pathogen to survive to persist in human populations, and proximity is usually directly responsible for the spread of the infection to humans (Ramenofsky 1987b, 1990). These infections had a higher diffusion potential than most of the directly transmitted diseases because it was unlikely that the period of communicability of measles and influenza would persist long enough to survive European voyages across the Atlantic Ocean. Smallpox, however, is a notable exception because it can remain viable in a dried state for more than a year (Upham 1986; Joralemon 1982; Ramenofsky 1987b). That being the case, it could have been transmitted from Mexico or Cuba to North America during the first pandemic of 1520–1524, for instance, and then been diffused widely across the continent, possibly reaching into the Caddoan Area. If the introduction of such a smallpox epidemic caused at least a 50 to 75 percent reduction in populations in which it has been documented (Dobyns 1983, 14; Upham 1986), the effects would have been disastrous to any native American group that was affected.

Relevant questions or research problems explored in this study that relate to the effects of European diseases on Caddoan groups include the following:

§ What is the historical significance of European-introduced diseases in the region? Did these diseases have a significant effect on population reduction or Caddoan social structure, and if so, when did the effect occur (Trubowitz 1984)?

§ Can demographic decline, stress, and health status among Caddoan groups be identified in the paleodemographic and bioarchaeological records, and if so, what were the biological and health consequences that can be detected?

§ Are there changes in settlement density and location or the tempo of abandonment that relate to episodes of epidemics? And if so, how does the process of regional abandonment relate to the development of Caddoan confederacies?

§ Ewers's 1973 analysis of epidemics among Caddoan groups indicates that the cumulative effects of recorded epidemics between 1690 and 1890 were a known 94 percent population reduction. What were the cumulative effects of disease introduced among Protohistoric period Caddoan groups?

§ Do the effects of European contact and the spread of European diseases engender the same types of responses by Caddoan groups living along major rivers as they do among those Caddoan groups inhabiting rural upland and hinterland areas?

§ Are there changes in mortuary practices, sociopolitical complexity, and mound building or use following the introduction of diseases indicating significant changes in hierarchical ranking?

In essence, the intent of these questions is to ascertain the impact of introduced European diseases in the Caddoan Area, the magnitude of Caddoan population declines, the timing of disease introduction and reintroduction, the likelihood of disease transmission and diffusion between Caddoan populations, and, most important, how disease transmission affected social, political, and ethnic affiliations over time.

Caddoan Area skeletal data for the Protohistoric and Historic periods (see Harmon and Rose 1989, 348–349; Burnett 1990a) are in many ways inadequate to systematically consider issues of depopulation or demographic stress because of the following factors: (*a*) unsystematic excavations and collection procedures, (*b*) poor preservation, and (*c*) a paucity of available diachronic information concerning possible intracommunity or regional variations in social complexity or status differentiation between 1520 and 1800.

Nevertheless, a Caddoan bioarchaeological data base of paleodemographics is being accumulated, particularly focusing on the Middle Ouachita River basin and pockets along the Red River (Burnett 1990a, 1990b; Harmon and Rose 1989). The research questions that can be addressed in a systematic way in Caddoan bioarchaeological assemblages dating to the Protohistoric and Historic periods include the following:

- § Are there elevated mortality rates among adults and adolescents in bioarchaeological assemblages from the Protohistoric and Historic periods?
- § Is there bioarchaeological evidence, such as fatal or healed gun and sword wounds, cuts, and punctures, of violent conflicts between Europeans and Caddoan peoples? Are there specific temporal and spatial patterns to the conflicts?
- § What was the local and regional adaptive efficiency of Protohistoric and Historic Caddoan populations? This may be measured by bioarchaeological indexes of nutritional status, childhood stress episodes, the frequency of infectious diseases and pathologies, and the mean age of death in regional and local bioarchaeological assemblages (e.g., Burnett 1990b, 11–49).

The hypothesis that a major demographic decline probably occurred among Caddoan populations prior to a documented and sustained European presence in the Caddoan Area has major implications for interpreting the nature of the archaeological record during the Protohistoric period and the periods following the first detailed European accounts of Caddoan peoples. Therefore, that fundamental changes in aboriginal Caddoan lifeways occurred during these periods but cannot be documented historically must be considered to be within the realm of possibility. Further, such changes as may have occurred in these "Dark Ages" need to be evaluated with respect to new and more reliable information. This includes information on the composition and formation of Caddoan sociopolitical entities described in the ethnographic record. Scholars also must interpret the possible extent of systemic continuities between the Caddoan archaeological and ethnological cultures during a period of rapidly changing conditions (Trigger 1981a, 1983, 1986b; Ramenofsky 1986; Wolf 1984). To do otherwise is to treat cultural entities in isolation from their historical context and contribute to a static, atemporal perspective, one "which can be sustained only as long as one abjures any interest in history"(Wolf 1984, 394). Wolf goes on to note that "in the majority of cases the entities studied by anthropologists owe their development to processes that originate outside them and reach well beyond them, that they owe their crystallization to these processes, take part in them, and affect them in their turn"(Wolf 1984, 395).

The archaeological record of the Caddoan Area between ca. 1520 and 1800 is critically examined further to study Caddoan-European interaction and Caddoan cultural changes following European contact. This assessment is carried out by comparing the archaeological record of the Protohistoric and Historic periods within each of the three subareas of the Caddoan Area: the Western Caddoan, Central Caddoan, and Arkansas Basin or Northern Caddoan (Schambach 1983). In particular, elements of settlement change, regional population densities, and sociopolitical and ceremonial activities are traced within these areas from 1520 to 1800 to understand better how these facets of the Caddoan archaeological record are informative about the effects of European contact on aboriginal cultural systems in the Trans-Mississippi South. While potentially many different avenues and dimensions could be explored to assess contact between these two autonomous cultural systems, the research issues of this study provide the best opportunity at this time for examining the multifaceted nature of the contact process in the Caddoan Area.

Settlement Changes Biases in local and regional settlement data in the Protohistoric and Historic periods of the Caddoan Area exist because of previous emphases on the excavation of cemeteries and mounds to the exclusion of acquiring archaeological data from associated settlements or of acquiring intrasite information on site structure or community organization. There has never been a comprehensive survey effort carried out within any part of the Caddoan Area to acquire the regional archaeological data to characterize the density and distribution of Caddoan sites that postdate 1520. It is difficult to define, much less describe, a settlement system or its changes through time without having essential knowledge of the parts that make up that system. Sampling problems of this nature, therefore, must obviate the consideration of even the most basic comparison—that of quantitative differences in Caddoan settlement frequencies through time. Of course, frequency changes can constitute one possible indication of population changes in the Protohistoric and Historic periods.

The dispersed nature of Caddoan settlement systems, the *rancherías* of the Spanish documents, also precludes using the type of routine demographic analyses employed in studies of other parts of North America that rely upon quantitative differences in aboriginal settlement frequencies through time (e.g., Ramenofsky 1987b; Snow and Starna 1984; Smith 1987). Counting the number of sites in a dispersed settlement system cannot be directly compared to counting sites in a nucleated or consolidated settlement system because of the differences in occupation span and the necessity of having appropriate regional settlement data for demographic inferences. In the archaeological record for the Caddoan Area, inferences about population or settlement change are made most appropriately at the regional scale. In this way, sampling problems (mentioned above) and differences based on probable shifts in settlement size, movements, and amalgamation of different groups over time (Ramenofsky 1984), which change the character of the record, are circumvented.

Regional Population Changes Population densities of Caddoan groups at initial contact must have been variably affected by epidemic diseases introduced by Europeans because of variations in settlement character of upland and/or rural communities compared with major riverine and/or town communities and their effect on the transmission and diffusion of epidemic diseases (Dobyns 1983; Ramenofsky 1990, Table 1). The higher the relative Caddoan population density in riverine/town communities at initial contact with Europeans in combination with their position along communication axes, the more rapid and pervasive the processes of depopulation probably were. That is, those groups who had the highest populations and were situated along major trade and communication routes would be the ones most adversely affected by European diseases. The trends previously noted toward denser populations and some settlement compaction at, or near, the civic-ceremonial centers of the 1520 Caddoan town communities on the major rivers suggest that the most apparent effects of population decline would be concentrated in these specific types of areas (although see Burnett 1990b for the Mid-Ouachita River area between 1500 and 1700).

Ewers (1973, 109) suggested that only rarely did Caddoan group size fall below about 150 people before merging with another group. Refusing to fall below this minimum most likely was an attempt to maintain stable population levels and population fertility within the group. Thus, amalgamation would follow the effects of introduced European diseases as the Caddoan breeding population, as well as the labor and defense forces, were diminished. Additionally, formerly discrete social and ethnic entities had to coalesce for that new social and ethnic unit to remain a viable social and economic system (see Milner 1980; Thornton 1987; Ramenofsky 1987b). As a result of this amalgamation, many original and traditional Caddoan settlements were likely to be abandoned and, conversely, areas where Caddoan social and ethnic remnants amalgamated actually may appear at times in the Protohistoric and Historic periods to have experienced local population increases.

The types of research questions that pertain to settlement changes and regional population densities in the Protohistoric and Historic periods and that have a reasonable degree of being addressed through the study of the Caddoan archaeological and ethnohistorical records include the following:

§ Is the development of Caddoan confederacies in the Red and Neches/Angelina rivers related to the processes of regional abandonment and population decline that followed the introduction of European epidemic diseases?

§ Were particular valleys or areas, such as the Cypress Creek basin in Northeast Texas (Thurmond 1990a, 1990b) or the Mid-Ouachita River basin in Southwest Arkansas (Early 1990), abandoned or emptied as the result of the initial and/or continued exposure of Caddoan groups to European-introduced diseases?

§ Were there enclaves of Caddoans along the major trails and portages that developed in the Protohistoric and Historic periods following significant population loss in the region?

§ What changes occurred in settlement density and location and in the tempo of abandonment among the Red River Caddoan groups, and how did these changes relate to episodes of epidemics?

§ Did the effects of European contact, including the spread of European diseases, engender the same types of adaptive responses by Caddoan groups living along the major rivers, such as the Red River, as they did among those Caddoan groups inhabiting rural, upland, and hinterland areas?

Finally, when population and community sizes decline significantly and/or continuously because of disease, population loss can be expected to influence considerably existing social, ceremonial, and community organization.

Sociopolitical and Ceremonial Complexity To focus on elements of the native American archaeological and ethnohistorical records that are informative about processes of social and political integration is to be con-

TABLE 6. Criteria for Social Differentiation

Major Categories of Differentiation	Vertical Differentiation	Horizontal Differentiation
Age/Sex	Skewed distribution	Normal distribution
Frequency	Hierarchical pyramid	Variable but of equal size
Spatial distribution	Restricted	Uniform
Symbolic designation	Differential energy expenditure in treatment and relative value of grave offerings	Equal levels of energy expenditure; inclusion of nonvalued symbols

Source: Adapted from O'Shea 1984, Table 4.3.

cerned with evidence of social differentiation and complexity (i.e., the existence of social ranking) in the economic, sociopolitical, and ceremonial spheres within communities. As O'Shea (1984, 4) points out, ranking and differentiation are key aspects of complexity in sociopolitical relationships.

In the simplest terms, egalitarian societies are simple societies; ranked or stratified societies are complex. A ranked society is one "regulated by mechanisms (i.e., inheritance) that fix the potential number of statuses an individual may aspire to beyond those dictated by personal characteristics" (Rogers 1983, 22). This means there is limited access to positions of prestige, and holding a position of rank confers privilege in different sociopolitical spheres of that society. Rank distinctions are those that tend to elevate certain individuals above others in the social system (O'Shea 1981, 41) and are referred to herein as *vertical differentiation. Horizontal differentiation* includes those sociopolitical differences that generally only cut across age and sex categories or rank distinctions.

From the archaeological record, there are two primary means of inferring matters of sociopolitical organization and complexity: (*a*) the study of mortuary practices and (*b*) the study of a hierarchical or ranked organization, specifically the internal hierarchy of civic-ceremonial centers, settlements, or other habitation sites and the external hierarchy of the civic-ceremonial centers themselves. How are these sociopolitical and ceremonial aspects of the archaeological record identified?

Burial assemblages from the Caddoan Area dating to between 1520 and 1800 are examined for systemic changes in sociopolitical differentiation, especially the key variable of vertical differentiation (Table 6). Important criteria to be considered include the diversity of grave offerings, the spatial segregation of the individuals, inclusion of valued symbols and trappings of authority (Rogers 1983, 67), and differences in the treatment of the burial (i.e., the complexity of the burial ritual).

A range of research problems may be explored with the Caddoan mortuary data from the Protohistoric and Historic periods. The issues include the following:

§ Regional or temporal changes in mortuary practices, sociopolitical complexity, and mound building following the introduction of diseases (and the initiation of European contact) that may indicate significant changes in Caddoan ideology and ceremonial activities

§ The role and significance of nonutilitarian European trade materials in traditional Caddoan ideological systems and their ritual symbolic and ceremonial values (Miller and Hamell 1986)

§ Archaeological and ethnohistorical evidence for the use of the calumet ceremony among Hasinai and Kadohadacho groups and its symbolic, ritual, and economic denotations (Brain 1989, 319; Sabo 1987)

In the Caddoan Area, hierarchical systems can also be identified in the archaeological record by the presence of civic-ceremonial centers and supralocal or multicommunity cemeteries. Both elements of the archaeological record occur in the Caddoan Area beginning as early as ca. A.D. 900 (see Story 1990; Rogers, Wyckoff, and Peterson 1989; Schambach 1990a), but it is their later postcontact manifestations that are important in the present study.

Civic-ceremonial centers are archaeological sites with structural mounds and burial mounds. The structural mounds—those "capping a structure and/or providing a platform for a structure" (Story 1990, 340)—have been characterized by Story (1990, 341) as "places where religious practitioners could perform sacred rites, where ritual paraphernalia could be kept, and around which members of the society could periodically congregate to reaffirm what was important and right." The burial mounds, on the other hand, at the civic-ceremonial centers served as the mortuaries for the elite members of Caddoan sociopolitical groups. The highest ranking elite members of these Caddoan groups were typically buried in the center of the burial mound, and they were accompanied by a multitude of grave goods, many of them having been obtained through long-distance trade networks. Thus, the civic-ceremonial centers are manifestations of a highly developed system of ceremonial activity.

Specialized facilities such as platform mounds, public buildings, plazas, and charnel houses are assumed to represent expressions of a regional and centralized sociopolitical structure, one that was maintained by an elite group of individuals to sanctify chiefly authority, political power, ritual, ceremonies, and supernatural prerogatives of the community (Knight 1986, 681). Traditions of ceremonial activity in a mortuary context include the processing and interment of individuals in specialized mound contexts that can be interpreted as a result of hierarchical differences in rank or status that exist within the larger society as a whole (Brown 1981).

Supralocal or community cemeteries are the product of interments from a number of communities in the vicinity (Story 1990, 338–339). These cemeteries usually contain at least seventy individuals (Story 1990; Perttula 1991). The community cemeteries contain excellent evidence for the existence of social differences within a Caddoan population and community. Since community cemeteries are recognized by the type of burial interment, their relative size, grave good associations, and their isolation from habitation sites, they are analogous in functional context to the civic-ceremonial centers. The civic-ceremonial centers and supralocal cemeteries also exhibit patterns of spacing and dispersion from associated habitation sites that are probably dictated in large measure by differences in the relative densities of the surrounding support populations (Brown 1984c, 54). Civic-ceremonial centers and community cemeteries of the Protohistoric and Historic periods are not present in each river basin or all subareas of the Caddoan Area but are concentrated along the major rivers, such as the Little, Red, and Ouachita, or in the Cypress Creek basin in East Texas (Story 1990, 339–340; Hoffman 1983; Early 1990). Presumably these areas had the most complex Caddoan sociopolitical organizations and/or the highest population densities during these times.

Therefore, a significant and/or continuous Caddoan population decline due to the effects of disease can be expected to exert a considerable influence on the scale and retention of traditional supracommunity organizations and the number of functions able to be performed by these integrative mechanisms in the Protohistoric and Historic periods. In addition, the loss of the support population for the elite in Caddoan society should be evidenced in a general collapse in complexity, or even abandonment, of the civic-ceremonial system during the Protohistoric period (1520–1685) of European contact. Were they replaced by newer and more viable forms of sociopolitical integration, such as confederation and annexation (Knight 1986, 683)?

What types of research questions can be explored that address how and in what ways sociopolitical organization and complexity changed as a consequence of European contact? Particularly important factors include demographic losses; aboriginal territorial movements; European political and economic machinations; and the differential persistence of traditional rituals, symbols, and ceremonies. Both archaeological and ethnohistorical records must be examined to understand aboriginal political organization—

its functions, its trappings—and its symbolic and ritual interconnection with other aspects of Caddoan lifeways.

- § The complexity and significance of mortuary practices (i.e., body positioning, types of interments, grave goods, and demographic characteristics) in Protohistoric and Historic Caddoan populations with civic-ceremonial centers and supralocal or community cemeteries
- § The form and content of Caddoan ceremonialism among the Hasinai and Kadohadacho groups, specifically the sacred ritual programs and ceremonies (Sabo 1987)
- § The impact of severe stress, population decline, and territorial dissolution on the maintenance of Caddoan sociopolitical organization and status positions among town and rural communities from the Protohistoric to the Historic Caddoan period
- § The persistence of regionally complex social hierarchies and levels of integration among Kadohadacho and Hasinai groups following sustained contact with Europeans
- § Shifts in bases of authority in Caddoan society from sacred to secular in nature following Caddoan interactions with the Spanish and French
- § The attainment of social status, from evidence in the Caddoan archaeological and ethnohistorical records, as a consequence of possession of European trade goods, technology, the horse, and other imports and their ever-increasing access by all Caddoan social strata after ca. 1740
- § Changes in Caddoan political and ritual organization and the incorporation of European political and economic concerns, that occurred with the development of dependable trade relationships with Europeans after ca. 1714.
- § The significance of Caddoan medal chiefs (Ewers 1974; Sabo 1988), European methods of promoting political dependency, and the impacts thereof on aboriginal tribal factionalism and the maintenance of traditional Caddoan systems of authority.

Population Estimates No overall estimates of aboriginal population for the Caddoan Area at the time of initial contact with Europeans (ca. 1520) have been made by archaeologists and ethnohistorians. Archaeological considerations (reviewed in chapter 2) suggest that prehistoric Caddoan societies had dispersed settlement systems generally characterized by relatively low regional population density compared with denser nucleated populations in the Mississippi River Valley and interior parts of southeastern North America (Steponaitis 1986; Smith 1986; Smith 1987). Relatively higher densities of people and archaeological sites may occur in the vicinity of the Caddoan civic-ceremonial mound centers in the town communities.

Generally, the civic-ceremonial centers were kept separated from the domestic habitations, and population compaction probably did not occur around them as it did with the nucleated and fortified Mississippi River Valley settlements (Brown 1984b; Smith 1990; Jeter et al. 1989).

Dobyns (1983, 42) estimates population densities of 2.53 persons/square kilometers ca. 1520 for horticultural peoples living along the Mississippi River Valley and its tributaries. Applying this estimate to the Caddoan Area, which seems reasonable since Dobyns (1983) included the Red and Arkansas rivers, a very general estimate may be proposed of 200,000–250,000 people living in the Caddoan Area at initial contact ca. 1520. This population estimate would be higher except that there was apparently only a minimal permanent settlement in large sections of the Ouachita Mountains and Ozark Highlands in the Late Caddoan period (1400–1520) (Early 1988; Perttula and McGuff 1985; Sabo et al. 1988). There is no way now to evaluate the accuracy of this population estimate. It is well to keep in mind, however, that Mooney's estimate of populations for all Caddoan groups during sustained European contact (ca. 1690) was only 8,500 (Mooney 1928; Ubelaker 1976).

Thornton (1987, 30) proposes another method of native American population estimation that is based on multiplying the population of an aboriginal group at its nadir in the historic record by a constant of twenty or twenty-five (see also Dobyns 1966). The two constants express varying estimates of the rate of population decline in the Contact era. The nadir in Caddoan population was reached ca. 1890–1900 when only 507 Caddo were counted on their Oklahoma reservation (Thornton 1986, Appendix E). With this method, the Caddoan population ranged between 10,140 and 12,675 during sustained contact with Europeans.

A population of about two hundred thousand at 1520 and 8,500 to 12,675 at ca. 1690 would argue for more than a 90 percent decline in the size of the Caddoan population over that time. This is congruent with the overall range in demographic losses seen elsewhere in the Southeast with aboriginal populations probably similarly episodically exposed to the same types of epidemic diseases (Dobyns 1983, 288). By the same calculation method, Caddoan populations also declined 95 percent 1690–1880.

Two opposing views of demographic change in the Caddoan Area may be proposed based upon presumptions concerning the introduction of European acute diseases between ca. 1520 and 1800. Although the specific population sizes of Caddoan groups cannot be accurately estimated at this time, it is assumed that the population estimate of 8,500 Caddoan peoples at 1690 is fairly realistic (Mooney 1928; Ubelaker 1976). The basic difference between the two demographic models is in their assumptions about when depopulation begins.

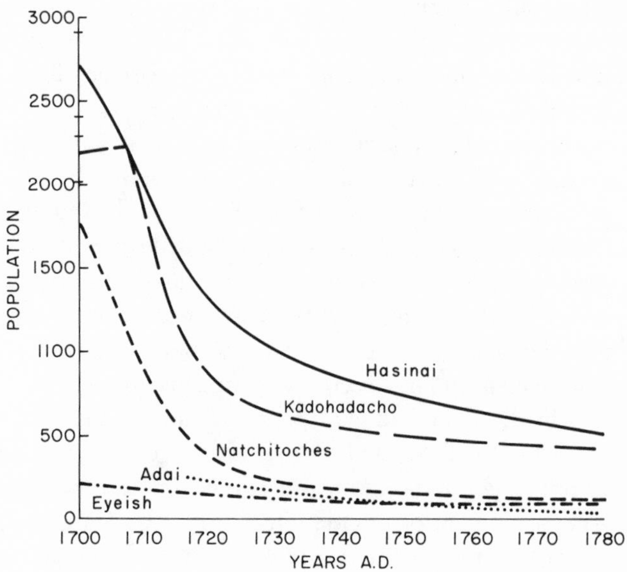

FIG. 11. Populations of Caddoan tribes, 1700–1780 (from Swanton 1942).

Differences in approaches to estimates of native American population depend primarily upon consideration of the impact of European diseases (Ramenofsky 1987b, 6–21). Such population estimates as Mooney's 1928 study of the Caddoan peoples are based upon dismissing acute infectious diseases as a significant factor in population estimation prior to sustained European contact ca. 1690. It is acknowledged that introduced epidemics after 1690 in the Caddoan Area severely reduced population (Fig. 11) (Swanton 1942, 17). When the introduction of European acute diseases is considered to be a major factor affecting the size of nonimmune populations from the period of initial culture contact, then assumptions of Caddoan population changes cannot be readily derived from population numbers during sustained and direct contact. That is, the overall Caddoan population structure or size at 1690 in the Caddoan Area must bear little correlation with Caddoan populations at ca. 1520 because of the different effects of each epidemic on population loss, and to project backward in time the 1690 population would be inappropriate.

In the first view, no epidemics would have taken place among any Caddoan groups until 1687–1691, based upon when the first historically recorded epidemic that affected the Caddoan people was described by the Spanish (see Table 4). The period between ca. 1520–1690 would, therefore, be one of continual Caddoan population growth (perhaps on the order of

3 percent annually [Upham 1987]), and the population maximum would have been reached about 1690 (Mooney 1928; Swanton 1942). Based on ethnographic records among Caddoan groups and following the major 1687–1691 epidemic, population then decreased 80 percent from 1700 to 1780 (from 7,000 to 1,400 individuals) and continued to decrease until ca. 1890–1900 (Thornton 1986, 1987:127–131; Swanton 1942, 24). The overall depopulation trend resembles the line based on Mooney (1928) in Fig. 12. The trend in depopulation is portrayed as a smooth monotonic decrease when in fact it would probably take a stair-step form, that is, one reflecting some population recovery or rise between epidemics and further population decline (Wood 1989).

The depopulation line based on Dobyns (1983) (see Fig. 12), conversely, assumes that the aboriginal Caddoan population reached its height near initial European contact (ca. 1520). Because of the possibility of a series of epidemics along frequented aboriginal trading routes, that population would have declined precipitously between ca. 1520 and 1690. The arguments of Dobyns (1983, Tables 1, 2, and 4) and Vehik (1989, Table 11) about disease diffusion suggest that in the Caddoan Area the initial epidemics of the sixteenth and seventeenth centuries were actually responsible for the greatest absolute declines in population.

Settlement Parameters Within the Caddoan Area differences in the dispersed settlement systems have important implications for differential population densities during the Protohistoric and Historic periods. The contrast is between major riverine town communities that had dense populations and the more sparsely populated rural communities located away from the major streams, along tributary streams and in the mountains (Dobyns 1983; Morey and Morey 1973). Therefore, it is possible to suggest rank-order relationships between Late Caddoan period phases in potential population density differences that have their basis in community or settlement variability, even though estimates of total numbers of people living in the Caddoan Area ca. 1520 to 1690 are unverifiable.

The de Soto narratives discussed in chapter 2 note variations in populations between major riverine and hinterland provinces. These differences appear to be reflected in the Late Caddoan period archaeological record (Story 1990; Jeter et al. 1989). The province Naguatex on Red River is illustrative of what is defined as a town community. It was described by one of the chroniclers as "the most populous of all the provinces through which the army passed during this expedition" (Swanton 1942, 32). Archaeologically, the Belcher phase is the most appropriate candidate for identifying the Naguatex province (Webb and Gregory 1978). Other Caddoan town community phases include the Texarkana, McCurtain, and Mid-Ouachita phases on the Red and Ouachita rivers (Fig. 13). Few particulars are avail-

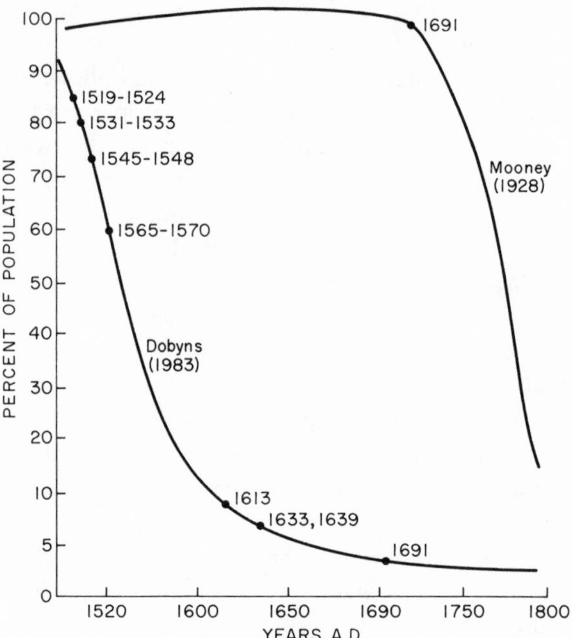

FIG. 12. Differences in depopulation trends among the Caddo based on differences in the assumed effects of European diseases, their appearances, and the period of maximum population.

able concerning the archaeological record of the Arkansas River Valley downstream from the area of the Fort Coffee phase. There are, however, indications that distinctive town communities were present ca. 1520 in the McClure and Carden Bottoms localities (Hoffman 1977a, 5–6, 1977b, 35). These types of communities seemingly resemble both Caddoan and Mississippian Quapaw phase systems in formal and functional content (Jeter et al. 1989; Hoffman 1986). Current thinking is that the east-central Arkansas occupations ca. 1520 are a pre-Quapaw Mississippian manifestation (Jeter et al. 1989, 226). The later Quapaw phase or Menard complex sites on the Arkansas River date after ca. 1600 in the late Protohistoric and Historic periods (Jeter, Cande, and Mintz 1990).

Rural Late Caddoan period community phases include the Frankston, Titus, Fort Coffee, Angelina, and Neosho phases (see Fig. 13). Absolute differences in population between the rural community phases cannot even be roughly estimated. However, the de Soto narratives do provide an illuminating discussion of recognizable differences in populations between the Guasco and Hais provinces (see Fig. 2) in East Texas that may approximate to some degree population rank differences between the Frankston and Late Angelina phases, respectively (Elvas, in Robertson 1933).

Differential population densities within the Caddoan Area have direct implications for the study of contact and assessing the impact of European epidemic diseases on Caddoan populations. Smaller and more highly dispersed rural communities may have had minimal direct contact with Europeans, giving them an adaptive advantage over the relatively more densely populated town communities by lessening the impact of epidemic diseases (Trubowitz 1984, 36). Therefore, while population densities in the Caddoan Area were probably not as high as those in the nucleated Mississippi period settlement systems in the Mississippi River Valley (see Fig. 3) and major eastern tributaries at the time of initial European contact, density patterns attested to in the archaeological and ethnohistorical records form the demographic constraints within which the consequences of European-introduced acute diseases must be considered.

The Temporal Framework Sustained and direct European contact is a quintessential aspect of the Caddoan Historic period and of the ethnohistorical and ethnographic descriptions of Caddoan peoples. However, intermittent, indirect, and unrecorded contact between Europeans and aboriginal groups is also important to consider in assessing changes in Caddoan lifeways before 1685. It is the contrastive nature of contact, namely direct and sustained versus indirect and intermittent, combined with differences in the behaviors and objectives of European colonization efforts as well as Caddoan-European exchange and trade relationships, that characterize and define the temporal units employed in this study.

If processes of aboriginal demographic change from exogenous diseases and the diffusion of European goods preceded actual European colonization efforts in the southeastern United States, the earliest native histories would have to be descriptions of cultural systems already experiencing the mitigating effects of European contact. As a result, an undue concentration on the period when direct and continuous face-to-face European contact and settlement began (after 1685) in studying the contact process in the Caddoan Area overlooks the ramifications of other forms of contact that preceded direct contact but that are not retrievable from historic and ethnographic documents. This period of intermittent and indirect European contact in the Caddoan area ca. 1520 to 1685 is necessarily considered from an archaeological perspective.

The two temporal periods forming the framework for all succeeding discussion in this book of the Caddoan archaeological record after 1520 are the Protohistoric or Early Historic Period (ca. 1520–1685) and the Later Historic period (ca. 1685–1800). The Protohistoric period is comparable

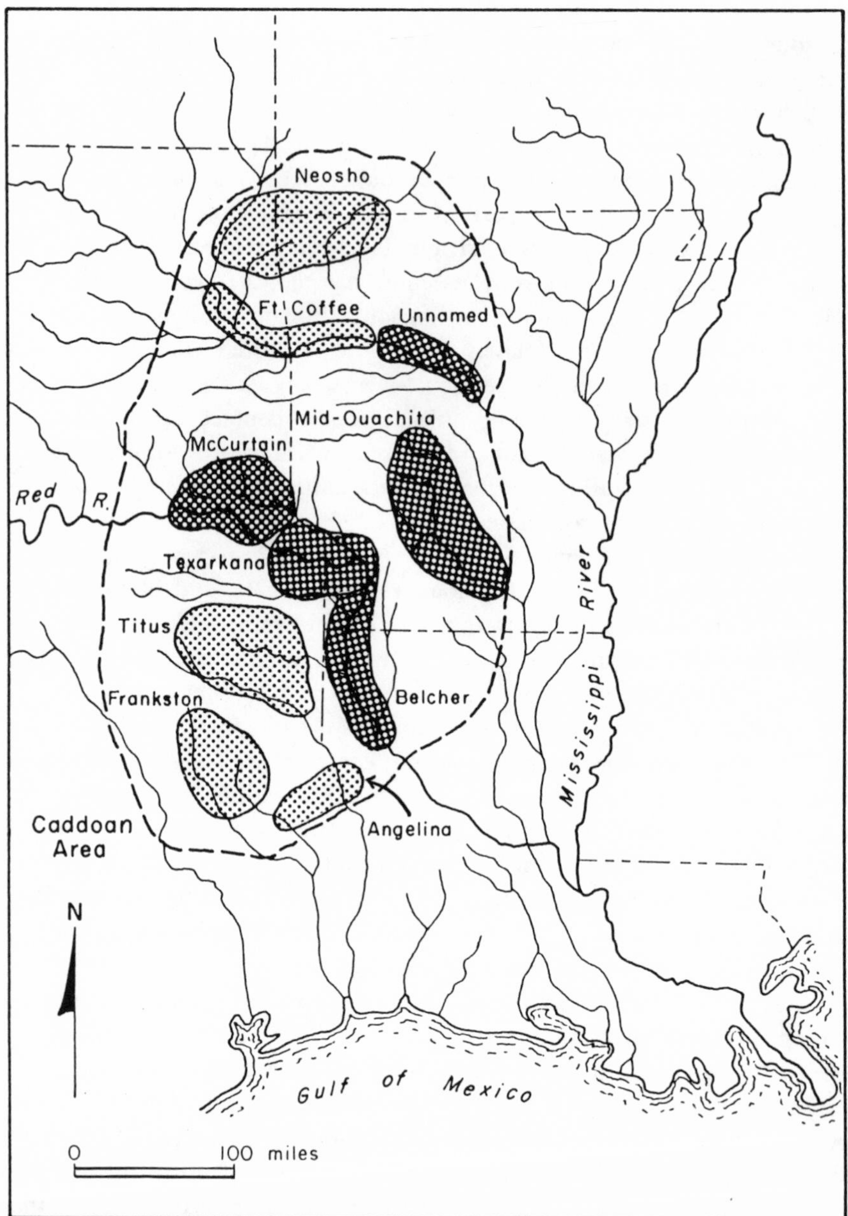

FIG. 13. Rural and town communities in the Caddoan Area, ca. 1520: *dots*, rural communities; *cross-hatching*, town communities.

to the Caddo IV period in Southwest Arkansas (see Schambach and Early 1983), the later portions of the Late Caddoan period defined by Story (1990, 334), and also corresponds to the time of initial European exploration and intermittent, stochastic contact with Caddoan peoples. The second period, the Historic period, corresponds to the Caddo V period, the Historic Caddoan period defined by Story (1990, 334), and to a sustained European presence in and settlement of the Caddoan Area.

The Archaeological Basis for Identifying Protohistoric and Historic Period Caddoan Sites

The archaeological record of the Protohistoric and Historic periods is organized using site stratigraphic sequences, dated by radiocarbon dates or other absolute methods, and the select seriation of time-sensitive artifacts, such as ceramic styles in vessel form and decoration, that can be extrapolated from one region to the other within the three Caddoan subareas. The combination of stratigraphy and seriation of selected archaeological components make up the basic means of temporal control and are used as baselines to place analytically relevant components within relatively narrow time spans (Schambach and Miller 1984; Story 1982, n.d.; Williams and Early 1990) given certain contextual conditions.

Radiocarbon dating has, unfortunately, only limited applicability in this study because few samples are available from these periods, sampling errors and ambiguity in corrections and calendrical calibrations exist, and precision is reduced when only a few isolated dates are available. The available radiocarbon dates are calibrated according to Stuiver and Becker (1986), and presented as a range of dates.[2] Archaeomagnetic and thermoluminescence dates are also used when they are available. They may be more reliable than radiocarbon dates because they are not dependent on natural or humanly modified fluctuations in rates of radiocarbon production (Browman 1981), and their use avoids problems in the nature of association since they are obtained directly on culturally significant events (Wolfman 1984).

For the period between ca. 1520 and 1685 the recognition of cultural-taxonomic units follows the diagnostic stylistic criteria (again, primarily decorated ceramics) outlined in current regional studies within the Caddoan area (e.g., Williams and Early 1990; Rohrbaugh 1984; Creel 1991b; Schambach and Early 1983; Story 1982; Thurmond 1985, 1990a). This period needs to be further subdivided to aid the study of Protohistoric and Historic period Caddoan cultural change, but current understandings of stylistic changes in ceramic decorative and arrowhead forms, for instance, as well as a dearth of absolute dates, does not presently allow further subdivision.

The same combination of stratigraphy and seriation is employed in identifying Caddoan archaeological components dating after ca. 1685. However, goods of European manufacture, which are well dated, such as glass beads (Brain 1979; Deagan 1987), bells (Brown 1979a), and gun parts (Hamilton 1980), are of considerable utility in verifying chronological identifications for this period (see further discussion in chapter 5).

SUMMARY

My concern here has been to establish the theoretical and methodological framework for examining the archaeological record in the Caddoan Area to document ways in which Caddoan peoples of the sixteenth through nineteenth centuries altered or maintained their ways as a consequence of European contact. The demographic issue is an important one to consider in the overall context of Protohistoric and Historic period changes, but one not likely to be firmly resolved until there are improvements in our understanding of the size of native American populations for all time periods, better descriptions of paleodemographic and bioarchaeological assemblages from both periods, and the development of ways by which Caddoan populations can be accurately measured from the archaeological evidence. While major demographic declines are considered critical factors in understanding the effects of the relationship between Caddoan populations and Europeans (Perttula and Ramenofsky 1982; Trubowitz 1984), social, cultural, political, and demographic factors must also be acknowledged as important in the culture contact process (see Gregory 1986, xii–xv). We will explore these various facets in more detail in Part 2 of this study; but remember that this is primarily an archaeological study of the effects of contact between the Caddoan peoples and Europeans, and the record sometimes falls short in some respects in providing consistent detail.

As understanding of the complexity of the contact era in the Caddoan Area and surrounding areas becomes increasingly more refined, a better appreciation of the consequences of European contact with Caddoan peoples (especially the effects of European-introduced diseases on aboriginal populations in the area) should result in a more comprehensive perspective on the nature of Caddoan life in Protohistoric and Historic times. This reconsideration challenges previous models of the nature of the Caddoan contact period and the assumptions of continuity on which they are based.

PART 2

Archaeological and Ethnohistorical Issues

4 / The Archaeological Record in the Caddoan Area, 1520–1685

Commanded by the voice of his people to know himself through knowing them, Jimmy had bared the buried history of the Caddoes, delving backwards in time from their end to their beginning. He had measured the antiquity of his lineage in countless shovelfuls of earth. The handiwork of his tribe had shown him the strangeness of his heritage, his own difference. . . . Digging down through layer upon layer, generation upon generation, he had come to know the importance to them of preserving the tribal continuity, the sacrilege it would be to them should ever the chain be broken, especially in its last link.

—*William Humphrey, "The Last of the Caddoes"*

Evidence of changes in Caddoan settlement density, location, and mortuary and sociopolitical complexity suggests that significant population declines and sociopolitical organizational simplification took place before 1650 in several regions and subareas within the Caddoan Area. These population declines may have led to episodic abandonment of major river valleys and/or the coalescence of different Caddoan groups in a few riverine settlements on the Red and Ouachita rivers. Local amalgamation of formerly separate Caddoan ethnic entities may also have occurred. After ca. 1685 Caddoan settlements were maintained on the major rivers only in close conjunction with European settlements and trading posts such as the French community of Natchitoches. Even though many minor river valleys were apparently also depopulated and abandoned, rural Caddoan communities do not appear to have experienced the same types of population declines as the town communities on the major rivers.

Caddoan occupations in the Protohistoric period predate direct and sustained European contact. Only the de Soto *entrada* in 1542 and the La Salle expedition in 1685 record actual face-to-face European contact with Caddoan groups in this period (see chapter 2). Therefore, understanding the character of the regional archaeological record, especially such dimensions as population and settlement density, geographic location, and sociopolitical organization, will be important in evaluating systemic changes in Caddoan lifeways. Are there systemic continuities in the Caddoan archaeological record that can be followed through the Protohistoric or Early Historic period? How are they manifested in the archaeological record, and what does their manifestation or persistence imply about the nature of the post-contact archaeological record?

As discussed in chapter 2, at the time of initial European contact, Caddoan groups lived in dispersed rural and town communities. By ca. 1400 the sociopolitical, ceremonial, and settlement patterns within these two Caddoan community systems had developed distinctive differences in size and sociopolitical complexity. However, economic pursuits were generally similar as Caddoan groups became more intensive agriculturists (Styles and Purdue 1984; Fritz 1989; Perttula 1990).

The rural Caddoan community systems, which were located in the Ozark and Ouachita highlands and the Texas and Oklahoma western Gulf Coastal Plain (see Fig. 10), were widely dispersed in functionally equivalent agricultural farmsteads and hamlets (Story 1981, 151; 1990). Each hamlet had an associated family cemetery. Demographic profiles from these small cemeteries appear to be representative of a family group (Rose 1984, 240). Larger community or supralocal cemeteries of up to 150 individuals (Thurmond 1981; Turner 1978), which are spatially isolated from the community's habitation sites, have interment forms and grave good associations that evidence internal mortuary ranking or status patterns. These patterns are the products of regionally recurrent use of the cemeteries over several hundred years by several related local communities. Only adult males and females were buried in these locations (Thurmond 1990a, 235).

Caddoan town communities were distributed along the major stream valleys in the Caddoan Area such as the Red, Ouachita, and Little rivers. These communities were hierarchically arranged. The first level in the settlement hierarchy consisted of the civic-ceremonial center, with platform and burial mounds. The civic-ceremonial centers are intimately associated with the towns, which consist of linear but dispersed farmstead compounds making up widely separate population clusters near the political and religious compounds within the town (Schambach 1983, 7–8). Outside the area of the town were the small isolated hamlets or farmsteads as well as the specialized processing and/or procurement locales. These small isolated settlements are thought to have been associated with the town through the exchange of economic goods and the participation in the sociopolitical and ceremonial activities of the respective communities (Thurmond 1990a; Brown 1984b; Perttula 1989c). Civic-ceremonial centers provided both intraregional and interregional social and political services for the communities, and they also facilitated the redistribution of goods, labor, and food resources when necessary.

Mortuary goods and other exotic artifacts suggest that intraregional contacts and the exchange of resources between both types of Caddoan communities flourished at the time of initial European contact (Brown 1983).

Interregional exchange and contact was also well developed between Caddoan polities and horticulturists living in the southwestern United States, the southern plains, and the Lower Mississippi River Valley (Baugh and Swenson 1980; Baugh 1986; Krieger 1946; Spielmann 1983, 1989; Kidder 1990a; Vehik 1988, 1990). The basis of this interregional exchange system rested in the interaction between the intermediary hunter-gatherers and farmers (Peterson 1978), and the key was exchange of salt and horticultural and game animal products between them.

THE WESTERN CADDOAN SUBAREA

The western Caddoan subarea includes archaeological phenomena in the Ouachita Mountains, in Northeastern Texas, and in southeastern Oklahoma outside the Red River Valley. Defined archaeological foci or phases present at ca. 1520 were the McCurtain, Titus, Frankston, and late Angelina[1] cultural units in the western Gulf Coastal Plain (Story 1990), a highland expression of the late Mid-Ouachita phase in the eastern Ouachita Mountains called the Buckville phase (Early 1983, 1988), and the McCurtain phase in the western Ouachita Mountains (Wyckoff 1967) (see Fig. 6).

Ouachita Mountains

In the western Ouachita Mountains of Oklahoma, McCurtain phase and Mountain Fork complex (Wyckoff 1967) Caddoan occupations were present between ca. 1300 and 1700. However, there was only limited use of these parts of the Ouachita Mountains after 1500 (Perttula and McGuff 1985; Wyckoff 1974). In the mountains west of Little River (Fig. 14), the evidence is basically restricted to surface/shallow subsurface scatters of Late Caddoan period–style triangular arrowheads along some minor mountain stream valleys and to components, such as the George site (34AT105) in the McGee Creek drainage, that contain a few hearths and processing features (Perttula 1987, 447–450). There are few archaeological deposits that can be interpreted as permanent residential settlements of Caddoan peoples, such as a farmstead or a hamlet.

In the lower Mountain Fork and Glover rivers of Southeast Oklahoma, however, Late Caddoan period settlements appear numerous. They are broadly contemporaneous with other Caddoan societies on Little River (outside of the mountains) in Southwest Arkansas subsumed by the Mineral Springs and Saratoga phases (Hoffman 1983). In both of these river valleys, habitation sites and mound centers were important components of the community settlement system at the time of initial contact with Europeans (Wyckoff and Fisher 1985).

The Beaver, Bill Hughes, Woods Mound, McDonald, and A. W. Davis

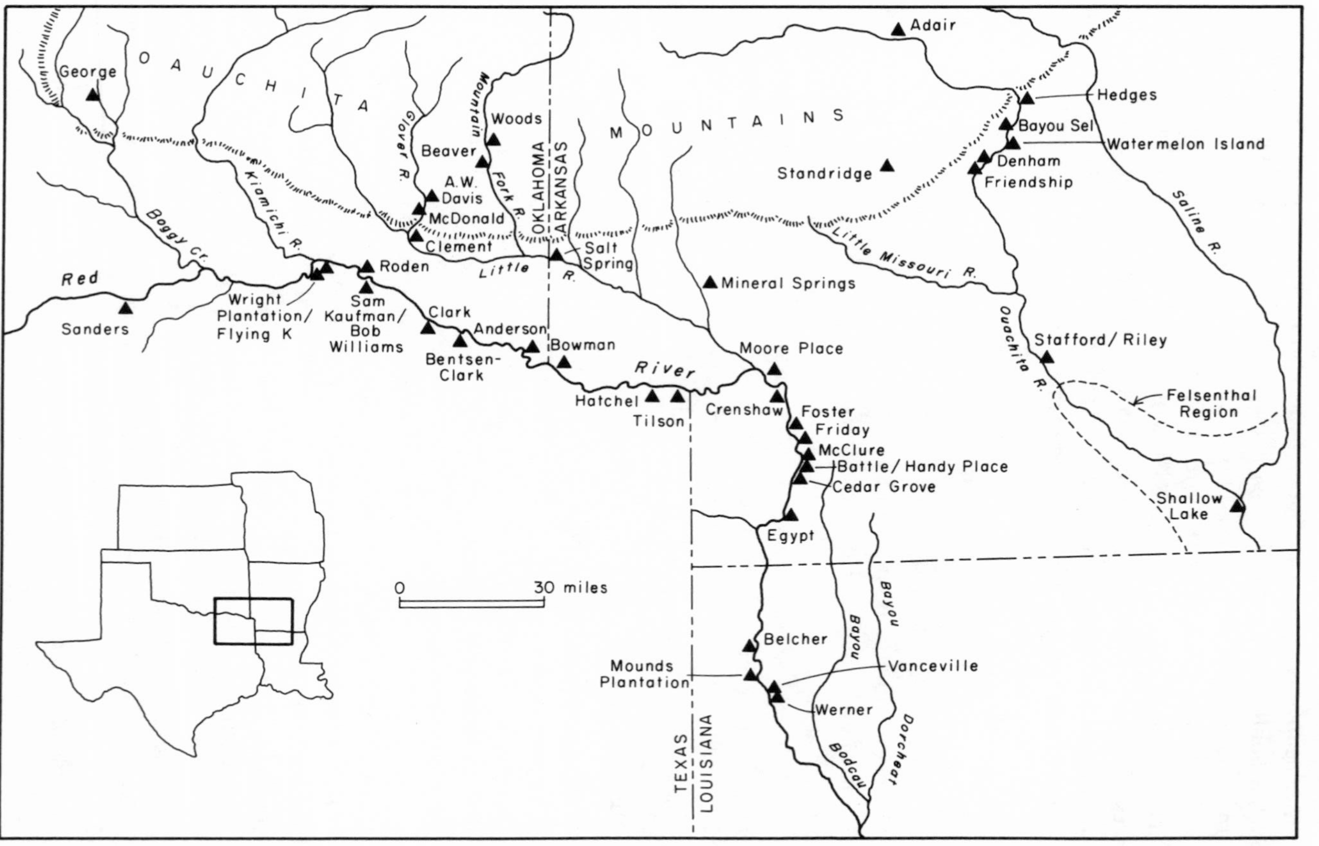

FIG. 14. The Red River, Ouachita River, and Little River drainages and the location of archaeological sites relevant

sites in McCurtain County, Oklahoma, attest to a post–1500 or Protohistoric period occupation in the southern Ouachita Mountains. The dating of the occupations at these McCurtain phase sites is, however, tentative at best given the limited number of absolute dates (Story 1990; Bruseth and Perttula 1991). Calibrated radiometric dates of 1495–1675 or 1618–1684 (M-1090), 1435–1685 or 1726–1810 (SM-887) and 1525–1665 or 1630–1954 (SM-888) obtained from these sites indicate both Protohistoric and Historic period Caddoan occupations, though the last two ranges are incongruent with other earlier radiocarbon dates from the same contexts (Wyckoff 1970). The calibrated dates for these sites range from 146 to 412 years B.P. (1538–1804), which are not generally comparable either with better dated archaeological phases to the north on the Arkansas River (Fort Coffee phase) or with Middle Red River McCurtain phase sites to the south.

The 1495–1675 or 1618–1684 ranges from the A. W. Davis site (Wilson 1962) were obtained from an in situ pine post from a round house of Caddoan construction in area A of the site. Its context appears reasonable given the cultural assemblage recovered from this part of the site. In association with the house was a cluster of five definite burials containing ceramics dating ca. 1500–1700, or the late McCurtain phase (including the following ceramic types: curvilinear Avery Engraved, Simms Engraved, Form B, Hudson Engraved, and Keno Trailed). The fact that the sherd assemblage from the site was primarily shell-tempered also suggests that the occupation postdates 1650 (Schambach and Miller 1984, 167). Natchitoches Engraved, a post-1685 horizon marker in the Caddoan Area (Schambach and Miller 1984, 124), was found on the surface and the plow zone in area A as well, but unfortunately no specific habitational or feature-related evidence can be related with it. A single construction phase pyramidal mound and adjacent midden area were found in area B of the A. W. Davis site (Wilson 1962, Plate 37). Excavations there were too limited to permit assigning the mound construction at the site to any particular temporal period within the McCurtain phase.

There is a regional gradient within the Ouachita Mountains in the scale and complexity of Late Caddoan period settlement. In the south-flowing streams in the Arkansas section of the Ouachita Mountains, Mid-Ouachita phase (ca. 1350–1500) Caddoan settlements consisted of hamlets and farmsteads, regional and/or local community centers with mounds, and limited activity sites of various kinds, including salt-making sites (Early 1982b, 1990). Early (1990, 13-4) has argued that the Mid-Ouachita phase represents the Caddoan cultural florescence in the Middle Ouachita River region. There were population increases and numerous mound centers were constructed during this phase; most of the mound centers were in the Coastal

Plain rather than in the Ouachita Mountains. The relative Caddoan population density in the Ouachita Mountains is thought to have been lower than in the coastal plain, and agriculture, the primary subsistence resource, was of lesser importance in the mountains.

Chronological estimates by Early (1990) suggest that mound construction and shaft/pit burials in this region do not postdate the mid–sixteenth century. The late component at the Hedges mound site (3HS60), situated on the Ouachita Mountains escarpment, is dated to 1450–1535+ by an archaeomagnetic date (Wolfman 1982, Table 11-1). Sequent mound/structure use at the Standridge site on the Caddo River, dated by archaeomagnetic samples, fall between 1375 ± 40 years and 1420 ± 30 years (Early 1978; Wolfman 1982). The last mound use after 1420 is contemporary with the interment of a multiple burial containing Maud-style triangular points; turquoise beads; and a ceramic assemblage of Woodward Plain, Bailey Engraved, Foster Trailed-Incised, black polished Avery Engraved bottle form, Nash Neck-Banded, and Simms Engraved Form A bowls (Early 1978, 25–26). These ceramic vessels in the closed burial context indicate that the grave dates to the latter part of the Mid-Ouachita phase, ca. 1450–1550 (see below). A black Avery Engraved bowl and a Simms Engraved Form A bowl are both diagnostic of McCurtain phase occupations of ca. 1500 on the middle Red River (Skinner et al. 1969, Table 8). Interestingly, a shaft/pit burial at the Clement site on the lower Glover River in southeastern Oklahoma also dates to the late fifteenth century (Wyckoff 1970, 111). The multiple burial was intrusive into the platform mound there.

Other than the Natchitoches Engraved sherds from the A. W. Davis site there is no substantive evidence of permanent eighteenth-century occupations by Caddoan groups of the Ouachita Mountains (Early 1988). Documentary evidence from the de Soto *entrada* reviewed in chapter 2 did support the notion that there was a sixteenth-century permanent Caddoan settlement in the Ouachita Mountains, but the relationship between ethnographically recorded seventeenth- and eighteenth-century Caddoan groups and Ouachita Mountain settlements recorded archaeologically is at best a vague one. European trade goods have not been found in association with Caddoan archaeological materials in the Ouachita Mountains, with the exception of a brass button, a piece of cut brass or tin, and a corroded copper fragment from undated contexts at the Adair site (Early 1988, 138).

Northeast Texas

In Northeast Texas the most reliable archaeological data from Protohistoric period Caddoan occupations derives from the Cypress Creek/upper Sabine and Neches river drainages (Fig. 15). The archaeological record for this

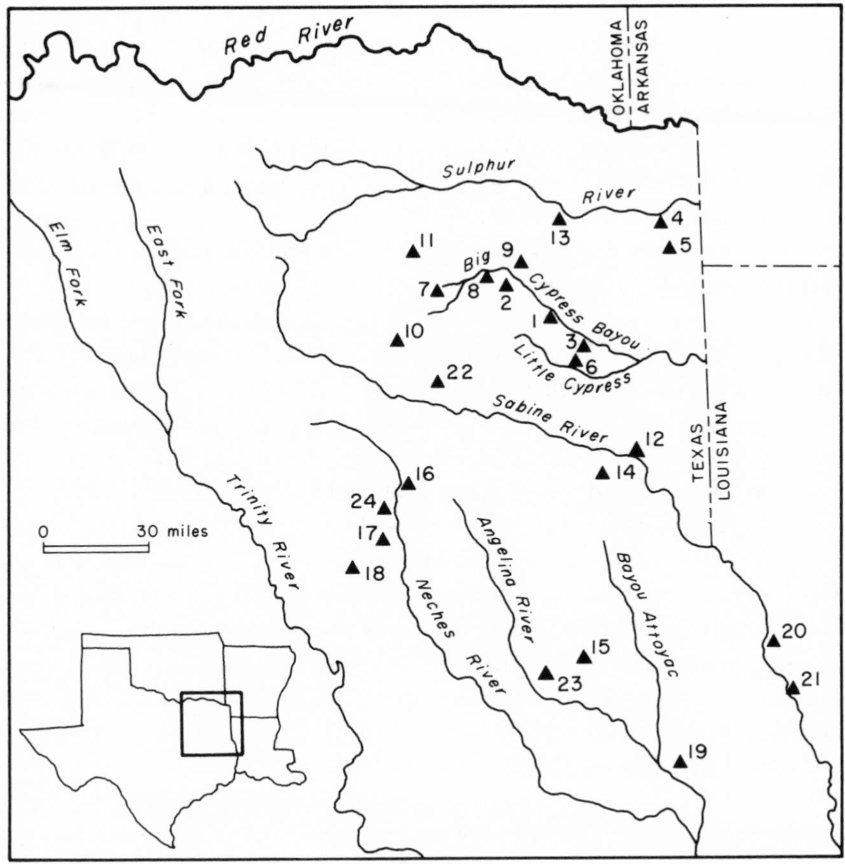

FIG. 15. The Neches, Angelina, Sabine, Big Cypress, and Sulphur river drainages and the location of archaeological sites relevant to ca. 1520–1685: (1) Harroun/Dalton; (2) Tuck Carpenter; (3) Roberts/Whelan; (4) Knights Bluff; (5) Clements and Goode Hunt; (6) H. R. Taylor; (7) Galt; (8) Lower Peach Orchard; (9) Alex Justiss; (10) Goldsmith/Reese/Steck; (11) Culpepper; (12) Resch; (13) 41MX5; (14) Musgano; (15) Washington Square Mound; (16) Ferguson; (17) A. C. Saunders; (18) Pace McDonald; (19) Wylie Price; (20) Bison "B"; (21) Salt Lick; (22) McKenzie; (23) Chayah; (24) Attaway.

period is known primarily from the 1930s' excavation of aboriginal cemeteries (Pearce 1932a) and less frequent present-day investigations (see Guy 1988, 1990; Story 1990, n.d.). Additionally, studies of the previously unanalyzed Caddoan collections from the Texas Archeological Research Laboratory by Thurmond (1981, 1990a) and Kleinschmidt (1982) provide a level of Caddoan assemblage descriptive completeness that is not paralleled by most other regions of Northeast Texas.

In the Cypress Creek/upper Sabine basins, the Whelan and Titus phases extend into the Protohistoric period. The Whelan phase begins around ca. 1350, based on calibrated carbon-14 dates of 1308–1392 or 1387–1425 (TX-240), 1327–1357 or 1389–1465 (TX-84), and 1327–1357 or 1391–1485 (TX-83) from the Harroun (41UR10) and Dalton (41UR11) sites, while the Titus phase begins ca. 1500 (Thurmond 1981, 1990a). Local chronological sequences for the region remain only partially developed because of the absence of absolute dates for the Protohistoric and Historic period sequences (Thurmond 1990a, Table 60; Story 1990, Table 81).

Turner (1978, Fig. 33) proposes a temporal arrangement of the Titus and Whelan phases (foci) that combines aspects of both occurrence and frequency seriations (Dunnell 1970; Renfrew and Bahn 1991). The temporal orderings are based on (*a*) the relative popularity of arrow projectile point types and (*b*) continuity in the presence or absence of defined ceramic types, decorative motifs, and vessel forms from associated Caddoan grave lots (Fig. 16). The temporal ordering proposed by Turner (1978) is facilitated by the presence of five sites with European goods in burial associations and a series of carbon-14 dates from the preceding Whelan phase (Thurmond 1990a, Table 60). Turner was able to identify general trends in the Caddoan ceramic assemblages that appear to be the result of temporal stylistic changes (see discussion in the appendix). Utility wares such as Bullard Brushed, Nash Neck-Banded, and Maydelle Incised (Suhm and Jelks 1962) are present throughout the entire sequence and thus do not exhibit temporally significant ceramic variation at meaningful 100- to 200-year intervals. Therefore, the Whelan and Titus phase ceramic types that exhibited distinct temporal changes of a directional and discrete nature are those depicted in Fig. 16.

Not all the ceramic decorative forms found in the Cypress, Sulphur, and Sabine river basins are locally produced wares. Wares imported from the Red River Caddoan groups as trade items are also present and include the types Belcher Ridged, Belcher Engraved, Glassell Engraved, and Hodges Engraved from the Belcher phase (Webb 1959, 153) and Avery Engraved and Simms Engraved pottery types of the McCurtain and Texarkana phases (Krieger 1946, Fig. 18). Their inclusion in the Whelan and Titus phase ceramic assemblages serves as a further check on the proposed temporal ordering by Turner (1978), since this can then be extended to independently established seriations on the Red River (Webb 1959; Skinner, Harris, and Anderson 1969; Schambach and Miller 1984; Creel 1991b). Ripley and Taylor Engraved are the dominant local decorated ceramic fine wares and as such are of major importance in distinguishing temporal differences between ca. 1400 to 1700 for Caddoan settlements and cemeteries in the region.

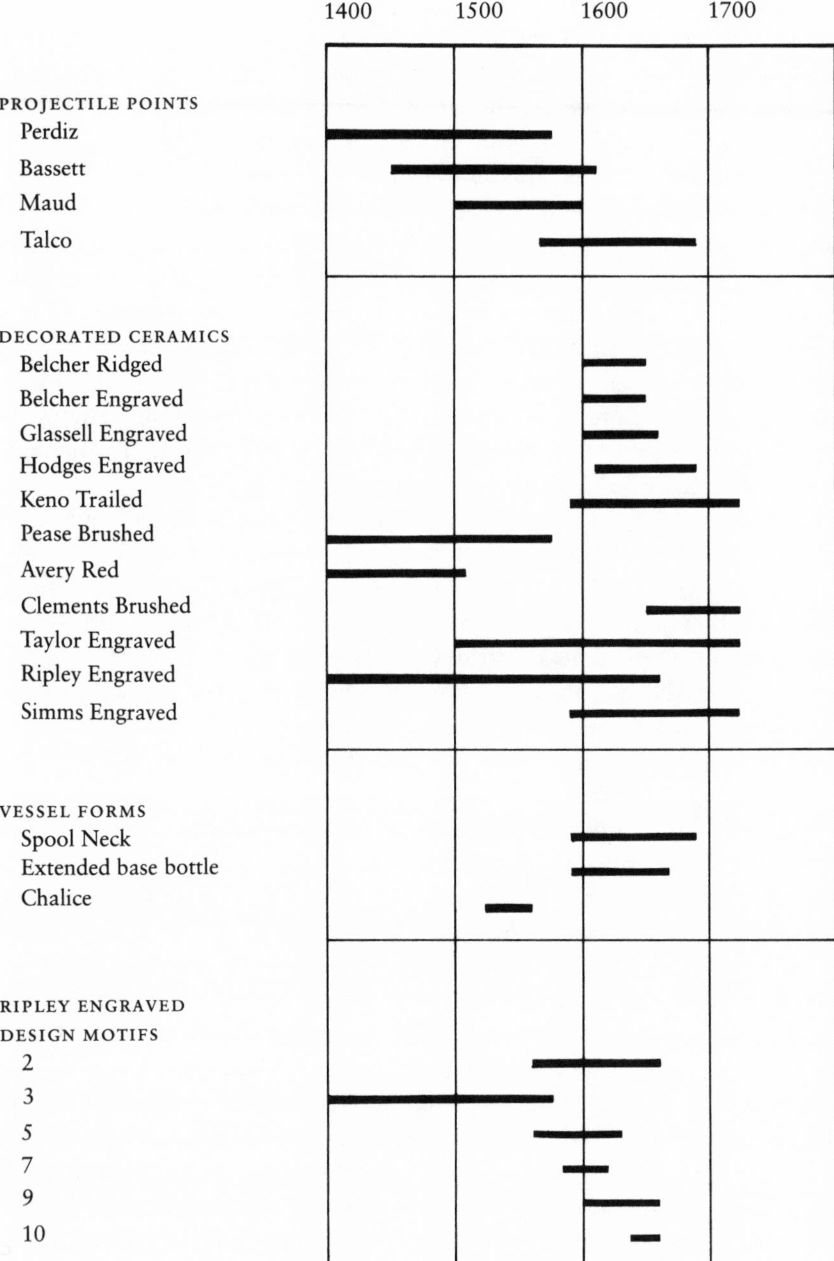

FIG. 16. Proposed temporal changes in projectile points and decorated ceramic types in the Cypress, Sulphur, and Sabine river basins, 1400–1700+. Bar lines represent periods of peak popularity (from Turner 1978, Fig. 33).

Ripley Engraved, in particular, exhibits considerable motif variation that is suggested by Turner (1978) to be temporal. Some vessel form differences in Ripley and Taylor Engraved types also apparently change through time, particularly the spool neck and extended base bottle, while others (such as the chalice form) have only a limited temporal distribution (see Fig. 16).

Unfortunately, a systematic series of Late Caddoan period and Protohistoric period radiocarbon dates are not available from the majority of components examined by Turner (1978) and thus the proposed temporal orderings have not been evaluated and tested through the use of absolute dating methods. Thurmond (1985, 191) has suggested, conversely, that the chronological subdivisions proposed by Turner for the Titus phase are really contemporaneous spatial groups of Caddoan components. These spatial groups are thought to denote tribes or subtribes integrated sociopolitically in an analogous manner to the confederacies known historically among the Hasinai or the Red River Kadohadacho groups.

The four contemporaneous spatial subclusters proposed by Thurmond (1981, 1985, 1990a)—the Three Basins, Tankersley Creek, Swauano Creek, and Big Cypress Creek (Fig. 17)—are defined on the basis of different Ripley Engraved bowl motifs or motif combinations, other shared pottery types, and different proportions of various arrow point styles (Thurmond 1985, 193–194). Each Titus phase subcluster is characterized by a distinctive constellation of ceramic and lithic stylistic forms.

Thurmond (1985, 196) states that the larger Cypress Cluster is "the archaeological manifestation of a series of social groups banded together in a sociopolitical structure analogous to and at least partially contemporaneous with that of the Hasinai to the south and the Kadohadacho to the northeast. Four subclusters . . . are believed to represent the individual component groups comprising this affiliated group."

The concept of the Cypress Cluster is an initial, pioneering attempt in Northeast Texas archaeology to relate archaeological units to regionally meaningful sociocultural variables. However, attempting to model archaeological contemporaneity for the Titus phase as a whole must mean the acquisition of a more comprehensive chronological data base than exists if these types of sociopolitical interpretations are to be seriously considered.

It is not possible to conclusively demonstrate that the differences in ceramic and arrow point styles between Titus phase subclusters are a result of temporal change or, instead, primarily reflect social and ethnic distinctions (Hodder 1982; Johnson 1987; Lemonnier 1986) within the Cypress Cluster. The suspected dating of the Cypress Cluster to between 1500 and 1700 (Thurmond 1985, 192; 1990a) has not been evaluated by absolute dating methods. Calibrated Titus phase radiocarbon dates of 1333–1339 or 1399–1453 (TX-3473) from the Steck site (Bruseth and Perttula 1981), 1440–

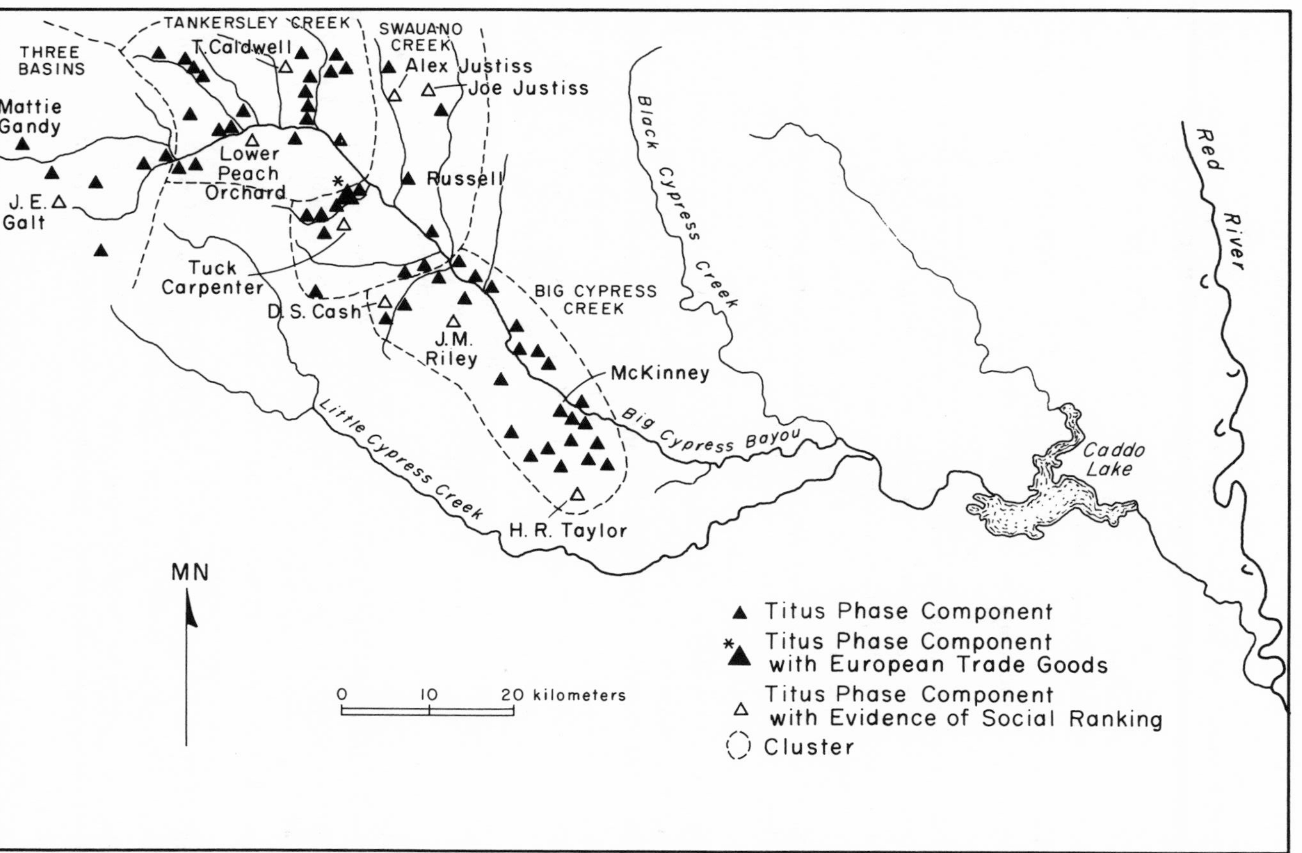

FIG. 17. Titus phase components—location, evidence of European trade goods, evidence of social ranking, and spatial clusters (after Thurmond 1981, Fig. 15).

1640 (TX-666) from the Tuck Carpenter 2 component (Turner 1978), and the 1476–1648, 1520–1580, and 1623–1681 (TX-199) ranges from the Sam Roberts site seem to indicate that these occupations occurred earlier than the current proposed chronological frameworks for the Cypress Cluster. Calibrated ages for these Titus phase components fall between 297 years B.P. and 521 years B.P., or from ca. 1429 to 1653.

From my perspective, the viewpoints outlined by Turner (1978) and Thurmond (1981, 1985, 1990a) are profitably subsumed by the notion that both spatial and temporal factors contribute to the archaeological character of the Titus phase and its subclusters. That is, the subclusters probably maintained a regional or local spatial integrity (i.e., spatial changes among them appear to be negligible), while at the same time there were diachronic changes in their formal composition that now permit establishing a detailed temporal sequence. As an example, preliminary investigations of changes in ceramic decorative treatments at several Three Basins subcluster Titus phase sites in the Dry Creek and Caney Creek localities of the upper Sabine River basin (Perttula et al. 1992, Table 10), using decorated sherds from trash middens at the Burks, Steck, Goldsmith, and Pine Tree sites (see Fig. 15), indicated that (*a*) trends in the relative frequency of ceramic decorative motifs for the fine wares in the two localities are best interpreted as temporally based, while (*b*) differences in the frequency of such techniques as brushing and neckbanding in the two localities are possible evidence for intrasubcluster differences across space. Thus, such discrete changes within a number of the Three Basins subcluster components, as these components are so interpreted by Thurmond (1985, Fig. 6), in decorative treatments of fine and utility wares cannot be accounted for strictly within the context of contemporaneity.

Further evidence to support such an intermediate position came from the analysis of the cooccurrence of decorated pottery types, design motifs, and certain types of vessel forms with Titus phase burials containing discrete sets of arrow point types. This analysis used discrete arrow point associations from different subcluster burials in the Cypress Creek basin (Thurmond 1981, 254–385; 1990a, 135–213) to ascertain if particular kinds of Late Caddoan period Titus phase pottery styles change with them in a regular, continuous sequence that could then be interpreted as an independent chronological ordering. The appendix describes this analysis in further detail.

From this analysis of burial lots, arrow point caches, and ceramic vessel associations, three temporal periods are proposed for the Cypress Cluster, along with a number of subphases (in the sense of Johnson [1987, 19]). The first period (period 1), including subphases a and b, dates from ca. 1350 to

1450. It appears to be equivalent to the Whelan phase (Thurmond 1985, 1990a).

Periods 2 and 3 belong to the Titus phase. Period 2, with subphases a and b, dates from ca. 1450 to 1600 and includes such major pottery types as Ripley Engraved (with the scroll and continuous scroll motifs [see the appendix]), Maydelle Incised, Bullard Brushed, and Harleton Applique. Period 3, the "classic" Titus phase, includes subphases a–c. This period began after ca. 1600 and certainly ended by the early eighteenth century (Thurmond 1990a, 1990b). Ripley Engraved, with the scroll and circle, scroll, and pendant triangle motifs (see Fig. A-1 in the appendix), is the most common fine ware in the grave lots. There are also a number of Red River Valley trade wares present in the period 3 burials, particularly in the latest subphase, subphase c.

This revision of Turner's (1978) proposed chronology permits the development of a more refined measure of change that is useful in understanding the temporal framework of the Late Caddoan and Protohistoric period Titus phase. Additionally, the inference of different spatially coherent social groups within the Titus phase and Cypress Cluster can then be employed further as a means of investigating changes in mound utilization, mortuary ritual, and social stratification on an intraregional basis.

Identifying cultural and material artifact changes within the occupation (ca. 1520–1685) of the area at temporal intervals of less than one hundred years is again primarily based on the character of the archaeological components under consideration. Information available for the Titus phase, as well as from the Frankston and Allen phases in the Neches basin, show that ideally "the relative duration of the hamlets (settlements) can be measured by the number of graves in the cemeteries and relative temporal placement of each hamlet can be determined by seriating mortuary assemblages" (Shafer 1981, 156). Therefore, the primary units of analysis for the Protohistoric period in Northeast Texas—the hamlet cemeteries—condition to a certain extent the precision and reliability of diachronic analyses within the period. The likelihood or possibility of frequent shifting of settlements on a generational basis would result in a large number of sites within the four subclusters of the Cypress Cluster, for instance, that are actually sequent to, rather than contemporaneous with, other known sites. Contemporaneity between subclusters becomes much more difficult to demonstrate with a series of archaeological components in this situation than intraphase diachronic changes, particularly if the assemblages being compared derive mainly from habitation contexts rather than mortuary contexts. Detailed temporal analyses and seriations depend on identifying distinctive ceramic motifs and vessel forms, and these are difficult to obtain and identify from the small and fragmentary ceramic sherds recovered in Late Caddoan or Protohistoric period trash middens or house floors. As a result, cemetery assemblages from these periods are absolutely essential to successful creation of temporal units refining perception of the rate and tempo of Caddoan cultural change.

Because these factors of archaeological context and analysis must be taken into account, it is important to discuss in detail the character and patterning of Late Caddoan and Protohistoric period cemeteries in Northeast Texas. Most cemeteries in the Cypress Creek and Sabine River basins contain less than twenty individuals (Thurmond 1981, 340). The small size of the cemeteries; their demographic profiles of roughly equal adult male and female representation, few adolescents, and no children (children were typically buried in subfloor pits within the household structures themselves); and limited evidence for internal rank differentiation—all are indicative of the type of mortuary population expected within egalitarian family units occupying the households for only short periods of time (Rose 1984, 240; Story 1990, 339).

Burials within the household cemeteries occur as single extended inhumations within a patterned arrangement of burials. The orientation and arrangement by spacing considerations can be duplicated within cemeteries from each of the Titus phase spatial clusters in that the burials are oriented roughly east-west and are extended, supine interments. According to Thurmond (1981, 455–456), artifact associations differ by age and sex, because "adolescents were buried with more offerings than children or infants, and with fewer offerings than adults. The graves of males often contain clusters of arrowpoints in patterns suggesting quivers of arrows, and those of females contain polishing stones or more numerous pottery vessels. Items of exotic material . . . are extremely rare. The occurrence of graves containing very large numbers of artifacts is also quite limited."

In contrast to the family household cemeteries, there also are the large community cemeteries, containing at least thirty-five to seventy individuals, that are not directly associated with settlements (see chapter 3). They reflect a wider community-based participation in ceremonial and mortuary activities (Story 1990, 339). The H. R. Taylor (41HS3), Tuck Carpenter (41CP5), and Lower Peach Orchard (41CP17) sites (Turner 1978; Thurmond 1981, 275–279, 301–312) are examples of these intraregional community mortuary centers. None of the Titus phase community cemeteries are associated with mound construction activities.

The larger community cemeteries themselves are internally organized by space and structurally divided by rank (Turner 1978, Fig. 3; Thurmond 1981, Fig. 20). There is little evidence for graves overlapping, but instead the cemeteries continually expanded over time. Thus, while the cemetery

TABLE 7. Relative Quantities of Grave Goods in Selected Titus Phase Cemeteries

Site	Ceramic Vessels (Mean)	Projectile Points (Mean)	Total Specimens (Mean)	Burials	Source
Tuck Carpenter	9.2	4.34	14.8	45	Turner 1978
Taylor	8.3	5.09	14.5	71	Thurmond 1981
Alex Justiss	7.3	6.88	15.4	25	Bell 1981
Goldsmith	8.3	3.33	13.7	3	Perttula et al. 1992

plan was consistently maintained, the cemeteries reflect community participation over many generations. The varying position of the higher status burials at the Tuck Carpenter and H. R. Taylor sites reflect this spatial expansion through time.

The rank or vertical differentiation apparent in the Cypress Cluster burials is based on certain criteria of the interments that differ from the kinds of treatment the remainder of the burials received:

1. High-status burials include multiple interments; all others are single, individual burials.
2. Quantities of grave goods are significantly higher than the mean average for the regional burial population as a whole (Table 7). First-rank or higher status burials differ from the population primarily in the frequency of arrow points and ceramic vessels placed as grave offerings (Table 8).
3. Certain kinds of artifacts are found only in first-rank or higher status burials. In the case of the Cypress and upper Sabine basins, this typically includes associations with Galt bifaces[2] (Thurmond 1981, 456).
4. They are always adult males.

At the Tuck Carpenter site, period 1 and 2 high-status burials (burials 21 and 23) are in the center of the cemetery, while the later (period 3, subphase c) high-status burials are along the outside cemetery boundaries (Fig. 18). Multiple interments such as burials 21 and 23 at the Tuck Carpenter site are apparently a rare part of the Titus phase mortuary program, having only been identified at two other Titus phase sites in Northeast Texas—W. A. Ford (Turner 1978, 33) and H. R. Taylor (Thurmond 1981, 311). Other

TABLE 8. Titus Phase Sites with Burials of Presumed High Rank

Site	Burial No.	Burial Treatment	No. of Speci-mens	No. of Arrow Points	No. of Ceramic Vessels	Period-Subphase							Source
						1a	1b	2a	2b	3a	3b	3c	
Galt	3	Extended supine	28	N/A	14	X							Thurmond 1981, Table 29
Caldwell	1	Extended supine	37	25	8				?	?			Thurmond 1981, Table 40
	4	Extended supine	35	25	9						X		
Lower Peach Orchard	N/A	Shaft tomb	N/A	N/A	N/A				X				Thurmond 1981, 277
Tuck Carpenter	1	Extended supine—M	35	21	13							X	Turner 1978, 12–49
	19	Extended supine—M	47	30	12							X	Thurmond 1981, Table 23
	21	Double extended—M/F	30	11	17		X						
	23	Double extended—M	36	22	11				X				
H. R. Taylor	2	Extended—M	41	29	8							X	
	11	Extended—M	28	20	8						X		Thurmond 1981, Table 35
	12	Extended—M	29	20	8						X		
	45	Double extended	72	23	26							X	
	59	Extended—M	39	28	11						X		
Joe Justiss	4	Extended	46	29	12						X		Thurmond 1981, Table 37
D. S. Cash	3	Extended	37	31	6							X	Thurmond 1981, Table 22
J. M. Riley	4	Extended	38	22	14							X	
	11	Extended	47	22	15							X	Thurmond 1981, Table 48
	15	Extended	31	24	7							X	

Abbreviations: N/A, not applicable; M, male; F, female.

single, extended interments were placed in the cemetery throughout the different periods in roughly aligned north-south rows. Most individuals who could not be assigned to particular occupational periods or subphases (see Fig. 18) were females or juveniles (Turner 1978, Fig. 16).

At the H. R. Taylor farm, seventy-one graves were excavated; at the Tuck Carpenter cemetery, seventy, including those excavated by collectors. For those, no further information is available about provenience or grave goods associations. The same type of burial program noted at the Tuck Carpenter site was in use at the H. R. Taylor site (Fig. 19). Mean values of ceramic vessels (8.3/individual), arrow projectile points (5.09/individual), and total number of specimens (14.5/individual) as grave goods at the H. R. Taylor farm are not significantly different from those for the Tuck Carpenter site (Thurmond 1981, Table 35). The segregation of interments by rank indicates that high-ranking individuals account for 8 percent to 9 percent of all the burials at the H. R. Taylor and Tuck Carpenter sites, respectively. Low-rank interments, namely those with quantities of grave goods two standard deviations below the mean average for the two sites (between 0 to 9.0 items at Tuck Carpenter and 0 to 6.7 items at H. R. Taylor), account for 19 percent and 23 percent of the burials at H. R. Taylor and Tuck Carpenter, respectively. Low-ranking individuals were usually adult females, juveniles, or children. Overall, in the Titus phase mortuary population, high-rank individuals account for less than 2 percent of all known burials (Thurmond 1990a, 235).

Based on criteria mentioned above for differences within the total Titus phase burial population (see Table 8), high rank can be assigned to five individuals at the H. R. Taylor farm—burials 2, 11, 12, 45, and 59 (Thurmond 1981, Fig. 20). All were adult males. The temporal ordering of these five burials based on the ceramic and arrow point lot analyses described in the appendix suggests that burials of higher status were made only in period 3, subphases b and c, after ca. 1630. The earliest burials were present in the center of the cemetery and along the outside cemetery boundaries (burials 11, 12, and 59). The later ranking burials, including one possible multiple burial (burials 2 and 45), are also along the outside cemetery boundaries (see Table 8 and Fig. 19).

Temporal differences in the total number of grave goods indicate that the later subphase burials at the H. R. Taylor farm had twice as many grave goods (X = 56.5, SD = 15.5) as did the earlier burials (X = 27.8, SD = 6.4). Most of the H. R. Taylor site burials apparently date to the last episode of cemetery use, period 3, subphase c. According to Thurmond (1981, Fig. 20), twenty-six females, twenty-five males, eight adolescents, and three children were buried at the H. R. Taylor site. As with the Tuck Carpenter site, it was primarily Caddoan children, adolescents, and females who were

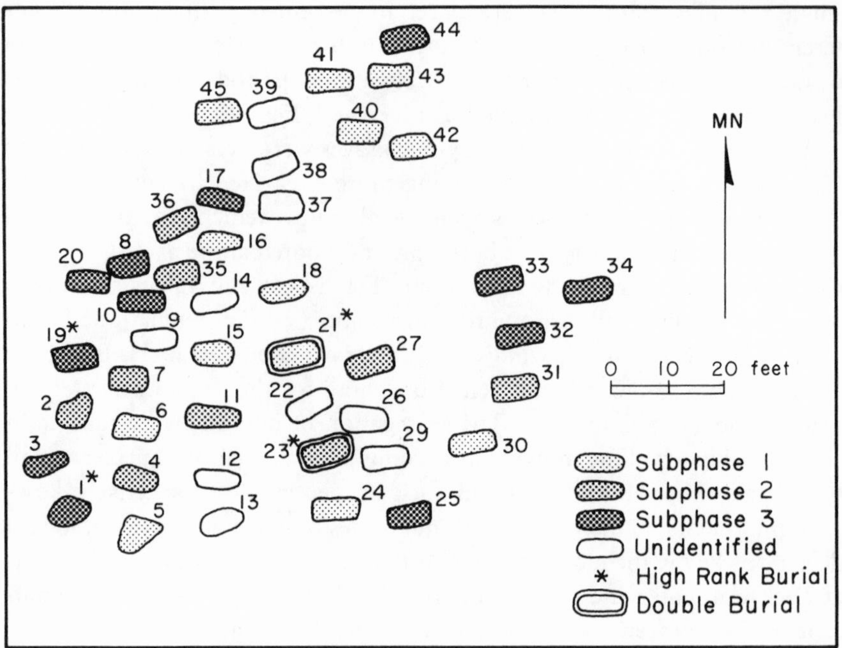

FIG. 18. Tuck Carpenter site (41CP5) cemetery plan.

not assignable to particular occupational periods or subphases within the Titus phase. This presumably relates to (*a*) the limited number of artifacts of any type in the burials and (*b*) the absence of arrow points—a prime marker for subphase assignments (see the appendix)—in many of the adult female burials. All of the child burials (three/three), half of the adolescents (four/eight), and about one-third of the adult females (eight/twenty-six) were not assigned to a subphase, compared to only one of the twenty-five adult males, at the H. R. Taylor site.

The majority of burials of presumed high social rank in the Cypress Creek basin date after ca. 1600, because they are most common in period 3, subphases b and c (see Table 8). Those individuals buried prior to that date demonstrate considerable intraregional variability in the manner of burial treatment as well as in the types of artifactual remains placed in the burials as offerings. In addition to multiple interments, shaft tombs are represented in a period 2 cemetery at the Lower Peach Orchard site. Included with the individual at the J. E. Galt site were such offerings as a large number of celt fragments and other native stone implements, rather than caches of arrow points (Thurmond 1981, Table 29). Galt bifaces were also recovered from the small cemetery.

Possibly more significant as an example of mortuary variability in the Protohistoric period, however, are the unique and deep (three- to six-meter) shaft burials known from the Lower Peach Orchard site on Big Cypress Creek (Herrington 1979, 4).[3] The five or six shaft burials were part of a large cemetery excavated by collectors in 1977, and information about the contents of the graves is quite incomplete (Thurmond 1981, 277). Associated caches of Maud and Bassett points from one shaft burial containing three individuals are consistent with the interpretation that it was an interment dating to period 2, subphase b, estimated to date from ca. 1550 to 1600 (see Table 8). This is the only shaft tomb from the site from which detailed artifactual information is available, unfortunately.

The large Titus phase cemeteries with individuals of high rank—considered herein the community, or supralocal, cemeteries—are distributed within each of the four spatial subclusters identified by Thurmond (1981, 1985) in the Cypress Creek basin. The earliest expressions of this type of community integration and organization occur in the Three Basins, Tankersley Creek, and Swauano Creek subclusters, with the latest being present in the Swauano Creek and Big Cypress Creek subclusters (see Fig. 17). Presumably after ca. 1650–1670 the Three Basins and Tankersley Creek subcluster areas were abandoned by resident Caddoan groups (Thurmond 1985, 198). It is not surprising, therefore, that it is in the Three Basins subcluster area that Norteno phase Wichita sites dating after ca. 1700–1760 are also found (see chapter 5).

In summary, these community cemeteries are primarily 1550–1650/1700 or Protohistoric phenomena of the Titus phase and Cypress Cluster. They do not extend into the later 1685–1800 Historic Caddoan period. The Caddoan cemeteries dating after 1685 do not have the type of coherence and structure noted in the Protohistoric period community cemetery centers. Rather, they are uniformly small, and each burial contains limited grave goods usually common only to household cemeteries, with the addition of European trade goods (see chapter 6). Community cemetery centers are thus short-term (ca. 150 years maximum), transitory phenomena characteristic of the Cypress/upper Sabine River areas during the Protohistoric period. The timing in the development of this form of community integration in the Cypress/upper Sabine basin is of considerable significance for this study because the Titus phase community cemeteries appear to have replaced mounds by the middle to late sixteenth century.

Sometime during period 2, mound construction ceased in the Cypress and Sabine basins. Calibrated radiocarbon dates from the Whelan phase components indicate that this occurred between roughly 1400 and 1550.

At the Sam Roberts site calibrated ages of 425 years B.P. and 387 years B.P. (about 1525 and 1563) derive from the single mound present (Thur-

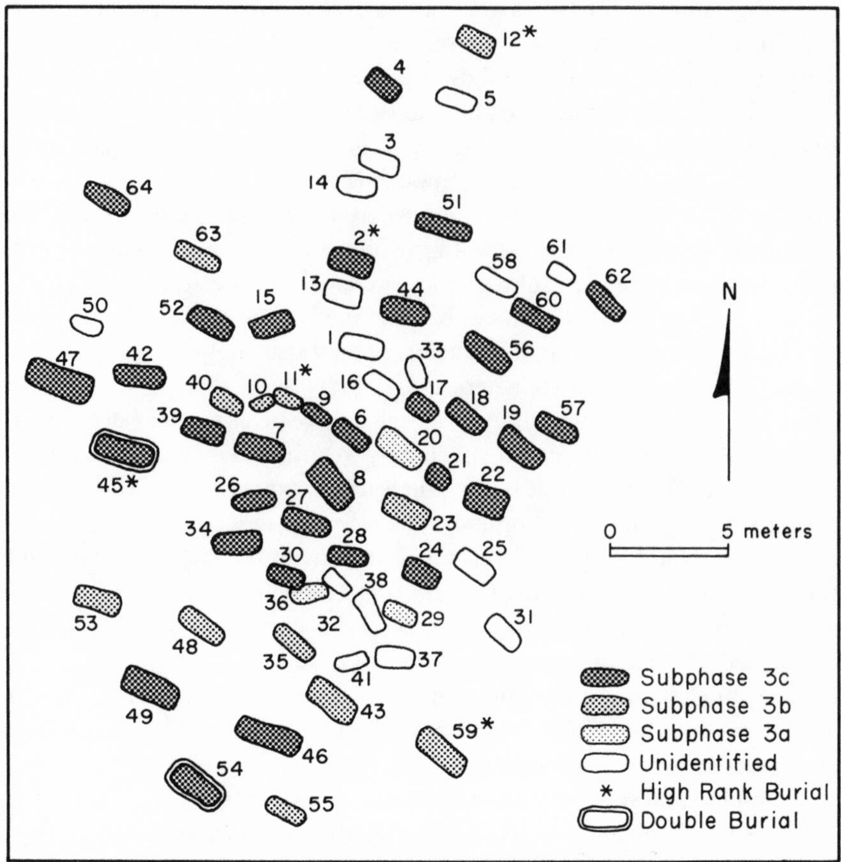

FIG. 19. H. R. Taylor site (41HS3) cemetery plan.

mond 1981, 428–451). At that site, little cultural material was recovered from the excavated mound or the substructure buried by the mound, but in house middens two hundred meters distant, both period 2 and 3 components were identified with which the period of mound construction may have been associated (Thurmond 1981, Table 24). Available evidence, therefore, suggests that mound construction did not last to 1600.

Unlike Protohistoric period mounds constructed in the major river valleys, Cypress basin mounds were substructural mounds; no pyramidal platform or burial mounds are known for this time period. Substructural mounds are restricted to those mounds that cap a burned structure constructed on the ground surface or in a small, shallow pit. Thus, a structure apparently never sat on the mound.

These changes in the sociopolitical and ceremonial aspects of Caddoan life are a reflection of a reduction in complexity and the scope of community integration between ca. 1400 and 1600. That the supralocal community cemeteries are not evenly dispersed throughout the region (see Fig. 14) implies a spatial coalescence, or a decrease in settlement density within particular parts of the two basins. This may indicate a systemic change in Caddoan rural communities at approximately the time of initial European contact. This reduction in sociopolitical and ceremonial complexity and means of community integration is related to differences in regional population and/or settlement density within the Cypress/upper Sabine basin that suggest a reorganization of Caddoan communities to only a few localities within the overall basins themselves. Subsequent to the discontinuation of community cemeteries ca. 1650–1700, most of the upper Sabine and Cypress Creek basins were abandoned (Thurmond 1990b). The only post-1700 Caddoan occupations that can be related to earlier use of the region are to be found in the lower Sulphur and Sabine Rivers at known trade portages or along trail crossings of these major streams (Harris, Harris, and Miroir 1980; Jones 1968).

There is an abundant Late Caddoan and Protohistoric archaeological record in the Neches River basin of Northeast Texas (Story 1990, 327; Perttula 1991). However, our understanding of that record in a detailed manner still awaits development of a means to identify short-term temporal episodes within the 1400–1700 time period and, thus, within the subdivision of the Frankston and Allen phases. The current understanding of the Protohistoric period in the Neches basin, specifically the upper Neches River area (Suhm, Krieger, and Jelks 1954, 184), derives from a literally undated view of the archaeological record (Story 1990, Table 83), thus foiling attempts to fully demonstrate or refine possible Caddoan change in ceramic assemblages, periods of mound construction, aspects of mortuary behavior, and intracommunity cemetery patterning.

There has been some recent progress along these lines, however. Shafer (1981) attempted to seriate ceramic vessels from five Frankston and Allen phase mortuary components (assemblages containing European goods) and "was able to demonstrate a general evolution from one assemblage to the other" (Shafer 1981, 176). This type of chronological analysis has recently been extended to include many other Frankston and Allen phase assemblages (Kleinschmidt 1984), and is based on the frequency of vessels with a Poynor Engraved, a Poynor-Patton Engraved hybrid, or a Patton Engraved motif.

Kleinschmidt (1982) employed the relative frequency of these types of engraved vessels to establish three temporal subdivisions of the Frankston phase (Frankston phase 1, 2, and 3), which is then followed by the Allen phase. Poynor Engraved is the dominant engraved type in Frankston phase

1 and 2 (accounting for 86–100 percent of the engraved vessels in sites belonging to these subdivisions), while Patton Engraved is the dominant engraved ware in the Allen phase (68 percent of the engraved vessels). The hybrid Poynor-Patton engraved motif is most common in the Frankston phase 3 subdivision, though Poynor Engraved and Patton Engraved are also both well represented. The temporal spans of the three Frankston phase subdivisions are not known, though Kleinschmidt (1982, 240) suggests that the Frankston phase 2 subdivision may begin in the early seventeenth century. These efforts have not yet been confirmed by chronological methods (see Corbin, Studer, and Nummi 1978).[4]

Relative estimates of the temporal span of the Frankston and Allen phases are that they date from about 1400–1600 and 1600–1750, respectively (Story and Creel 1982, 34). Each phase is reliably recognized on the basis of a distinctive ceramic and lithic assemblage (Fields 1981; Suhm, Krieger, and Jelks 1954, 220; Story n.d.), along with the occasional association of European goods with post-1700 Allen phase occupations (Cole 1975; Story n.d.).

Story and Creel (1982, 32) use the available archaeological data from the Neches and Angelina river drainages concerning settlement patterns, community structure, and the organization of cemeteries to hypothesize that Frankston and Allen phase populations were organized in a "weakly hierarchical structure" analogous to what has been called in ethnographic terms the Hasinai confederacy. The empirical basis for the existence of the hierarchical structure, called the "temple-residence complex" by Wyckoff and Baugh (1980), is primarily based on the ethnohistorical record for the Hasinai groups (Swanton 1942, 170–173, 210–233; Bolton 1987, 70–91, 138–169) and excavations at the A. C. Saunders (41AN19) mound center (see Fig. 15). This site is suspected to represent a fire-temple, associated with the grand xinesi in the historical record, and was thus one of the major centers of the Frankston and Allen phase sociopolitical structure defined by Story and Creel, that of the "affiliated group" (Story and Creel 1982, 32 and Fig. 8).

The Anderson Cluster is defined by Story and Creel (1982, 33) as the archaeological correlate of the "affiliated group" in the Neches/Angelina river drainages. The Late Caddoan and Protohistoric period Frankston phase and the Historic Caddoan period Allen phase represent the main temporal subdivisions or subphases (Johnson 1987, 19) within the cluster. Accordingly, Story and Creel (1982, 34) state that "the Allen phase is believed to have developed out of the Frankston phase, and more importantly, to have shared the same form of organization, kinds of intergroup interaction, and settlement patterns."

While it would appear sui generis, the Protohistoric period Caddoan development in the upper Neches River basin does share certain aspects of sociopolitical and ceremonial change with the contemporaneous Titus phase. Frankston phase mound centers such as the A. C. Saunders and Pace McDonald sites, both of which were apparently structural mounds without accompanying mortuary events (Story 1981, 149), are not used after 1600. Kleinschmidt (1982, 240) places the A. C. Saunders site in the Frankston phase 2 subdivision, "probably just prior to the historic contacts in the early 17th century."

Changes in cemetery size and limited internal social differentiation in the Allen phase (Cole 1975) are comparable to the structural patterns noted in post-1600 cemeteries in the Cypress Creek basin (see also chapter 6). However, it appears that community-oriented cemeteries are not present in the Neches River basin, and there may have been different forms of community integration developed in the region after initial European contacts (Story 1990, 339–342). As with the Cypress/upper Sabine basin Titus phase occupations discussed above, most of the Caddoan cemeteries in the Neches/Angelina river basin are rather small and were not utilized for long periods of time. The Omer and Otis Hood cemetery (Suhm, Krieger, and Jelks 1954) with twenty burials is roughly of comparable size to a few of the larger Cypress Creek cluster cemeteries. It dates to the Frankston phase 2 subdivision (Kleinschmidt 1982, Table 19).

The cessation of mound construction and little evidence for forms of community integration in the Allen phase archaeological record permit the tentative identification of a Protohistoric period change in the sociopolitical and ceremonial complexity of community organization. The change is toward a more regionally localized sociopolitical system generally compatible with the 1680–1720 ethnohistorical records from the East Texas Hasinai tribes (Wyckoff and Baugh 1980, 246–249), where ritual and ceremony were conducted in nonmound structures or plazas and cemeteries were strictly for extended family use.

THE CENTRAL CADDOAN SUBAREA

The central Caddoan subarea during the Protohistoric period includes Southwest Arkansas, Northwest Louisiana, and Southeast Oklahoma within the Red, Little, and Ouachita river valleys. Defined archaeological phases of ca. 1520 include the Belcher, Texarkana, Saratoga, McCurtain, Mid-Ouachita, and Social Hill phases (see Table 3 and Fig. 14).

In the Great Bend area of the Red River, which is the Red River alluvial valley between the mouths of the Little and Sulphur rivers in Southwest Arkansas, the Protohistoric period is represented by the contemporaneous Belcher and Texarkana phases. While both phases are known primarily from cemetery excavations, all the known Caddoan mound groups in the Great Bend area contain at least limited evidence for a Protohistoric period occupation. In some instances, burials were found in mounds used only for that purpose, but excavations at the Hatchel, Battle, and Belcher sites (only the Belcher site excavation has been published [Webb 1959]) indicate that significant mound construction and/or expansion took place during both the Texarkana and Belcher phases (Creel 1991b). The Battle Mound, a multiple platform edifice 205 meters long, 98 meters wide, and 10.4 meters high (Hoffman 1970, 163), was primarily built in the Belcher phase over a Haley phase (1200–1400) platform mound 1.8 meters high. The Battle Mound is not only the largest known Caddoan mound, but it is one of the largest platform mounds in the southeastern United States (Muller 1978, 321).

Ceramic stylistic differences between the Belcher and Texarkana phases reflect the development of relatively consistent, localized, and homogeneous complexes composed of fine wares and utility wares. The fine wares, typically shell-tempered engraved vessels of multiple forms, tend to have a wider spatial distribution than the utility wares as well as a more restricted temporal character, generally on the order of fifty to one hundred years (Schambach and Miller 1984, 166). The utility wares, which are incised, brushed, plain, or punctated jar forms, do not exhibit the same patterns of ceramic decorative variation as the fine wares and consequently may be of lesser importance in delimiting in detail the temporal character of the two phases. The utility wares are, of course, most common in habitation contexts, but the closed context of burials accompanied by mainly fine ware engraved ceramics provide the best opportunity of detecting temporally significant ceramic stylistic changes during the approximately two hundred–year interval of the Protohistoric period (Schambach et al. 1983; Schambach and Miller 1984; Williams and Early 1990).

The temporal sequence of grave lots from the Cedar Grove site near Spirit Lake in Southwest Arkansas provides the most comprehensive chronological framework for the Protohistoric period in the Great Bend area (Table 9). Beginning with the ceramic types and varieties defined by Schambach and Miller (1984), the vessels from the different grave lots were then arranged and grouped into components based on the frequency distributions of nine defined ceramic types and recognizable varieties within each of the types. Early, Middle, and Late components were defined from Schambach and Miller (1984, Table 11-12 and 164–168).

The Early and Middle components (Schambach and Miller's group 1 and group 2 burial lots) make up different but sequent Belcher phase occupations at the Cedar Grove site. Six thermoluminescence (TL) dates from features 17 and 18, features within a Belcher phase house contemporary with the Middle component burials, range between 1520 ± 50 years and 1710 ± 40 years (Wolfman 1984, Table 17-3). Averaging the TL dates produces a weighted average of 1621 ± 28 years with an overall error of twenty-seven years (Wolfman 1984, 260). A calibrated radiocarbon date of 1450–1674 or 1748–1800 (GX-6745) and calibrated ages of 412 and 310 years B.P. (1538 and 1640) from the Belcher phase Cox site in the Great Bend area (Schambach 1983) corroborate the estimated age of the Belcher phase occupations at the Cedar Grove site. The Early Belcher phase component dates prior to 1600 (Schambach and Miller 1984, 167), though no radiocarbon or TL dates were obtained from these Cedar Grove grave lots. Belcher Engraved var. Belcher and var. Ogden and Foster Trailed-Incised var. Foster are the primary ceramic types in the Early Cedar Grove component of the Belcher phase. For the Middle Belcher phase component, estimated to date from ca. 1593 to 1644, the primary ceramic types in the grave lots include Karnack Brushed-Incised var. Karnack, Foster Trailed-Incised var. Dobson, Keno Trailed, Hodges Engraved, and Glassell Engraved var. McGee.

Because of differences in the frequency and occurrence of varieties of Foster-Trailed Incised and Hodges Engraved within the Chakanina phase component at the Cedar Grove site (Schambach and Miller's group 3 burial lot), it is subdivided here into two sequential Late components: Late A and Late B (see further discussion in chapter 5). Both components are presumed to belong to a Chakanina phase occupation dating from ca. 1700 to 1730 (Trubowitz 1984, 262). Three TL dates from the Chakanina phase midden average 1749 ± 22 years, with an overall error of twenty-one years (Wolfman 1984, 260).

The accuracy of the temporal ordering of grave lots from the Cedar Grove site indicates that the Protohistoric period in the Great Bend area can be successfully partitioned into more discrete temporal units. The recognition of the different ceramic varieties by Schambach and Miller (1984) has created a more reliable chronology than others in which much of the stylistic variation (and hence potential temporal information) has been subsumed within the larger type category. Only one sequence error is apparent in the temporal ordering, and that is in the lack of continuity in the Hodges Engraved var. Armour and var. Candler between the Middle and Late A and B components (see Table 9). This discontinuity may be the result of both the small sample sizes and the high percentage of untyped engraved ceramics in the Late A component as well as from the possibility that some of the grave lots in these components are incomplete (Schambach and Miller 1984, 166). In any event, the clear association of specific varieties of the ceramic decorative types with particular discrete and short-term temporal intervals serves

TABLE 9. Temporal Ordering of the Mortuary Ceramic Vessels from the Cedar Grove Site (Percentage Ceramic Type per Period)

Ceramic Types/Varieties	Early	Middle (1593–1644)[a]	Late A[b]	Late B (1725–1770)[c]
Foster Trailed-Incised				
var. Foster	18			
var. Dobson		17		
var. Red Lake		8		
var. Undetermined			12	
var. Dixon				7
var. Moore				11
var. Finley				4
var. Shaw				7
Belcher Engraved				
var. Belcher	36			
var. Ogden	27			
var. Owen		8	12	7
Natchitoches Engraved				
var. Lester Bend			6	4
var. Unknown				4
Keno Trailed				
var. Undetermined		8		
var. McClendon		8		
var. Phillips			12	
var. Glendora			6	
var. Scott's Lake				4

as a key in helping to create the framework for interpreting changes in other aspects of Caddoan life in the central Caddoan subarea during the Protohistoric period.

At the Belcher civic-ceremonial site in northwestern Louisiana, two conjoined mounds and an adjacent mound platform (Webb 1959, Fig. 4) were utilized during the Belcher phase occupation. Mounds A and B were originally separate earthworks that were conjoined in the final periods of site use. Mound A, approximately 30 meters in diameter and roughly 4.5 meters in height, had contained two houses (nos. 7 and 8) as well as several large burial pits. The mounds grew by accretion as the structures placed on each of the mounds were eventually burned and large pit or shaft burials were excavated through the house floors. Each episode of structure destruc-

TABLE 9. (*Continued*)

Ceramic Types/Varieties	Early	Middle (1593–1644)[a]	Late A[b]	Late B (1725–1770)[c]
Hodges Engraved				
var. Sentell			6	4
var. Kelley's Lake				4
var. Armour		8		11
var. Candler		8		11
Karnack Brushed-Incised				
var. Karnack	9	17		
var. Fish Bayou		8	6	
var. Unknown			6	
Avery Engraved				
var. Graves	9			
var. Unknown				4
Cabaness Engraved				7
Glassell Engraved				
var. McGee		8		
Belcher Ridged				
var. Undetermined			6	
Percentage Untyped			29	11

Source: Adapted from Schambach and Miller 1984, Table 11-12.
Note: Totals vary from 100% because of rounding.
[a]Based on six thermoluminescence dates (Wolfman 1984).
[b]Burials 1, 2, 3, 5, and 7.
[c]Based on three thermoluminescence dates (Wolfman 1984). Includes Burials 4, 9, and 10.

tion and interment was followed by capping the mound with earthen fill and subsequent construction of another structure on the renewed earthen platform.

For Mound B, four structures and eight burials were recorded. The two latest and sequential episodes of mound construction and/or shaft burials, the Belcher III and IV components, are attributable to the Belcher phase (Webb 1959). Houses 2 (and Burials 2, 3, 5–10), 5 (Burials 14 and 15), 6 (Burials 16–19), and 7 (Burials 22–25) make up the Belcher III component, and House 1 (with no burials) makes up the Belcher IV component defined by Webb (1959). It is significant that the use of shaft burials were discontinued at the end of the Belcher III occupation. Belcher III and Belcher IV stratigraphic changes, episodes of house and mound use, and ceramic stylistic changes have allowed the development of a relatively tight internal chronological ordering quite comparable to that of the Cedar Grove site upriver (Table 10).

Five carbon-14 dates were obtained from the Belcher phase components at the Belcher site. The earliest dated Belcher III occupation, House 7, has calibrated radiocarbon date ranges of 1532–1542 or 1640–1890 (O-322), 1302–1414 or 1386–1434 (TX-142), and 1503–1631 or 1617–1659 (TX-473), while a calibrated date of 1484–1650 (TX-477) derives from the House 2 period of mound use. One calibrated date from the Belcher IV occupation, 1484–1650 (TX-476), came from House 1. The calibrated dates overlap between the house construction periods and are not consistent with the Belcher site ceramic seriation. In any event, changes in the frequencies of decorated ceramics at the Belcher site do generally correspond to those at the Cedar Grove site, which is much better dated by absolute methods.

The Belcher Engraved bowls from the Belcher site are the Belcher Engraved var. Belcher (Schambach and Miller 1984, 120). At the Cedar Grove site, the var. Belcher is common only in the Belcher phase component (Early Cedar Grove in Table 9), dating earlier than 1593. The higher frequencies of Belcher Engraved in House 5 and its subsequent decrease in frequency in House 2 and 1 deposits are comparable to the changes in the frequency of Belcher Engraved between the Early, Middle, and Late A components at the Cedar Grove site. The Hodges Engraved category is best represented at the division between the Belcher III/IV components, which is contemporaneous with the Middle Belcher phase component at the Cedar Grove site, dating ca. 1593–1649 (see Table 9). Finally, the low absolute frequency of Keno Trailed, the presence of an unnamed but early variety of Keno Trailed at the Belcher site (Schambach and Miller 1984, 124), and the absence of Natchitoches Engraved suggests that the Belcher IV component ended prior to 1700, probably around 1670. This estimate is based on percentage changes in the representation of the major ceramic types within the Belcher III and IV components. There was not much type replacement or frequency changes between the predominant wares (Hodges Engraved and Belcher Engraved) in the two Belcher site components, which implies that little time actually separates them. The Belcher III component is estimated to date ca. 1500–1650, and the Belcher IV component to date ca. 1650–1670.

At the Belcher site, therefore, periods of mound use and the aboriginal excavation of mound shaft burials evidently predate 1650. The ceramic assemblages recovered from Belcher phase mound pit burials from the Friday (3LA28), Foster (3LA27), and McClure (3MI29) civic-ceremonial sites excavated by Moore (1912) predate 1650 as well (Schambach and Miller 1984, Table 11-2). The identification of Foster Trailed-Incised var. Foster

TABLE 10. Seriation of Belcher Phase Occupations at the Belcher Site (16CD13), Caddo Parish, Louisiana (Percentage of Decorated Ceramic Type per House)

	Belcher III				Belcher IV
Ceramic Types	House 7[a]	House 6	House 5	House 2	House 1
Belcher Engraved	19	23	47	22	11
Hodges Engraved	8	9	11	23	22
Glassell Engraved	11	3	6	5	11
Belcher Ridged	23	21	6	8	11
Cowhide Stamped	8	3	6	13	
Foster Trailed-Incised		12	6	5	
Simms Engraved	4				
Keno Trailed		3	5	2	11
Karnack Brushed	4	9		4	

Source: Adapted from Webb 1959.

[a]Corrected radiocarbon dates from House 7 are 1717 ± 116 (0–322) and 1572 ± 46 (Tx-473). House 2 has a corrected radiocarbon date of 1540 ± 57 (Tx-477), and House 1 has a corrected radiocarbon date of 1540 ± 57 (Tx-476).

from each of these sites indicates that these shaft burials probably predate 1593 (see Table 9), because this variety dates to the Early Cedar Grove component of the Belcher phase. Later off-mound cemeteries at these sites, as well as others in the Boyd Hill and Spirit Lake localities (Schambach et al. 1983, 93–94), postdate the Belcher IV component at the Belcher site because they contain Natchitoches Engraved var. Lester Bend and Keno Trailed var. Scott's Lake (Schambach and Miller 1984, Table 11-2). These ceramic types are good markers for post-1700 Caddoan occupations in the Great Bend area of the Red River (see chapter 5 for further discussion).

The discontinuation of elite mound shaft burials in the Belcher phase coincides with the regional cessation of mound construction as well. The shaft burials share a number of characteristics: (*a*) they are only found at civic-ceremonial centers; (*b*) they contain multiple primary burials; (*c*) within the multiple primary burials only one individual, always an adult male, appears to be of paramount significance with the others being placed with the paramount individual at his death; and (*d*) all burials, including those of children, were associated with artifacts of exotic origin (conch shell, pearls, gorgets, columella pendants, and beads) denoting high social rank or status (Webb 1984; Trubowitz 1984; Story 1990). The survival of this type of social organization—a ranked class structure—to ca. 1650 in the Great

Bend area indicates that there was no apparent diminution in mortuary complexity through most of the Belcher phase. However, a simple comparison of the presence or absence of shaft burials in the Belcher phase may be less illuminating regarding the persistence of mortuary complexity than are significant changes within the Belcher phase mortuary program at the Belcher site itself in this respect.

During the 150 years when mound shaft burials were used by the Belcher phase inhabitants of the Belcher site and vicinity, approximately thirty-four individuals were interred. Among those thirty-four individuals were four to five adult males, eight to ten adult females (the numbers of adult burials where the sex is known are approximate because the burials in House 5 could only be identified as adults), two juveniles, eleven children, and five infants. If each of the four episodes of house construction and destruction and burial interment was a generational event, triggered by the death of a paramount adult male, the number of individuals per burial and per mound episode might reflect short-term differences in ranked class composition and grave goods associations through the Protohistoric period. Examining the grave goods data provided by Webb (1959), one finds that the number of associated grave goods per burial varied through time, though they were also dependent on the frequency of multiple burial interments because multiple burials usually contained the most grave goods. Nevertheless, the general trend in the mortuary program within the Belcher phase occupation at the Belcher site was toward (*a*) an increase through time in the grave goods per individual, (*b*) an increase in primary individuals interred during the period (ca. 1500–1625), and (*c*) decreases in these same factors after ca. 1625–1650, when the shaft burial mortuary program was abandoned. Although it is hard to generalize on the basis of the information from one Caddoan site, the available data appear to indicate an initial persistence and subsequent intensification of hierarchically differentiated social rituals and ceremonies in the Protohistoric Belcher phase. This was followed by a diminution in social organization and status roles, which preceded the abandonment of complex Caddoan mortuary practices. All these changes occurred prior to the onset of sustained European contact with Caddoan peoples in the Red River Valley, but surely they reflect significant and rapid changes in Caddoan ideology and ceremonial activities in the Protohistoric period.

The absence of ceramic markers in the Belcher phase for occupations postdating sustained European contact—particularly Natchitoches Engraved and Keno Trailed (including var. Scott Lake and var. Glendora)—indicates that this diminution in mortuary complexity took place prior to the period of direct European contact. Only one site in the northwestern Louisiana section of the Belcher phase is known to contain Natchitoches Engraved (Harris and Harris 1980, 225), but investigators found no European goods at the site. Only in the Boyd Hill and Spirit Lake localities were these varieties of Keno Trailed and Natchitoches Engraved found together on several aboriginal Caddoan sites (Schambach and Miller 1984, Table 11-2). Their distribution denotes that post-1685 Historic period Caddoan settlements existed in only two small stretches of the seventy-kilometer Great Bend segment of the Red River. Both localities and aggregates of settlement are more than seventy kilometers distant from the Louisiana sections of the Belcher phase, and more than forty kilometers distant from other post-1685 Caddoan settlements farther upstream on the Red River, namely the Little River phase (see Story 1990).

For the Texarkana phase most of the information on Caddoan settleent, mound construction, and mortuary practices comes from unpublished Works Progress Administration reports of excavations in Bowie County, Northeast Texas (Krieger 1946), and from amateur excavations at the Bowman site on the Red River in Southwest Arkansas (Hoffman 1971, 814). The Texarkana phase occupations primarily have been recognized by ceramic grave associations, with the principal local pottery types including Barkman Engraved, Avery Engraved, Simms Engraved, Hatchel Engraved, Bowie Engraved, McKinney Plain, Nash Neck-Banded, and Foster Trailed-Incised.

Texarkana phase mortuary components are contemporary with the Belcher phase components at the Belcher site and the Cedar Grove site, and the burial plots at the Hatchel and Mitchell sites are estimated to date from ca. 1300 to 1700 (Creel 1991b). Both Avery and Simms Engraved vessels were found in all four mound or burial episodes at the Belcher site (Webb 1959, Table 2). Indeed, Texarkana phase ceramics comprised between 1.2 percent and 8.9 percent of the ceramic grave goods in the Belcher III component, but (based on data in Table 9) were most common there before ca. 1593. No Texarkana phase ceramics were recovered in the Belcher IV component (Webb 1959, Table 2).

The low frequency of shell-tempered pottery in the known Texarkana phase sites, primarily in the utility wares such as McKinney Plain and Nash Neck-Banded (Suhm, Krieger, and Jelks 1954, 206), may indicate that many of the Texarkana phase occupations date prior to 1600–1650, as might the high frequency of compound Avery Engraved bowls with flaring rims in the Texarkana phase sites (Davis 1970, 51). These types of vessels are also found in contemporaneous McCurtain phase occupations farther west up the Red River in contexts that suggest they date prior to ca. 1600 (Prewitt 1969; Skinner, Harris, and Anderson 1969, Fig. 8; Perino 1983). Creel (1991b) presents data from a seriation of the burial lots from the Hatchel and Mitchell sites that constitutes good evidence for Texarkana phase occupations at them ca. 1550–1700. Ceramic types found in the last part of the Texarkana phase include Keno Trailed, Simms Engraved, Foster Trailed-Incised, Avery Engraved, Belcher Engraved, Hodges Engraved, Nash Neck-Banded, and McKinney Plain. Their association at these sites aligns them with the Belcher IV and Late Chakanina phase components at the Belcher and Cedar Grove sites, respectively (see Tables 9 and 10). Unfortunately, there are no radiocarbon dates for the latter part of the Texarkana phase that would verify the temporal extent of the phase or discriminate which cultural materials are associated with the Historic Caddoan period Little River phase in the same locality. Mound construction in the Texarkana phase is coincident with the main period of Caddoan settlement at the Hatchel site, ca. 1400–1700. Two radiocarbon dates from the mound are 1450 ± 50 years and 1450–1600 (Creel 1991b).

There is a possibility that the mound at the Hatchel site (41BW3) was used after 1680 (Wedel 1978, 8). The Terán map of 1691–1692 shows an upper Nasoni community on the Red River composed of a number of farmsteads, and at the western end of the community was a platform mound with a structure on the top (see pp. 159–160). In documentary studies by M. M. Wedel, this Caddoan community has been identified as having been located in the Great Bend area of the Red River northwest of Texarkana and the platform mound as being in all likelihood the Hatchel Mound (Wedel 1978, 10). Sherds of Natchitoches Engraved and Keno Trailed have been found in a mantle of refuse at the Hatchel Mound, and a number of burials dating to this period have been excavated in the village and burial plots (Creel 1991b); but no new mound construction stages were added to the Hatchel Mound in the Historic period (Davis 1970, 50; Schambach et al. 1983, 93). Deep shaft burials have been reported from the roughly contemporaneous Tilson site (41BW14) at Summerhill Lake, but insufficient information on grave goods prevents determining its specific placement in the Protohistoric and Historic Caddoan period sequence (Perttula 1991).

Little River Region

In the Little River region the Protohistoric period is represented by the Saratoga phase (Hoffman 1971). This phase is known primarily from mound shaft burials and cemeteries at the Mineral Springs site (Bohannon 1973), but platform mound construction also took place at this time. The culmination of mortuary complexity in the Little River region occurred during this phase (Bohannon 1973, 40; Hoffman 1983).

The end of the phase (designated the Mineral Springs VI component at the Mineral Springs site [Bohannon 1973, 13–14]) marks, however, a possible diminution in mortuary complexity (Hoffman 1983, Table 5), after which the region was apparently abandoned. There is no substantial evidence in the Little River region for the presence of permanent Caddoan occupations later than ca. 1550, contemporary with much of the Texarkana phase occupation to the south on the Red River. Ceramic seriation by Bohannon (1973, Table 3) of the grave lots from Mound 6 at the Mineral Springs site places the diminution in mortuary complexity about the same time as the Belcher III component noted at the Belcher site (see Table 10), which is estimated to date from ca. 1500 to 1650. The most frequent ceramic association in the Mineral Springs VI component is the Haley Engraved var. Adams form (Hoffman 1971, 777). This Caddoan bottle form is intermediate in the manner of decorative treatment between both Haley Engraved and Belcher Engraved, which is the later form (Schambach and Miller 1984). The incipient spool necks on var. Adams bottles are also temporally diagnostic of the Protohistoric period, which further suggests that the Saratoga phase ends in the sixteenth century.

Two sites in the Little River area, one a salt-producing site on the Rolling Fork River (3SV29) and the other a small habitation site on the Little River (Hoffman 1971, 782–783), contained shell-tempered assemblages dominated by Nash Neck-Banded and Emory Punctated-Incised (A. M. Early, Ph.D., personal communication, 20 March 1987). The dominance of shell tempering on these sites indicates at least some Caddoan use of the Little River region after ca. 1650 (Schambach et al. 1983). The specialized use of salt licks in the Caddoan Area appears to have begun about 1400–1500 (Gregory 1973, 260; Early 1990) but became increasingly emphasized by the Caddoan peoples in the seventeenth and eighteenth century along with the development of the deer hide trade.

Middle Red River

The middle Red River region extends from approximately the Oklahoma and Arkansas state line to the mouth of the Kiamichi River and includes the Red River Valley in both Northeast Texas and Southeast Oklahoma. The Protohistoric period archaeological record in this part of the Red River Valley is known in cultural-taxonomic terms as the McCurtain focus or phase (Bell and Baerreis 1951; Story 1990). Dominated by fine-ware red-slipped ceramics, including Clement Redware or Roden ware (Perino 1981), Avery Engraved, Simms Engraved, and coarse-tempered utility jar forms such as Nash Neck-Banded and Emory Punctated-Incised, this particular Caddoan phase was rather long-lasting, ranging from ca. 1250 to 1700. Within that long span of time there were certain specific ceramic stylistic changes (especially in the fine wares) but also notable differences in mound construction, settlement intensity, and mortuary practices that are analogous to the record of change seen in the Great Bend and Little River Protohistoric period archaeological records.

The occurrence seriation of the ceramic vessels from the burials from the

Sam Kaufman–Bob Williams site indicates that there are differences in ceramic body form and design element variability through time and that these relate to more discrete temporal and/or geographical contexts within the McCurtain phase (Table 11). Additional temporal refinements, which have not been incorporated in the Sam Kaufman–Bob Williams seriation, utilizing decorative changes in the Nash and Emory types, also seem likely with further investigations (Perino 1981, 33, 37).

From these data, three periods or subphases (in the sense employed by Johnson [1987]) have been established within the McCurtain phase along the middle Red River. The earliest, Period III, includes the ceramic types red Avery Engraved with the chevron and semicircular motifs, black Avery Engraved bottles, the carinated form of Simms Engraved, Nash Neck-Banded, and Emory Punctated-Incised. Period II, estimated to date from ca. 1500 to 1700 (the Protohistoric period), primarily includes red Avery Engraved vessels with the scroll curvilinear motif, the hubcap form of Simms Engraved, Hudson Engraved, Keno Trailed, and the utility wares. Period I, which has European trade goods in association with the Caddoan archaeological deposits, has a minimal amount of red Avery Engraved, more Hudson Engraved, Nash Neck-Banded, and Emory Punctated-Incised vessels with distinctive incised scrolls on the body of the vessel (Perino 1979, 1981, 1983). Taylor Engraved, Hodges Engraved, and Foster Trailed-Incised may also occur in Period I features, and in fact Perino (1983, 72–74) suggests that Taylor Engraved replaced Avery Engraved bottles in the Historic Caddoan Period I ceramic assemblages of the McCurtain phase. The periodization of the McCurtain phase permits a somewhat more detailed investigation of Caddoan cultural changes over time in the region.

Like other Late Caddoan occupations on the Red River, the McCurtain phase settlement pattern includes large villages with substructural mounds, household cemeteries, the utilization of shaft tombs for multiple burials, and house sites scattered along major and minor drainages. Of the three McCurtain phase periods, Period III of the McCurtain phase is characterized by a high level of social complexity and hierarchical differentiation. Mound and off-mound shaft tombs and multiple pit burials containing Gulf Coast shell gorgets, tools manufactured of exotic lithic raw materials, and a wide variety and number of other grave goods are exclusively found during this McCurtain phase period.

The McCurtain phase component at the Roden site, where two shaft tombs were excavated, lasted to 1424–1466 (UGA-2177, calibrated), and the shaft tombs at the Sam Kaufman (Skinner, Harris, and Anderson 1969) and the Clement (Bell and Baerreis 1951) sites are contemporary with it. Later in McCurtain phase Period II, however, multiple shaft burials were discontinued, and individual extended burials in such large household cemeteries as those at the Roland Clark and Sam Kaufman–Bob Williams sites became the dominant form of mortuary interment (see Loveland 1987; Perino 1983). A calibrated date of 1440–1522 or 1580–1624 (UGA-2178) from the Period II or late McCurtain phase occupation at the Roden site does indicate that this diminution in mortuary complexity on the middle Red River coincides with the earliest segments of the Protohistoric period in the Caddoan Area. Only at the Roden site were substructural mounds apparently still in use on the middle Red River during that period of time (Perino 1981, 13). However, since there is no actual documentation in Perino (1981) of the stratigraphy, context, or association of particular ceramic stylistic classes with the Area G Mound at the Roden site (Perttula 1982), a conclusive assessment of Perino's conclusion that the mound was constructed sometime between 1500 and 1600 is not possible.

The development of less complex mortuary rituals as well as the cessation of mound construction in the McCurtain phase on the Red River occurred in Period II perhaps as early as 1550. The Caddoan peoples in this region maintained a settlement and territorial continuity, however, at least in the Mound Prairie area,[5] which is a fifteen- to thirty-kilometer section of the Red River downstream from the mouth of the Kiamichi River (Skinner, Harris, and Anderson 1969, 7). Both the Sam Kaufman–Bob Williams and Roden sites contain several household/cemetery clusters that were apparently rebuilt and continuously used from the end of Period III and spanning Period II of the McCurtain phase.

At the Roden site, the majority of the thirty-eight child and adult burials that were excavated were found associated with evidence of at least six Period II houses in Area A (Perino 1981). More than six house/cemetery clusters are known from the Sam Kaufman–Bob Williams site that were utilized during Period II (Perino 1983), and this includes household cemeteries containing more than twenty burials each. The individual settlements were not large, being apparently limited to associated farmstead compounds with household cemeteries, and included salt-making sites (Bruseth and Perttula 1991).

In the context of the overall McCurtain phase settlement of the middle Red River, the apex of the phase in sociopolitical and mortuary complexity was reached during Period III. After ca. 1500 Caddoan mortuary rituals and ceremonies became less complex, and the settlement hierarchy was simplified as a consequence of the cessation of mound construction and mound and/or nonmound shaft burial interments. This was apparently accompanied by an overall regional decrease in population and, perhaps, a decreasing intensity of occupation.

Period I in the middle Red River, estimated to date after ca. 1700, cannot be easily distinguished from Period II of the McCurtain phase solely on the basis of the ceramic occurrence seriation (see Table 11), though Hudson Engraved does appear to be more common at this time (Perino 1983). This problem is most likely the result of the short temporal span of Period I in the middle Red River, and the continued manufacture of some of the same types of Caddoan fine ware ceramics. The specific association of European bead types (Brain 1979) with a few European metal artifacts and the presence of Keno Trailed var. Phillips at the Anderson, Bowman, and Sam Kaufman–Bob Williams sites are evidence that Period I lasts only to ca. 1730 (Schambach and Miller 1984, 123). Natchitoches Engraved is totally absent from the middle Red River region. The Sam Kaufman (Harris 1953), Bob Williams (Perino 1983), and Roden (Perino 1981) sites all contain at least one Historic Caddoan burial post-dating 1700, based strictly on the types of European goods that are present in the graves. Another burial at the Sam Kaufman–Bob Williams site had a Quapaw phase or Menard Complex teapot (Perino 1979, 26) dating to the same time period. Several other burials from these sites can also be included in this late subphase of Historic Caddoan period settlement because of a specific variety of decorative motif present on Emory Punctated-Incised jars from other burials at the three sites (Perino 1979; Perttula 1980). This undefined variety of Emory Punctated-Incised may be restricted in use to the early part of the Historic Caddoan period, from ca. 1680 to 1730 (see also chapter 5).

Middle Ouachita River

The middle Ouachita River region extends from the Ouachita Mountains escarpment south to Camden, Arkansas, where the Felsenthal region of the Lower Mississippi Valley subarea begins (Rolingson and Schambach 1981). The physiographic and biogeographic boundary between the lower Mississippi Valley and the Gulf Coastal Plain also has cultural implications because the middle Ouachita River area was occupied by sedentary Caddoan-speaking agriculturists (Early 1990; Burnett 1990b), while the southeastern forest floodplains south of Camden were occupied by hunting-gathering-fishing foragers who lived in permanent settlements, constructed mounds, and made ceramics that are clearly affiliated with Tunican-speaking peoples (Schambach 1991; Kidder 1990a).

The cultural taxonomy of the middle Ouachita River area was refined in the late 1980s and early 1990s in part because of the extensive investigations at the Hardman site (3CL418) by the Arkansas Archeological Survey (Williams and Early 1990), the Standridge site by the Arkansas Archeological Society (Early 1988), and the reanalysis of skeletal materials by Burnett (1990b) from a number of Late Caddoan and Protohistoric sites in the region. The Late Caddoan and Protohistoric Caddoan period in the middle

TABLE 11. Seriation of Burials from the McCurtain Phase Occupations at the Sam Kaufman–Bob Williams Site

Ceramic Types/ Vessel Forms	Period III (1250–1500)	Period II (1500–1700)	Period I (1700+)
Avery Engraved Red			
Chevron motif	X		
Semicircular motif	X		
Scroll curvilinear		X	X
Compound Bowl	X		
Miniature Simple Bowl		X	X
Avery Engraved Black	X		
Sims Engraved			
Carinated A	X		
Hubcap B		X	
Hudson Engraved		X	X
Keno Trailed		X	
Nash Neck-Banded	X	X	X
Emory Punctate-Incised	X	X	X[a]
European Trade Goods			X

Source: Adapted from Skinner, Harris, and Anderson, 1969, Table 8.
Note: X indicates presence.
[a]See Perino 1979; Perttula 1980; Harris 1953.

Ouachita River basin includes the Mid-Ouachita phase (ca. 1350–1500), the Social Hill phase (ca. 1500–1650), and the Deceiper phase (ca. 1650–1700) (Early 1990). The Social Hill and Deceiper phases replace the Late Period Mid-Ouachita phase taxonomic unit proposed by Early (1982a) in a preliminary assessment of the archaeology of the middle Ouachita River region.

According to Early (1990, 13-4), the Mid-Ouachita phase represents the florescence of Caddoan lifeways in the region because it is represented by numerous mound centers (where sociopolitical and ceremonial activities occurred) and large, dense populations distributed in town communities, farmsteads, and salt-making sites. Although mound centers are common at this time, there is no archaeological evidence for the use of mound shaft burials or other elaborate mortuary practices in the region (Early 1990, 13-

25). The Mid-Ouachita phase Caddoan populations were intensive agriculturists (Burnett 1990b, 11–109), but bioarchaeological analyses indicate that they were a healthy and well-adapted population of farmers.

In the succeeding Social Hill phase, the understanding of the archaeology for the region is that Caddoan settlements were still extensive, though there probably were a fewer number of mound centers being constructed or used (Early 1990, 13-5). Bioarchaeological data continue to suggest that these Caddoan populations were well-adapted and intensive agriculturists, but there is evidence from Copeland Ridge (3CL195) Social Hill phase component skeletal remains that osteomyelitis variola was present as a manifestation of smallpox that had been introduced into the region by the diffusion of the European disease (Burnett 1990b, 11-14). The mean age at death of the Caddoan adults also dropped from 35 years of age in the Mid-Ouachita phase to 27.6 years of age in the Social Hill phase (Burnett 1990b, Table 11-10), and this was accompanied by some evidence for chronic anemia (Burnett 1990b, Table 11-26). Nevertheless, based on the preponderance of the bioarchaeological and archaeological evidence from the Middle Ouachita River region, Burnett (1990b) and Early (1990) argue that the Caddoan Social Hill phase populations suffered no adverse impact by contact with Europeans or by the introduction of European diseases.

In the Deceiper phase, there was a smaller number of sites, fewer mound centers, and a decrease in Caddoan population levels (Early 1990, 13-26). Most of the known Deceiper phase sites cluster on the Ouachita River upstream from the Hardman and Bayou Sel sites (see Fig. 14). According to Early (1990, 13-6), the Deceiper phase comprised a "resident regional population with a coherent social identity," and the bioarchaeological evidence appears to support these claims. That is, during the Deceiper phase the mean age at death increased to 37.0 years of age, the mean age of female death was comparable, the skeletal infection rates had decreased by 60 percent from the Social Hill phase, and there was little evidence for chronic anemias or high levels of subadult mortality (Burnett 1990b, 11-87). Stable carbon isotope data from the Deceiper phase indicates that the consumption of maize by these Caddoan peoples had decreased some 20–30 percent over that seen in the earlier Mid-Ouachita and Social Hill phases (Burnett 1990b, Tables 11–23).

The mortuary data from the Deceiper phase is also illuminating about the nature of protohistoric Caddoan societies in the middle Ouachita River region. Cemeteries contain extended inhumations with "modest grave goods" (Williams and Early 1990, 5-31), and based on the diversity and amounts of grave goods within these cemeteries there is no evidence for vertical differentiation.

The Deceiper phase represents the final Caddoan settlement in the middle

Ouachita River region. Significantly, "there is no evidence to support the continuing presence of Caddoan groups in the area after A.D. 1700" (Early 1982a, 217). Caddoan occupations with European trade goods are not known in the Arkansas portion of the Ouachita River Valley, except for one Deceiper phase burial from the Hardman site with a glass trade bead (Williams and Early 1990, 2-12–2-13).

Mid-Ouachita phase (or now referred to as the Deceiper phase?) occupations identified as being affiliated with the Cahinnio Caddo (Hodges and Hodges 1945; Hodges 1957) may be plausible for some area sites with post-1685 occupations since the Cahinnio Caddo were living in the vicinity of Camden, Arkansas, when Joutel ([1713] 1906, 171–172) and his party first encountered them in 1687 (see discussion in chapter 5). Dickinson (1980) further suggests the possibility that the town of Cayas described by the de Soto *entrada* in the Tanico province (see Fig. 2) might be associated with the Cahinnio Caddo, who then moved farther down the Ouachita River during the seventeenth century and later moved out of the Ouachita River Valley to amalgamate with the Kadohadacho on the Red River (Swanton 1942). More recent consideration of the de Soto *entrada* route by Hudson (1990), however, places the Tanico province on the Arkansas River (the river of Cayas) rather than the Ouachita River, which suggests affinities between Tanico and proto-Tunican speakers (Jeter 1986; Jeter et al. 1989, 226).

As noted above, for the Social Hill and Deceiper phases above Camden, Arkansas, Early (1982a, 223; 1990, 13-5) contends that there were no significant differences in settlement pattern complexity and sociopolitical organization from the preceding Mid-Ouachita phase, except that during the Deceiper phase the population was lower in density. This strongly implies that there were no substantial changes in sociopolitical organization or settlement hierarchy in the Protohistoric period.

Instead, settlement pattern data suggest that there were several contemporaneous clusters of "town" communities present above the junction of the Little Missouri and Ouachita Rivers during this period (Early 1982a, Fig. 8-4). Each town community may have had several civic-ceremonial centers, as little as one or two kilometers apart from each other. A related cluster of Caddoan settlement is apparently present in the Camden, Arkansas, locality (Verley 1964), but in this area the evidence of settlement is restricted to Protohistoric burials intrusive into earlier constructed mounds. Limited excavations by Verley (1964, 42) at the Stafford (3OU13) and Riley (3OU1) sites indicated that the mounds were composed of midden deposits accumulated contemporaneously with the Felsenthal region Gran Marais phase (Rolingson and Schambach 1981, Table 21; Schambach 1991) and the Mid-Ouachita phase, rather than the product of Protohistoric construction. The pattern of mortuary treatment described by Verley (1964) is very similar to that seen in the Protohistoric Caney Bayou phase downstream on the Ouachita River, where bundle burial cemeteries were placed intrusively in the tops of earlier mounds (Schambach 1991, 122–123). Until further exploration of the Protohistoric period is carried out in this part of the middle Ouachita River region, it would be premature to directly associate mound construction (or the presence of mounds) with nearby cemeteries or burial interments on mounds that contain Protohistoric period ceramic assemblages.

There is relevant information in the non-Caddoan Protohistoric period archaeological record in the Ouachita River basin that needs to be introduced, since evidence of cultural changes noted here amplifies the discussion for the Caddoan Social Hill and Deceiper phases of the Mid-Ouachita region. Contemporaneous with these Mid-Ouachita phases is the Caney Bayou phase (ca. 1550–1700) in the Felsenthal region (Rolingson and Schambach 1981; Schambach 1991). Rolingson and Schambach (1981, 210) have noted "that during the Caney Bayou period, occupation in the Felsenthal region was very light, perhaps due to the impact of European diseases introduced by De Soto. . . . The picture that seems to be emerging here, is one of small groups, perhaps refugees, with a ceramic complex that suggests a recent mixing of diverse groups."

Included in the ceramic assemblages were Baytown Plain, Baytown Plain var. Shallow Lake, Coleman Incised, Cowhide Stamped, Cowhide Stamped var. Blackwell, Glassell Engraved, Parkin Punctated, Parkin Punctated var. Boeuf Brake, and Winterville Incised (Rolingson and Schambach 1981, 193). These ceramics share similarities to those found in Caddoan complexes on the middle Ouachita River (Early 1990), to Mississippian assemblages in the Yazoo and Natchez Bluffs areas (Jeter et al. 1989), and to late Tunican assemblages in Southeast Arkansas (Jeter, Kelley, and Kelley 1979) and Northeast Louisiana (Kidder 1988, 1990b; Jones 1985). Since Keno Trailed, Hodges Engraved, and Natchitoches Engraved have also apparently been found in a Caney Bayou phase context (Schambach 1991, 122), the phase must continue into the early part of the 1700s.

By the time of the Caney Bayou phase in the Felsenthal region, mound construction had ceased, and these sites "were now serving a mortuary function for what seems to have been small population aggregates" (Weinstein and Kelley 1984, 45). The tops of mounds were used only for the intrusive interment of bundle burials. Some small habitation sites for the Caney Bayou phase are known, but overall levels of population are much lower than noted for the preceding Gran Marais phase. The preexisting sociopolitical organization of the Gran Marais phase included at least a three-tiered settlement hierarchy of large multiple-mound centers, small single-mound sites, and permanent hamlets in the Felsenthal region of the Ouachita River, along with seasonal hunting and fishing camps. By the middle of the sixteenth century, the Caney Bayou phase was composed simply of a nonhierarchical social and settlement system in which populations lived only in small habitations along the Ouachita River and its tributaries. While the ethnic identities of the Caney Bayou or Gran Marais phases are not clearly known, the available archaeological and ethnohistorical evidence suggests they were probably Tunican and Koroan groups, with the possible admixture of some Caddoan groups (Jeter 1986; Jeter et al. 1989; Kidder 1990a; Rolingson and Schambach 1981; Schambach 1991).

For the Central Boeuf basin of northeastern Louisiana (see Belmont 1985, Figs. 1 and 3), Kidder (1988) has defined the Jordan phase as the local Protohistoric period occupation. The Jordan phase populations are protohistoric Mississippians (Jeter et al. 1989, 222 and Fig. 22), with ethnic affinities to the Koroa and Tunican groups (Kidder 1988, 1990a).

With no apparent prehistoric antecedents in the area, the Jordan phase occupation in the Central Boeuf basin appears to represent a sixteenth-century movement or "flight response" of lower Mississippi River Valley groups, possibly remnants of the Wilmot and Transylvania phase peoples, into the area (Kidder 1988; Jeter et al. 1989). One of the more notable cultural features of the Jordan phase was the construction of a multimound civic-ceremonial center, along with a series of ponds and ditches presumed to control and channel water, between ca. 1540 and 1680 at the Jordan site (Kidder 1988). Jordan phase sites appear to have been abandoned by the end of the seventeenth century, by which time the Protohistoric period mound-building activities ceased.

The diverse ceramic assemblage from the Jordan phase and other contemporaneous phases in the Southern Ouachita River basin provides some evidence for the ethnic assimilation of groups throughout the larger Ouachita, Tensas, and Bayou Bartholomew basins between ca. 1550 and 1680, followed subsequently by a post-1680 movement of these new ethnic units to areas within the basin where profitable trade and exchange relationships could be conducted with the Europeans in the region (Kidder 1990a, 74–76). Both Caddoan and Natzchean ceramics are present in what is otherwise a Protohistoric Mississippian shell-tempered assemblage (Belmont 1985, 280; Kidder 1990a).

Sometime after ca. 1650 in the middle Ouachita River region, the area was reoccupied by people of the Quapaw phase or Menard complex (Schambach and Early 1983, SW133–SW137; Jeter, Cande, and Mintz 1990). Precisely when that took place is unclear, but the assemblage from One Cypress Point (3AS286) in the Felsenthal region appears to date to between 1600 and 1700 (Hemmings 1982, 182), which is roughly contemporary with the ethnohistorically documented 1680s Quapaw villages on the lower Arkansas River (Ford 1961; Jeter et al. 1989). A Quapaw phase component has additionally been identified at the salt-making Bayou Sel site in the middle Ouachita River region (Schambach and Early 1983, SW134). Whether this was contemporary with the Caddoan Protohistoric period occupation of the region is not known, although Joutel ([1713] 1906) had commented on the mutual Caddoan and Quapaw use of the area in 1687 to gather salt for trade. Jeter (1986) hypothesizes that the Quapaw began to displace the native Caddoan and Tunican groups in this region around the turn of the eighteenth century.

THE NORTHERN CADDOAN AREA

The northern Caddoan subarea includes the Arkansas Valley lowlands from roughly Carden Bottom on the east to the confluence of the Neosho and Arkansas rivers on the west and to the confluence of the Neosho and Elk rivers on the north, as well as the western Ozark Highland in Northeast Oklahoma, Northwest Arkansas, and Southwest Missouri (Fig. 20). Post-1500 or Protohistoric period archaeological sites in the northern Caddoan area are not well known but appear to be concentrated in two localities: the Carden Bottom along the middle Arkansas River and in the Braden Bottoms in eastern Oklahoma. Additionally, Hoffman (1977a, 28) notes that "there are undescribed (late) Caddoan phases . . . along tributaries of the Arkansas River . . . the Fourche la Fave and Petit Jean Rivers," but, unfortunately, they have not yet been studied by professional archaeologists.

The Fort Coffee phase in the Braden Bottoms of the Arkansas River in eastern Oklahoma lasts from about 1450 to 1600 (Rohrbaugh 1984, 267) and is known principally from a few habitation and cemetery sites that were excavated by the Works Progress Administration in the 1930s (Orr 1946). When compared with communities of the preceding Spiro phase in the same area (Rogers, Wyckoff, and Peterson 1989; Peterson 1989), the Fort Coffee phase community is less complex in matters of sociopolitical and settlement hierarchy, in mortuary treatment and cemetery organization, in interregional exchange, and in being "composed of fewer and more mobile peoples" (Rohrbaugh 1984, 272). No mounds of any type were constructed during the phase, nor were any specialized public or community buildings (Rogers 1982) used during this time.

The Fort Coffee phase ceramic assemblage includes fine wares of the Hudson Engraved and Womack Engraved types and common shell tempered utility wares such as Woodward Plain, Woodward Applique, Braden Incised, Nash Neck-Banded, and Emory Punctated-Incised (Rohrbaugh 1984, 280). The latter two ceramic types are probably imports from the Texarkana

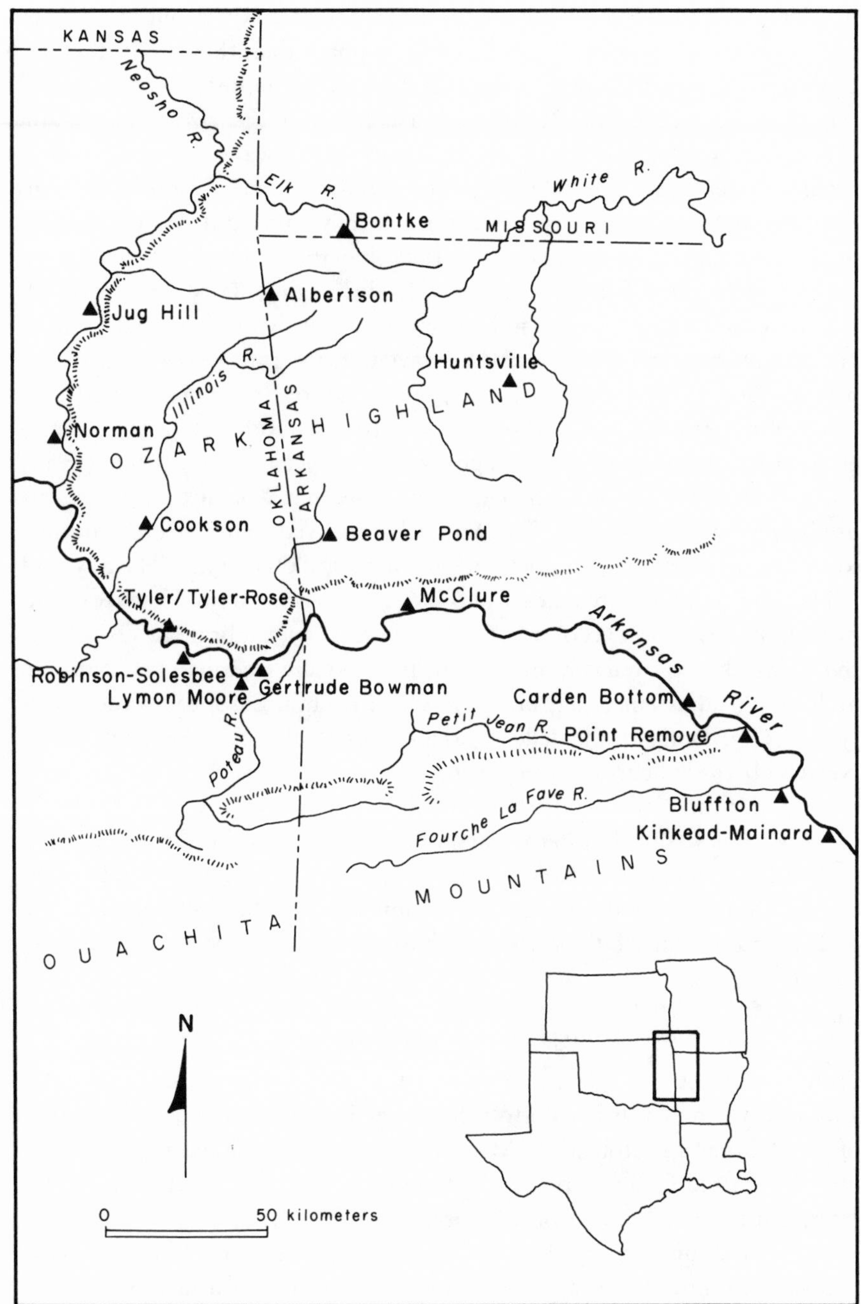

FIG. 20. Significant sites of the northern Caddoan subarea, ca. 1520–1685.

or McCurtain phase groups living on the middle Red River, but these types are much more frequent in the Fort Coffee phase than they are in the preceding Spiro phase (Brown 1984a, 262). Another import, a spool-necked Hudson Engraved bottle (Rohrbaugh 1984, Fig. 12.3b) from the Lymon Moore site (34LF31), is a McCurtain phase ceramic ware commonly manufactured after 1500 (see Table 11). The Womack Engraved ceramics from the Lymon Moore cemetery represent a locally produced Arkansas basin ware that clearly is an earlier dated variety than the Womack Engraved from the middle Red and Sabine river basins (Rohrbaugh 1982, 57; Story 1967).

Differences in vessel shape and decorative motifs between the Fort Coffee and the Norteno phase Womack Engraved (Story 1967) appear to be the product of stylistic change. At the Lymon Moore site the calibrated date range of ten radiocarbon dates is 1385–1593 (see Rohrbaugh 1984; Sabo et al. 1988), with the calibrated ages falling between 616 years B.P. (1334) and 310 years B.P. (1640). These dates indicate that Womack Engraved was used there ca. 1340–1640. The Womack Engraved found at the Protohistoric Wichita Bryson–Paddock site in northern Oklahoma (Hartley and Miller 1977) apparently dates 1442–1644 or 1617–1659 (TX-2360, calibrated) and 1650–1690 or 1725–1809 (TX-2359, calibrated). Elsewhere, the Womack Engraved ceramics occur in post-1680 Caddoan and Norteno archaeological assemblages, many of which contain European trade goods (Jelks 1967; Duffield and Jelks 1961; Harris et al. 1965; Bell, Jelks, and Newcomb 1967; Scurlock 1962, 296).

No European trade goods have been found in northern Caddoan sites in the Arkansas basin of eastern Oklahoma. The latest calibrated carbon-14 date ranges from the Fort Coffee phase—1597–1619 (TX-3927) and 1598–1619 (TX-3915)—indicate that the termination of the Fort Coffee phase and abandonment of the Arkansas basin may have been completed by ca. 1600–1650.

Carden Bottom Archaeology and the Quapaw Phase

From a point of view of ceramic styles, the archaeology of the middle Arkansas River and Carden Bottom localities is a distinctive amalgamation of Caddoan and Protohistoric Mississippian period ceramics that has been linked with the Quapaw phase (Hoffman 1977a, 1986; Jeter et al. 1989; Jeter, Cande, and Mintz 1990; House 1991). The Quapaw phase (Phillips 1970) was thought to represent the archaeological remains of the Quapaw people who moved into the lower Arkansas River region in Protohistoric times. Its affiliation with the Quapaw people has been recently called into question by Jeter, Cande, and Mintz (1990) and House (1991), because it appears there is a significant continuity in material culture between the Quapaw phase and Protohistoric Mississippian period occupations in the lower

Arkansas River region. Consequently, Jeter and colleagues (1990) propose the use of the taxonomic term *Menard Complex* rather than the taxonomic term *Quapaw phase* because the relationship between the historically known Quapaw peoples and the Quapaw phase remains unestablished (Jeter et al. 1989, 224), and in fact the Menard Complex may be more representative of a Tunican-Koroan group. Nevertheless, the Protohistoric period archaeology in Carden Bottom represents a Protohistoric occupation with a significant importation of Caddoan ceramics from the middle Ouachita River region, which were used locally as mortuary goods (Early 1990; House 1991; Hoffman 1986), but a contact record that is much different from that of the Caddoan Protohistoric sites to the south and west.

In terms of the settlement hierarchy, Protohistoric Menard Complex sites on the lower Arkansas River are compact villages, some of which have fortifications (Jeter et al. 1989, 229). Fortified Caddoan sites are unknown throughout the Prehistoric, Protohistoric, or Historic periods in the Caddoan Area. Civic-ceremonial centers of the Menard Complex include such sites as the Greer and Menard sites (Ford 1961; Phillips 1970) on the lower Arkansas River. They have plazas ringed by house mounds with a flat-topped platform mound at one end. However, above the Ozark escarpment at Little Rock, the contemporaneous Carden Bottom phase community system (Hoffman 1986, 25) appears to be a less complex version of the lower Arkansas River settlement system. That is, while there are compact villages on the Arkansas River above Little Rock, only one civic-ceremonial center, the Point Remove site (Davis 1967), is known above Little Rock and the Braden Bottoms in the Arkansas basin in eastern Oklahoma. It is unclear, moreover, to what time period the Point Remove site mound construction pertains to or what its cultural and taxonomic affiliation is (Hoffman 1986, 30).

Rock art area styles (Fritz and Ray 1982, 252) and specific ceramic vessel forms such as the Mississippian "head pots" (Mills 1968, vii) help to delimit the approximate extent of the Menard Complex (the Quapaw phase). It extends from the mouth of the Arkansas River to the Carden Bottom. From the ceramic associations seen in the burial clusters at the Kinkead-Mainard site (Hoffman 1977a, Fig. 1), the Goldsmith Oliver 2 site (Jeter et al. 1990), and those found at the Menard site and its vicinity (Ford 1961:171–180; House 1991), Protohistoric and Historic period occupations clearly are both present in the Carden Bottom locale and near Little Rock (Table 12).

The occurrence seriation of the five burial clusters at the Kinkead-Mainard site (3PU2), each cluster being associated with individual houses, is based on the presence or absence within each of the clusters of specific diagnostic ceramic types and stylistic mode dichotomies. Clusters 3 and 4 were combined in this analysis because they were not different in the pres-

TABLE 12. Occurrence Seriation of the Burial Clusters from the Kinkead-Mainard Site, Pulaski County, Arkansas

Types and Forms	Cluster 1 (5 burials)	Cluster 5 (4 burials)	Cluster 2 (10 burials)	Cluster 3/4 (35 burials)
Ceramic Types				
Keno Trailed	X	X	X	X
Natchitoches Engraved			X	X
Wallace Incised		X	X	X
Old Town Red	X	X	X	X
Vessel Forms				
Spool-neck bottle	X	X		
Hourglass-neck bottle			X	X[a]
Plain bottle				X
Plain effigy				X

Source: Adapted from Hoffman 1977a.

Note: X indicates presence. Clusters proceed left to right in estimated chronological order.

[a] A Type A, subtype 3, head pot (Mills 1968, 3).

ence or absence of specific ceramic types, though the percentage frequency differences between Keno Trailed and Natchitoches Engraved versus Wallace Incised and Old Town Red suggests that Cluster 3 is later, but not significantly later, than Cluster 4. The absence of Natchitoches Engraved in Clusters 1 and 5, in combination with the presence of Keno Trailed, support a general chronological estimate of 1600–1700 (see Table 9 and Jeter, Cande, and Mintz 1990). The broad stylistic similarity between household and burial clusters in the types of ceramic vessels used as grave goods evidences the apparently short time separating them.

The other burial clusters are subsequent to Clusters 1 and 5, but because of the lack of European goods, it is likely each probably lasted at the most only until ca. 1730–1740. The association of each of the burial clusters with individual houses and the number of burials with each cluster suggest that before sustained European contact domestic structures at the Kinkead-Mainard site may have been inhabited for shorter periods of time than they were after ca. 1680 or that mortality rates more than doubled after that time (Burnett 1990b, 1990c). Burial Clusters 1 and 5 contain three times fewer individual burials than do the later house structure cemeteries. Perhaps this represents a change in the size of the social unit inhabiting the structures; a reuse of particular structure areas for several succeeding generations; or, conversely, the result of major differences in burial practices between the two periods of occupation. Whether similar changes can be documented from other Menard Complex or Quapaw phase settlements is unclear, but post-1700 mass burials at the Douglas, Old River Landing, and Wallace Field sites (Ford 1961, 169 and Table 3) do point to significant changes in mortuary practices on the lower Arkansas River in Historic times.

Bioarchaeological analyses by Burnett (1990c) also indicate that Menard Complex populations experienced high subadult mortalities, a diminished adult longevity, and were characterized by chronic stress and nutritional deficiencies, all of which reduced the adaptive efficiency of these peoples. Burnett (1990b, 11–135) argues that these bioarchaeological data represent the cumulative effects of cultural disruptions and depopulation caused by contact and interaction between the Menard Complex populations and Europeans and from significant droughts in the area between 1549 and 1577 (Burnett and Murray in press).

Archaeological sites in the Carden Bottom area are too poorly known to discuss more specific Protohistoric and Historic period cultural changes. The infrequency of Natchitoches Engraved and/or European trade goods in the Carden Bottom locality (Hoffman 1986, Table 3.1) might be appropriate evidence to show that occupations there principally do not postdate the Protohistoric period. Brain (1985a, Fig. 5-3) reports that Clarksdale bells, artifacts considered to be good clues to the route of the de Soto expedition, have been recovered from the Carden Bottom, and Hudson (1990) places the Tanico province in this vicinity. Hoffman (1986, 28) also reports that copper wire bracelets, copper tinkling cones, and glass beads have been found in small amounts in Carden Bottom phase sites. The Protohistoric archaeological context of these apparent mid–sixteenth-century Spanish trade goods has not been clearly established, however.

Western Ozark Highland

In the western Ozark Highland, the Protohistoric period is represented by the Neosho phase (Freeman 1962). This phase is broadly contemporaneous with Fort Coffee phase settlements on the Arkansas River. Caddoan peoples in the western Ozark Highland during this time developed a seasonally mobile settlement system primarily around residential settlements where agricultural activities were concentrated (Wyckoff 1980, 343). From these agricultural settlements, Neosho phase peoples made seasonal forays into the more rugged interior country to hunt and collect available plant and animal foods, including bison on the nearby prairies. Rock shelters were used at these times for habitation and then later for storing edible foods.

These residential settlements were located in the larger river valleys along the Arkansas, Grand, and, perhaps, White rivers (Sabo et al. 1988, 90–92, 235–236).

Excavations at the Huntsville Mound (Sabo 1982, 1986) indicated that the final clay cap on the mound dated to the Neosho phase (date ranges calibrated to 1430–1674 or 1761–1795), but this is the only evidence for Late Caddoan or Protohistoric period mound construction on the western flanks of the Ozarks (Perttula 1984, 62). No information is available on what kind of Caddoan settlement, if any, was associated with this final episode of mound utilization.

Chapman (1980, 226) has argued that Neosho phase cultural materials in the western Ozark Highland strongly resemble cultural remains (particularly the ceramic assemblages) found in eighteenth-century Osage sites along the Missouri River. He postulates that there may be a cultural relationship between the development of the Osage tribe and the Neosho phase utilization of the western Ozark Highland. However, radiocarbon dates for the Neosho phase do not clearly extend into the eighteenth century. Relevant calibrated radiocarbon dates from the Neosho phase range from 1333 to 1339 to 1598 to 1618 (Table 13).

The carbon-14 dates reflect the fact that most of the western Ozark Highland was abandoned before the eighteenth century and probably even as early as 1600 in some areas. Therefore, the known Neosho phase occupations clearly date to before the earliest hunting and raiding incursions of the Osage in the Arkansas basin, which were characteristic of the mid-1700s (Chapman 1974). The Osage did not actually settle in the Arkansas River basin until ca. 1790 (Chapman 1982), which was a generation or two after the Arkansas River basin Wichita villages had been abandoned and settlements shifted to the Red River to avoid Osage harassments (Bell 1984b). Considering these data, there is little likelihood that the Neosho phase is related to the Osage tribe, but rather is instead more closely linked with the Fort Coffee phase settlements in the Arkansas River basin.

The identification of watermelon seeds (*Citrullis vulgaris*) from deposits in the Bontke Shelter in Southwest Missouri and the Beaver Pond Shelter in Northwest Arkansas (Cobb 1976; Fritz 1986a) may be more circumstantial evidence for the Protohistoric Neosho phase use of the western Ozark Highland. Watermelon, domesticated in the Old World, was introduced by Europeans to North America prior to 1680 (Blake 1981). The Caddoan tribes of East Texas were cultivating this crop at least by the late seventeenth century (Swanton 1942, 131). The contextual associations of these seeds are ambiguous (Fritz 1986a), but provided that the seeds are not intrusive they may have been deposited during the Protohistoric period utilization at these shelters by Neosho phase peoples.

TABLE 13. Radiocarbon Dates from the Neosho Phase

Laboratory Number	Site	Calibrated Age	Calibrated Range (A.D.)	Source
WIS-724	Bontke Shelter	536 B.P.	1338 ± 9, 1410 ± 20	Cobb 1976
O-2162	Jug Hill	544 B.P.	1365 ± 75	Wyckoff 1980
WIS-714	Bontke Shelter	617, 610, 549 B.P.	1343 ± 38, 1404 ± 17	Cobb 1976
UGa-3942	Albertson	513 B.P.	1455 ± 30, 1608 ± 10	Sabo 1986
O-2126	Jug Hill	427, 378, 324 B.P.	1547 ± 107	Wyckoff 1980
Beta-3973	Huntsville	429, 369, 327 B.P.	1552 ± 122, 1778 ± 17	Sabo 1986

SUMMARY

There are broad and basic similarities in the Protohistoric, or Early Historic, period (1520–1685) archaeological record in Northeast Texas and the Ouachita Mountains region of the western Caddoan subarea. During this period, both mound construction and shaft burials, marks of sociopolitical and ceremonial activities considered representative of vertical differentiation and hierarchical ranking in Caddoan societies, are discontinued shortly after the middle of the sixteenth century. Because absolute and relative means of chronological control are not refined for these areas, the best estimate is that these sociopolitical, religious, and status activities ceased by the end of the sixteenth century.

For the Protohistoric period in the Ouachita Mountains no evidence exists indicating that other forms of community sociopolitical integration evolved to replace the civic-ceremonial centers. Indeed, not much archaeological proof suggests that the Ouachita Mountains were even permanently inhabited by Caddoan peoples after ca. 1600, except along widely separated riverine locales draining into the Red River or in the Ouachita River valley itself.

In Northeast Texas, discontinuation of mound construction generally seems to be contemporaneous with formation of Caddoan supralocal or community cemeteries and with possible short-lived utilization of shaft burials at nonmound centers, especially in the Cypress Creek basin (Fig. 21). These differences in sociopolitical, ceremonial, and mortuary practices from ca. 1400 to 1700 point to a decrease in the overall complexity of community organization. This rearrangement in community organization is accompanied by a localization of these rural Caddoan settlement systems to fewer areas within the region. Examination of the detailed archaeological record in the Cypress Creek/upper Sabine River basin (see the appendix) suggests that these rural Caddoan communities may have been maintained to only around 1730 at the latest (Perttula and Skiles 1989; Thurmond 1990a). None of the communities in the Cypress Creek/upper Sabine River basin appear to have been ethnographically described, though, and most of what is known from ethnographic and archival documents pertains to the Nadaco or Anadarko Caddo. The groups who during the Allen phase occupied the Neches River drainage were direct ancestors of the Hasinai tribes who were living near the Spanish missions ca. 1691–1772, and they continued to maintain residence there until the 1830s. The Hasinai groups are the best-known Caddoan tribes from an ethnographic perspective (Swanton 1942; Griffith 1954), and the ethnographic and archival information about them is usually a major source of analogs for interpreting the regional archaeological record. The Protohistoric period archaeological record documents

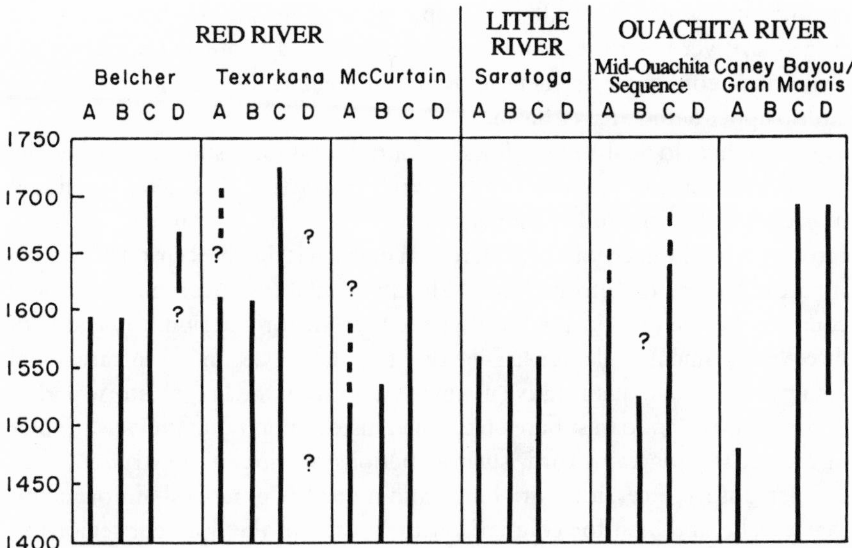

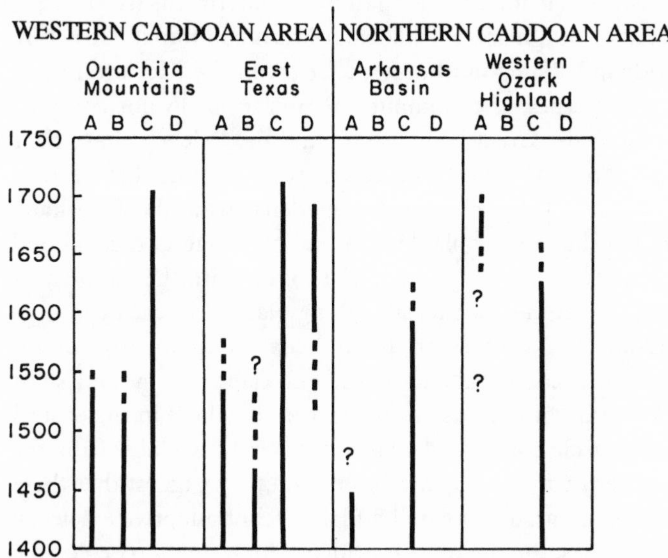

FIG. 21. Temporal trends in the archaeological record: *A*, mound construction; *B*, mound shaft burials; *C*, family cemeteries; *D*, community cemeteries.

significant changes in Caddoan sociopolitical complexity in the Neches and Angelina River basins. Mound construction ceased about 1600, but no supralocal or community cemeteries replaced them as they did in the Cypress Creek/upper Sabine River basin.

The archaeological record for the central Caddoan subarea during the period between ca. 1520 and 1685 reveals distinctive civic-ceremonial and mortuary behavior and prompts theories about how their uses changed through time in each of the different regions within the central Caddoan subarea. Not much information is directly available concerning settlement counts either before, during, or after the Protohistoric period, to be able to directly document or demonstrate either population decline or intraregional amalgamation in a quantitative manner. Analysis of the Protohistoric period in the central Caddoan subarea has relied instead upon qualitative variables in the archaeological record, such as periods of mound construction and use, the observed ceramic variability, and mortuary practices—information that can be obtained for comparison from each of the different regions to some extent. As measures of sociopolitical integration and vertical differentiation, mound construction and mound shaft burial interments (see Fig. 21) reflect the maintenance of a hierarchial sociopolitical community structure in the central Caddoan subarea until only ca. 1650. In the McCurtain and Saratoga phases, these types of community organization do not continue past ca. 1550, while in the Great Bend region and the Belcher phase their use evidently went through several phases of reorganization before they were finally discontinued. The archaeological evidence from the Texarkana phase is more limited, but the available information suggests that mound use in the phase continued to ca. 1690 (Creel 1991b), with the majority of the mound construction at the Hatchel site taking place after ca. 1500.

In the middle Ouachita River region, mound centers apparently continued to be used between ca. 1500 and 1650, but elaborate mound shaft burials were not a feature of their use as they were elsewhere in the central Caddoan subarea. Bioarchaeological data are fortunately available from the middle Ouachita River region (Burnett 1990b), and they suggest that these Caddoan populations maintained overall a high level of adaptive efficiency in the Protohistoric period, though there is evidence for a smallpox epidemic in the Social Hill phase (ca. 1500–1650) and increased adult mortality rates. By the Deceiper phase (ca. 1650–1700), the mean age of death by Caddoan adults had risen significantly and evidence of stress had declined.

The last periods of mound construction in the Saratoga phase are followed by the Protohistoric Caddoan abandonment of the Little River drainage. All other areas continued to be settled by Caddoan populations, typically in the form of small hamlets or farmsteads. Archaeological evidence suggests that Caddoan settlement began to be restricted to widely separated locales along the Red River and other drainages within what had once been a continuously and densely populated region. This type of regional settlement is consistent with a diminution in population during the Protohistoric period. In the middle Ouachita River region, intraregional community cemeteries of the Protohistoric period were intrusive burials in nonfunctional mounds. This type of mortuary practice was also seen in the Protohistoric Mississippian period in Northeast Louisiana, Southeast Arkansas, and the Felsenthal region of the Ouachita River drainage (Jeter et al. 1989; Schambach 1991).

In the northern Caddoan subarea archaeological sites postdating 1520 are restricted to only a few regions, most notably in the Arkansas River basin Fort Coffee phase in eastern Oklahoma. Radiocarbon dates and ceramic associations from the Fort Coffee phase suggest that much of the area was abandoned shortly after 1520, with total abandonment by ca. 1620. Limited archaeological evidence from the western Ozark Highland also points to the intermittent Caddoan use of the area during the Neosho phase, but again middle to late seventeenth-century assemblages are absent there as well.

Protohistoric period occupations in the general area are best documented from the non-Caddoan Menard Complex, or Quapaw phase, cultural materials on the Arkansas River (Hoffman 1977a; Jeter et al. 1989). A seriation of the burial clusters from the Kinkead-Mainard site indicate it was occupied generally ca. 1600–1700. The Keno Trailed ceramics from the earlier clusters (Hoffman 1977a, Fig. 10) resemble Keno Trailed var. McClendon (Schambach and Miller 1984, 123). This is the earliest defined Keno Trailed variety at the well-dated Cedar Grove site on the Red River and was found in a good Belcher phase context there in a burial lot dating ca. 1593–1644.

Hoffman (1977a, 21) had also noted that Keno Trailed vessels have been found in other sites on the Arkansas River north of the Kinkead-Mainard site that belong with the Carden Bottom phase. They cannot be definitively associated with a defined Caddoan, Mississippian, or Quapaw ceramic assemblage (Hoffman 1986, 28–29), and thus it is not possible to correlate them with relevant archaeological features and contexts. Between Historic period Quapaw phase occupations on the lower and middle Arkansas River and Wichita or Norteno phase occupations four hundred kilometers away near the Kansas and Oklahoma state line, no aboriginal sites on the Arkansas River contain European goods or can be demonstrated to have been occupied after 1730.

The trends in seasonal settlement mobility noted in the Fort Coffee phase (Rohrbaugh 1984; Wyckoff 1980) during the Late Caddoan period culminated in the abandonment of the area within a hundred years of initial and indirect contact between Europeans and Caddoan peoples. The temporal and spatial distribution of Womack Engraved in the Caddoan Area in the seventeenth and eighteenth centuries appears to reflect that the remaining Fort Coffee phase inhabitants were by this time already moving out to the prairies and south toward the Red River from the Arkansas Valley in eastern Oklahoma.

5 / The Archaeological and Ethnohistorical Record in the Caddoan Area, 1685–1800

The great Caddo Chief . . . is a man of more importance than Any other ten Chiefs on this Side of the Mississippi within my Agency.

—*Dr. John Sibley, 30 January, 1810*

This man (the Caddo Chief) is a very important Character & his Nation generally well behaved people, & the Nations to the West as far as River Grand Almost Entirely Under his Influence.

—*Dr. John Sibley, 29 May, 1813*

The Alibami Chief Unalabahola Said he was but a Young Chief & had But little to Say; But should look up to his Older Brother the Caddo Chief & should always be advised by him.

—*Dr. John Sibley, 6 October, 1813*

The archaeological and ethnohistorical record of the Caddoan Area between ca. 1685 and 1800 discloses the initial period of sustained and direct contact between Europeans and Caddoan populations. A key factor during this period is the overall process of regional abandonment and the redispersion of Caddoan populations, which relates to the development of the Hasinai, Natchitoches, and Kadohadacho confederacies. These confederacies represent areas where a number of ethnic entities joined together to forge and maintain a new and different Caddoan cultural identity. The process of aggregation may have begun before 1600 in some places, based on the regional Caddoan archaeological record, but because of the increasing importance of the French fur trade in the early to middle eighteenth century, Caddoan groups began to redisperse in the early eighteenth century to better hunting areas. After that time the remaining population aggregates on the Red River and in East Texas decreased further in size and complexity.

THE EUROPEAN PRESENCE

Direct European contact with Caddoan peoples begins at the time when Europeans actually lived among the Caddoan populations and/or had regular face-to-face meetings with them. Because the initiation of direct and sustained contact varied from place to place across the Caddoan Area, this phase of contact and interaction is only generally dated to ca. 1685–1800.

(Contact with Anglo-American settlers after ca. 1800 is discussed in chapter 2.)

The Spanish established a number of missions in East Texas between 1691 and 1722, with the last manned mission being abandoned by the Spanish government in 1772 (Gilmore 1978). The French established trading posts and forts on the Red River in the years 1714 (Natchitoches) and 1719 (Fort de St. Louis). In addition to these permanent settlements, traders, adventurers, and coureurs de bois lived among the Caddoan peoples, but their general illiteracy left little information to help us better understand the scope and range of their activities. By the 1750s it was reported that there was a French trader living at each of the different Caddoan settlements, even in Spanish Texas. Pichardo noted (Hackett 1931–1946, 3: para. 670), for instance, in commenting about the 1750s along the Spanish-French frontier "that in Natchitoches there are few inhabitants other than the French soldiers. . . . From Natchitoches to Cadodachos . . . it is about fifty leagues toward the NW. Between them are French settlements, as there are likewise at the said place of Cadodachos, though these French do not have fixed habitations, but only come and go to sell muskets and other things needed by the Indians, from whom they obtain annually about 100,000 lbs. of furs, as well as tallow and the oil of bears, buffaloes, and deer."

European populations were rather small throughout this period of sustained contact in the Caddoan Area. The 1690 establishment of missions among the Hasinai tribes in the Neches-Angelina river valleys in East Texas included only fifty soldiers, fourteen missionary fathers, and seven lay brethren (Morfi 1935, 152). The second phase of mission establishment in 1716 was accompanied by 125 soldiers and fewer than twenty religious authorities. In the French settlement of Natchitoches, the population as late as 1771 numbered less than one thousand, including over three hundred black, mulatto, and Indian slaves (Archivo General de Indias, Legajos 2357). The French garrison at the Natchitoches post did not exceed one hundred men until after 1730 (Morfi 1935, 247). Throughout the Spanish mission period the Los Adaes garrison was continually being reduced, and after 1730 the majority of the missions were abolished and the Spanish personnel removed to San Antonio. In the period between ca. 1685 and 1730, therefore, there were probably fewer than four hundred French and Spanish residents living in the Caddoan Area.

After 1730 the relative density of Europeans increased, but unlike earlier times, European settlement was concentrated along the Red River in the vicinity of Natchitoches and Los Adaes (Fig. 22). During the remainder of the eighteenth century and on into the early nineteenth century, European population increased primarily in the Red River Valley, particularly after

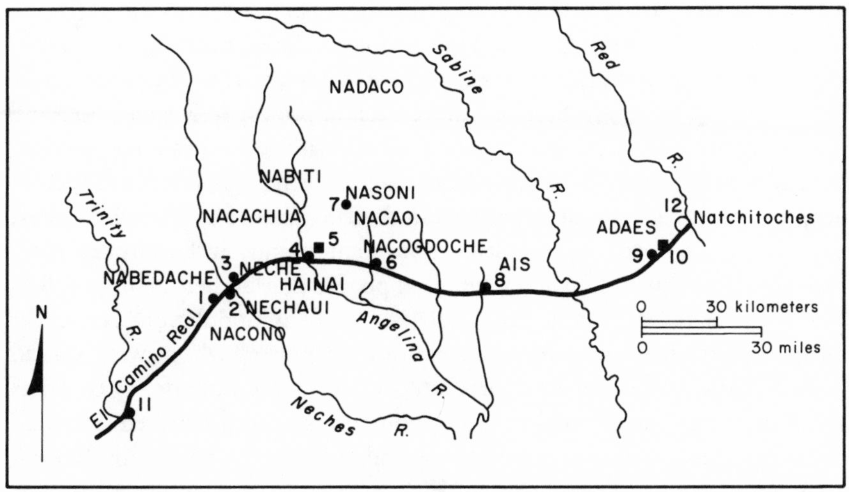

FIG. 22. European settlements and Caddoan groups in East Texas and Northwest Louisiana, 1690–1779: (1) Mission San Francisco de los Tejas, 1690–1693; (2) Mission El Santísimo de Nombre María, 1690–1692; (3) Mission Nuestra Padre San Francisco de Tejas, 1716–1719, 1721–1730; (4) Mission Purísima Concepción, 1716–1719, 1721–1729; (5) Presidio Nuestra Señora de los Dolores de los Tejas, 1716–1719, 1721–1730; (6) Nuestra Señora de los Nacogdoches, 1716–1719, 1721–1772; (7) Mission San José de Nazones, 1716–1719, 1721–1730; (8) Mission Nuestra Señora Dolores de Ais, 1716–1719, 1721–1773; (9) Mission San Miguel de los Linares de los Adaes, 1716–1719, 1721–1773; (10) Presidio Nuestra Señora del Pilar de los Adaes, 1721–1773; (11) Nuestra Señora del Pilar de Bucareli, 1773–1779; (12) Natchitoches, 1714–present.

the Anglo-Americans began settling in Louisiana and Texas (Strickland 1937; Steely 1986; Watkins 1984). In Spanish East Texas European populations after 1730 were living mainly at Nuestra Señora de los Nacogdoches and from 1773 to 1779 at the civil settlement of Nuestra Señora del Pilar de Bucareli on the Trinity River. After 1779 and the abandonment of the Bucareli settlement, the Spanish community of Nacogdoches became an important fur and livestock trade center, because many Indians preferred to do business there instead of in Natchitoches (Bolton 1914, 1:75; Jackson 1986). Nacogdoches became the distribution point for most of the Caddoan groups in Spanish East Texas of the annual presents given by the Spanish after 1767 in the Louisiana and Texas provinces (John 1975, 622).

In terms of absolute numbers of people and number of settlements, therefore, the Europeans' presence was a moderate one; however, their presence was unfortunately accompanied by the continual introduction of acute epidemic diseases, at least one every generation from 1739 to 1877 (Ewers 1973, Table 1), among the Caddoan peoples. These epidemic diseases reduced their population about 80 percent between 1691 and 1772 (see Figs. 8 and 9). In 1691, there may have been approximately eight thousand Caddo living in the Caddoan Area compared with fewer than one hundred Europeans. By 1772, there may have been only half that many Caddoan peoples living and about fourteen hundred Spanish and French settlers. Even as late as 1830, the largest European community in East Texas, Nacogdoches, had fewer than seven hundred people (Berlandier 1969, 10). Berlandier estimated the Caddo and Tejas (i.e., Hasinai) populations in 1828 at thirty-two to thirty-three hundred, more than half of whom were Caddo or Kadohadacho and living near Caddo Lake on the boundaries of Texas and Louisiana. The Hasinai groups' populations ranged between sixty and three hundred, with the Nacogdoche and Ais groups having the largest populations.

The Caddoan Historic Period from Archaeology and Ethnohistory

The archaeological and ethnohistorical records of the late seventeenth and eighteenth centuries document patterns of cultural change in Caddoan lifeways during the period of initial direct and sustained contact with Europeans and Anglo-Americans. The Historic Caddoan archaeological record, however, is less comprehensive and systematic than the record for the period between 1520 and 1685,[1] and consequently, I rely here on such archaeological components as the Deshazo and Cedar Grove sites (Story 1982, n.d.; Trubowitz 1984), which are well known, to examine processes of cultural change that have broad regional and systemic implications. The ethnohistorical record is also selectively explored for trends in colonial and Caddoan economies, changes in colonial Indian policy, and population and settlement differences noted among Caddoan groups. My purpose is to use those means available to understand and describe Historic Caddoan lifeways and to explore the archaeological record to determine how and when significant changes in Caddoan societies occurred.

Initially important is establishing from the archaeological record the temporal parameters of Historic period Caddoan occupations. Caddoan archaeological sites postdating 1685 can theoretically be identified by three methods: (*a*) using radiocarbon, archaeomagnetic, and thermoluminescence (TL) measures for absolute dating of the archaeological deposits, (*b*) using ceramic seriations from closed contexts (Table 14), and (*c*) using direct contextual association from temporally diagnostic European trade goods found with the aboriginal Caddoan assemblages. By itself, no one method is sufficient to identify Caddoan archaeological sites dating after 1685.

Excavations at Caddoan settlements dated reliably after 1685 by absolute

TABLE 14. Ceramic Stylistic Forms Present in Post-1685 Archaeological Assemblages

Region/Phase	Keno Trailed	Natchitoches Engraved	Foster Trailed-Incised	Simms Engraved	Hudson Engraved	Womack Engraved	Patton Engraved	Head Pots and Human Effigies	Teapot Forms	Fatherland Incised	Nodena or Old Town Red on White	Emory Punctate	Avery Engraved	Estimated or Absolute Age
Quapaw	X	X	X					X	X	X	X			1650–1800
Middle Arkansas[a]	X	X						X			X			1700–1730
Upper Arkansas[b]	X							X						1700–1730
Glendora	X	X	X			X	X		X	X	X			1700–1760
Tunica/Trudeau	X	X	X							X		X[c]		1731–1764
Lawton	X	X							X	X		X		1714–1800
Chakanina	X	X	X	X									X	1700–1750
Little River	X	X	X	X								X		1719–1780
Middle Red	X	X	X	X	X	X			X			X	X	1700–1730
Hunt	X			X										Pre–1730
Kinsloe	X	X		X			X					X		1700–1835
Norteno		X		X		X						X		1700–1780
Allen				X			X						X	1650–1750

Note: X indicates presence.

[a]Based on the Kinkead-Mainard site (Hoffman 1977a).

[b]The Carden Bottom phase (Hoffman 1977a, 1977b, 1986; Mills 1968).

[c]Winterville Incised var. Tunica (Brain 1979, 234–235) and Emory Punctate-incised are post-1700 stylistic developments of Foster Trailed-Incised (Schambach and Miller 1984, 121–122).

methods suggest that European goods are uncommon among Caddoan peoples as late as 1730 and, hence, that their presence or absence cannot be relied upon to conclusively identify post-1685 Caddoan occupations (Trubowitz 1984). Caddoan aboriginal ceramics remain the most common artifact found in late seventeenth- and eighteenth-century occupations in Spanish Texas and French Louisiana, even at settlements established by the Europeans (Corbin 1989; Corbin, Alex, and Karlina 1980; Corbin et al. 1990; Miroir et al. 1973). The presence of distinctive horizon-marker Caddoan ceramic styles in the Historic period archaeological record, the occasional association of these ceramic styles with European goods, and the employment of absolute dates can create a reliable chronology (Schambach and Miller 1984, Table 11–12; Williams and Early 1990). The Cedar Grove chronology, in particular, is of considerable utility in ordering Protohistoric and Historic Caddoan assemblages in such locales outside the Great Bend of the Red River as the Mid-Ouachita region of southwest Arkansas.

Stylistic varieties of Natchitoches Engraved and Keno Trailed are the most common ceramic markers for the post-1685 period (Schambach 1983), but there are also regional and temporal differences within the Caddoan Area and adjacent regions in the Historic period ceramic assemblages. The lower Arkansas, Ouachita, and Red rivers share certain ceramic types with post-1685 archaeological sites in the Natchez bluffs and Yazoo basins of the lower Mississippi Valley (see Phillips 1970; I. Brown 1983; Brain 1978b, 1989; Kidder 1990b; Jeter, Cande, and Mintz 1990). Caddoan sites post-dating 1685 from the Great Bend of the Red River to the Neches River in East Texas contain Simms Engraved or Emory Punctated-Incised with the local Historic period horizon markers Patton Engraved (in the Allen phase), Natchitoches Engraved, or Keno Trailed types (Suhm, Krieger, and Jelks 1954, 219–227), but the common Red River domestic ware Foster Trailed-Incised is absent (see Table 14).

The presence of ceramic stylistic forms that are dominant in one region but found in only limited quantity in another is good evidence of intraregional contact between contemporaneous Caddoan groups. It helps establish a Historic period chronological sequence of wider applicability. Absolute duration of archaeological phases in the post-1685 Caddoan period are, however, still poorly differentiated.

Nature of the Record

The Historic period archaeological record in the Caddoan Area can be characterized as (*a*) low in regional density and (*b*) spatially discontinuous as compared with the distribution of 1520 archaeological phases and 1520–1685 Caddoan settlements (Fig. 23). Approximately seventy post-1685 Historic period components are described in the literature, but only a few are known from other than a burial context (Story 1990, Table 85; Jeter et al. 1989).[2] Excavations at the Deshazo (Story 1982), Cedar Grove (Trubowitz 1984), and Kaufman-Williams (Perino 1983; Skinner et al. 1969) sites indicate that Historic period Caddoan settlements were typically small, dispersed farmsteads and hamlets with an associated household cemetery (Figs. 24 and 25).

Most sites were apparently occupied for only short periods of time, perhaps an average of twenty to forty years, based on the analysis of structure rebuilding episodes at more intensively studied sites (Good 1982, 67–69). Cemeteries are generally not large either, containing fewer than ten individuals at both the Deshazo (Story 1982) and Cedar Grove (Trubowitz 1984, 97–108) settlements and seventeen to twenty-two individuals at the Clements and Hunt sites (Lewis 1987; Jackson n.d.a, n.d.b). At a few Caddoan sites on the Red River, such as Sam Kaufman–Bob Williams or Hatchel-Mitchell, larger cemeteries dating as late as ca. 1700 indicate that other Caddoan groups established larger and/or more continuously and intensively occupied settlements.

While a single farmstead might only include one or two structures, the community (or *ranchería*) was composed of many farmsteads, as described by Father Douay in 1687: "It is at least twenty leagues long, not continuously settled, but with rancherias of ten or twelve huts" (quoted by Pichardo in Hackett 1931–1946, 1: para. 361). Joutel ([1713] 1906, 141–142) also noted among the Hasinai this type of settlement: "By the way, we saw several cottages at certain distances, straggling up and down, as the ground happens to be fit for tillage. The field lies about the cottage."

Among the Hasinai, individual families lived in their farmstead, or *ranchito,* and a number of *ranchitos* were organized into *rancherías* spread out over about fifteen to thirty leagues (about forty to eighty miles—a league is equivalent to 2.76 miles or 4.44 kilometers [Wedel 1978, 2]) around public buildings used by the tribal leaders. For example, as described by Morfi (1935, 87), in 1716 the Nacogdoche Indians were "divided into 22 rancherias . . . which spread for a distance of 10 leagues from South to North . . . the Ais, consisting of 70 families, settled in 8 rancherias occupying a distance of two leagues."

Each *ranchería* was separated from the others by unoccupied lands and hunting territory. When the Spanish established their missions among the Hasinai tribes they were always placed in the center of the *ranchería* where most of the people lived in an attempt to consolidate the aboriginal populations in the vicinity of the mission.

On the Red River, archaeological evidence suggests that Historic period

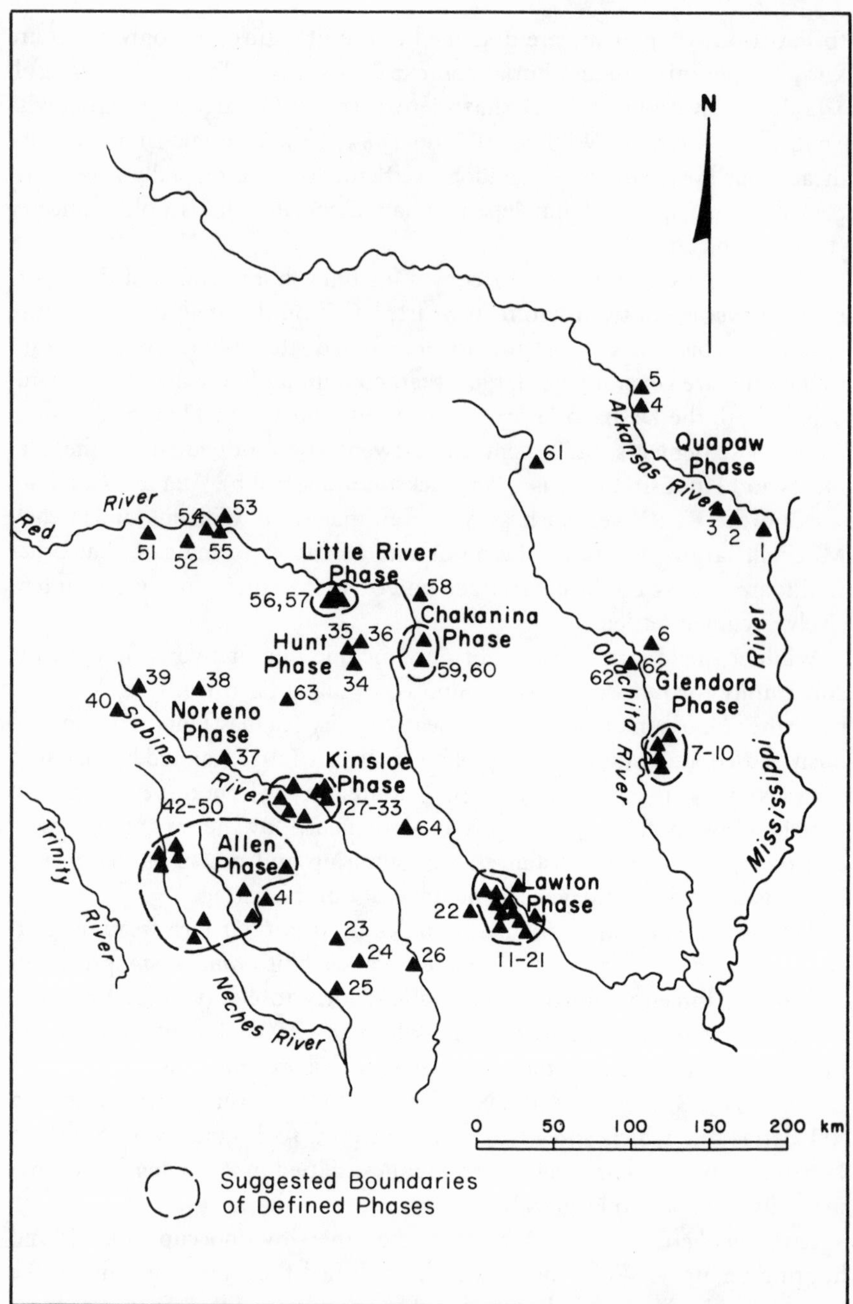

FIG. 23. Post-1685 Caddoan settlements and suggested boundaries of defined phases.

FIG. 23 KEY

Key (asterisk indicates Quapaw phase settlements [Hoffman 1986])

1. Menard* (Ford 1961)
2. Douglas* (Ford 1961)
3. Greer* (Phillips 1970)
4. Moore's Bayou* (House and McKelway 1983)
5. Kinkead-Mainard* (Hoffman 1977a)
6. Gee's Landing (White 1970)
7. Moon Lake (Gregory 1973)
8. Keno (Moore 1909)
9. Glendora (Moore 1909)
10. Pargoud Landing (Gregory 1973)
11. U.S. National Fish Hatchery (Walker 1935)
12. Southern Compress and Oil Mill (Gregory and Webb 1965)
13. American Cemetery (Gregory 1973)
14. Lawton Gin (Webb 1945)
15. Natchitoches Country Club (Gregory 1973)
16. Settle's Camp (Gregory 1973)
17. Drake's and Little Cedar Creek (Gregory 1973)
18. Chamard (Gregory 1973)
19. Wilkinson (Ford 1936)
20. Allen (Ford 1936)
21. Bois d'Arc Creek (Gregory 1973)
22. Los Adaes (Gregory 1973)
23. Mission Dolores de los Ais (Corbin, Alex, and Karlina 1980)
24. Buckley (Jelks 1965)
25. Wylie Price (Jelks 1965)
26. Coral Snake (Jensen 1968)
27. Ware Acres (Jones 1968)
28. C. D. Marsh (Jones 1968)
29. Susie Slade (Jones 1968)
30. Brown (Jones 1968)
31. Cherokee Lake (Jones 1968)
32. Millsey Williamson (Jones 1968)
33. Taylor (Clark and Ivey 1974)
34. Atlanta State Park (Harris, Harris, and Miroir 1980)
35. Clements (Jackson n.d.a; Dickinson 1941; Lewis 1987)
36. Hunt (Jackson n.d.b)
37. Woldert and 41WD331 (Woldert 1952; Perttula et al. 1986; Perttula and Gilmore 1988)
38. 1973S (41WD206) (Skiles, Bruseth, and Perttula 1980)
39. Gilbert (Jelks 1967)
40. Pearson (Duffield and Jelks 1961)
41. Deshazo (Story 1982)
42. San Pedro (Newell and Krieger 1949)
43. Allen (Cole 1975)
44. Mayhew (Story 1982; Kenmotsu 1987a)
45. King (Story 1982)
46. Patton (Cole 1975)
47. Jewell (Cole 1975)
48. Owens (Cole 1975)
49. Cecil (Cole 1975)
50. Freeman (Cole 1975)
51. T. M. Sanders (Krieger 1946)
52. Womack (Harris et al. 1965)
53. Roden (Perino 1981)
54. Old Wright Plantation (Skinner, Harris, and Anderson 1969)
55. Sam Kaufman–Bob Williams (Skinner, Harris, and Anderson 1969; Perino 1983)
56. Roseborough Lake (Miroir et al. 1973; Gilmore 1986a)
57. Eli Moore, Hatchel, Mitchell (Wedel 1978; Jackson 1932)
58. Crenshaw (Gregory 1973)
59. Spirit Lake (Hemmings 1983)
60. Spirit Lake locality: Cedar Grove, Friday, Shaw-Russell, McClure, Battle, Rube Russell, Lester Bend (Schambach et al. 1983; Trubowitz 1984)
61. Watermelon Island, Gum Springs, Friendship (Hodges and Hodges 1943, 1945; Hodges 1957)
62. Shallow Lake (Rolingson and Schambach 1981; Hemmings 1982)
63. 41CP71 (Thurmond 1981; Bell 1981)
64. Louis Procello (Espey, Huston, and Associates, Inc. 1983)

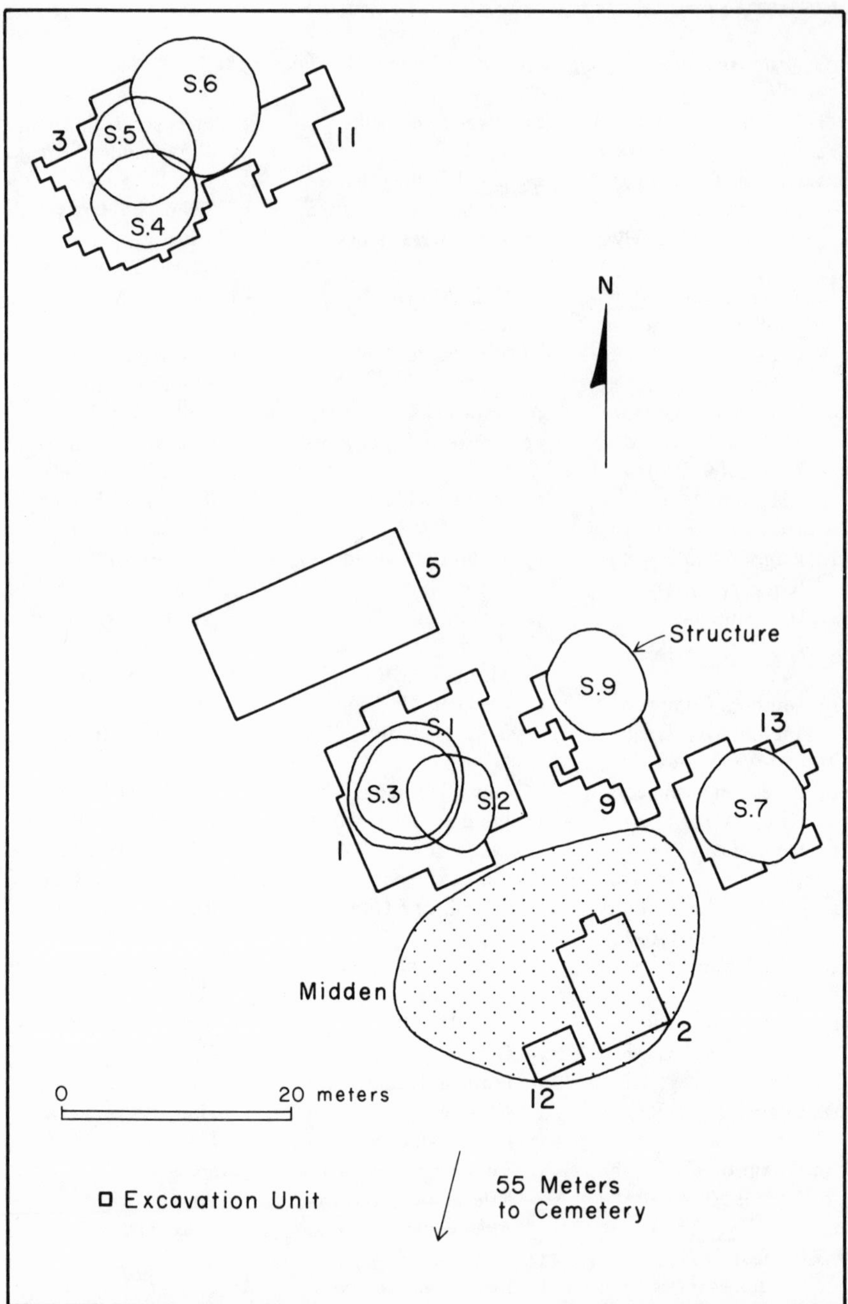

FIG. 24. Settlement plan at the Deshazo site, Nacogdoches County, Texas (after Story 1982, Fig. 11).

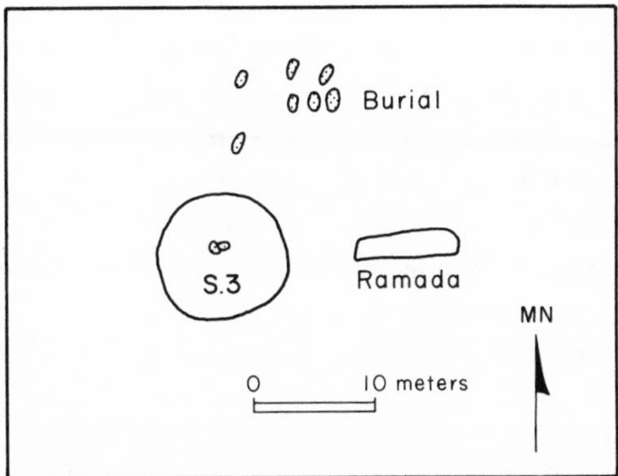

FIG. 25. Chakanina phase settlement at the Cedar Grove site, Lafayette County, Arkansas: *S*, structure; *MN*, magnetic north.

Caddoan dispersed farmsteads were associated together in a manner similar to that of the small communities described above. One such community mapped by Domingo Terán de los Ríos in 1691 covered an area on the order of five to fifteen kilometers on either side of the river (Schambach et al 1983, 120–121). The Spirit Lake locality (see Fig. 23) is about fifteen kilometers in length; ten Caddoan habitation sites dating to the Historic Caddoan period are known in that locality (Schambach and Miller 1984). The Hatchel-Mitchell-Moore-Tilson complex and the Kaufman–Roden–Wright Plantation complexes are similar Historic period *rancherías,* with settlements extending for about ten kilometers in length along the river (Creel 1991b; Bruseth and Perttula 1991). Other such communities may well have existed in other parts of the Caddoan Area, where clusters of sites dating after 1685 have been found (Story and Creel 1982, 30–33; Perttula 1991, Table 4; Williams and Early 1990), but their presence has not been documented archaeologically.

This type of settlement was actually mapped in 1691–1692 by Don Domingo Terán de los Ríos during his expedition to the Kadohadacho (Hatcher 1932). This particular *ranchería* settlement has been identified by Wedel (1978) as corresponding to the Hatchel-Mitchell-Moore-Tilson archaeological locality in Bowie County, Texas. The settlement covered between four to nine kilometers on both sides of the Red River, and was divided into individual compounds (analogous to *ranchitos*) each containing one to three structures, an above-ground granary, and an outdoor ramada or arbor (Fig. 26). Thirty-six structures, family and caddi[3] residences, were present, though some may have been abandoned or were of temporary construction. Scrutiny of Figure 26 indicates that there were several compounds with no granaries, which would be an unlikely occurrence if the farmstead were a permanent residence then in use by a Caddoan family. If there were indeed thirty-six families contemporaneously occupying this *ranchería* on the Red River, then it was much larger than those previously described in East Texas. Only five to ten families per *ranchería* were noted for the Hasinai tribes in East Texas (see above). This is a significant difference, given the probability of population amalgamation in the Historic period for the large Red River Caddo communities.

If this type of extended settlement was present before 1540 (see discussion of the Terán-Soule model in Schambach et al. 1983), differences in the absolute size of the *ranchería* between precontact, Protohistoric, and Historic period Caddoan occupations can be expected to have changed and/or varied as a reflection of regional population densities and processes of aggregation. Thus, the difference in the number of families in East Texas versus Red River Caddoan *rancherías* ca. 1690–1720 does not necessarily imply a greater regional population on the Red River. Rather, the ethnohistorical records suggest that there were actually more separate but smaller *rancherías* among the Hasinai groups, as opposed to fewer, but larger communities among the Kadohadacho and aggregated tribes on the Red River. Two factors can probably account for the larger size of the Red River Caddo *rancherías;* (*a*) the population amalgamation of groups within the Kadohadacho "confederacy" and (*b*) village nucleation in response to Osage harassments along the exposed frontier of French Louisiana and Spanish Texas (Williams 1964, 550).

While these types of discrete communities or extended settlements of Caddoan peoples can be identified in the archaeological record for the late Historic period, they appear to represent the archaeological remains of what were only widely separated groups between other areas already abandoned and devoid of settlement at ca. 1685 (Fig. 27). Of the Historic period cultural phases recognized in the Caddoan Area, only the Lawton, Allen, Little River, and Chakanina phases can be reasonably affiliated in any degree with eighteenth- and nineteenth-century Caddoan groups mentioned in the French and Spanish ethnographic descriptions (see Swanton 1942):

Lawton phase	Natchitoches confederacy
Allen phase	Hasinai confederacy
Little River phase	Upper Nasoni village in Kadohadacho confederacy
Chakanina phase	Kadohadacho confederacy

There is some evidence that there are also clusters of Historic Caddoan sites in such areas as the upper Neches, upper Sabine, and Cypress Bayou drain-

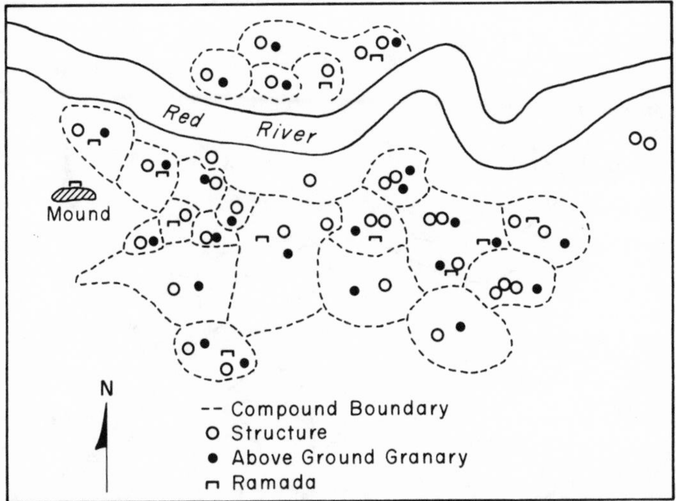

FIG. 26. Detail of a Caddoan community, or *ranchería,* on Red River, mapped 1691–1692 by Don Domingo Terán de los Ríos. Community covers no fewer than four kilometers and as many as nine kilometers along Red River (Schambach 1983, 7).

ages, which have no apparent ethnographic or ethnic associations (Perttula 1991, Fig. 5). That is, there are no specific ethnographic descriptions that appear to be applicable to these clusters of Historic Caddoan Indian period settlements (Bolton 1908).

REGIONAL EXPRESSIONS

Arkansas and Ouachita River Basins

The Arkansas and Ouachita river basins outside of the lower Mississippi River Valley appear to have been emptied or abandoned by ca. 1680. In the Arkansas basin, Wichita groups such as the Taovayas, Tawakoni, and Yscani had begun to migrate downstream from south-central Kansas by 1600 (M. Wedel 1982, 1988). By 1700 the Mento Wichita band was only a six day's journey from the Quapaw (who lived near the mouth of the Arkansas River), perhaps being located near present day Tulsa, Oklahoma (M. Wedel 1981, 21, 30). These Wichita bands[4] were horse dealers and bison hunters, and they had developed a mobile if seasonally sedentary settlement system by the eighteenth century. Their movement into this part of the Arkansas River basin was to lead to further French exploration of the

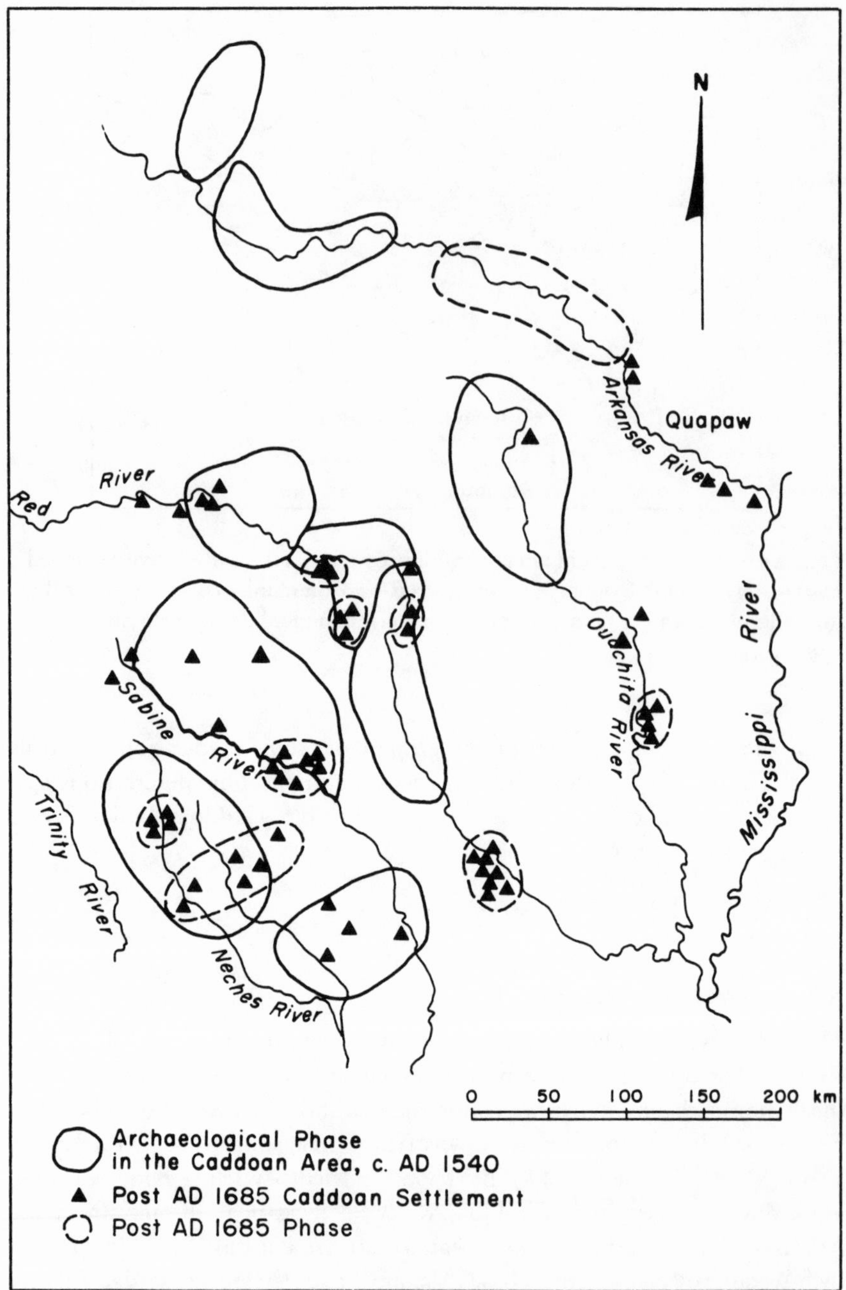

FIG. 27. Spatial relationship between archaeological phases and post-1685 Caddoan settlements: *solid lines* enclose Caddoan Area archaeological phases, ca. 1540; *dotted lines* enclose post-1685 phases; *triangles* indicate post-1685 Caddoan settlements.

upper Arkansas basin, starting with Bénard de la Harpe and Du Tisne in 1719 (M. Wedel 1971, 1972, 1973), and to attempts to institute regular and profitable trade relationships with these Wichita tribes.

There is no eighteenth-century map or documentary evidence that suggests that Caddoan groups were still living on the Arkansas River or its tributaries between Little Rock and Fort Smith, and the Kichai (or Quidehais) (M. Wedel 1979, 190) had apparently already moved out of eastern Oklahoma by then as well (Rohrbaugh 1982, 60–61). Du Rivage in 1719 noted that the Kichai spoke a Caddoan dialect but were nomadic bison hunters possibly living on the upper Red River at that time. The ready ability of these Wichita groups to occupy the Arkansas River basin in eastern Oklahoma was considerably facilitated, then, by the fact that previous Caddoan residents of the region had already abandoned it (Rogers in press).

Whether there was an eighteenth-century Caddoan occupation in the middle Ouachita basin is unknown because of unit definition problems, multicomponent occupations, and the overall lack of systematic archaeological research until very recently (Williams and Early 1990). Published reports of burial excavations (Hodges and Hodges 1943, 1945; Hodges 1957) indicate that diagnostic eighteenth-century ceramic types are present at a few sites, but the occupational context is unclear. For instance, Keno Trailed, Natchitoches Engraved, and Hodges Engraved (see Table 14) do occur in burials with Mid-Ouachita phase ceramics (Friendship Engraved, Military Road Incised, Blakely Engraved, and the Watermelon Island seed jar) (Hodges 1957, fig. 1). Keno Trailed var. McClendon and var. Glendora have also been identified (see Webb 1959, Fig. 112a,c,h), as have Hodges Engraved var. Armour and var. Candler (Webb 1959, Fig. 108a,c,e,h), from Mid-Ouachita basin collections. As previously noted, the last three varieties are common at the Cedar Grove site in the eighteenth-century Chakanina phase occupation.

In the Deceiper phase occupation at the Hardman site, shell-tempered Keno Trailed, Hodges Engraved, Simms Engraved, and Karnack Brushed-Incised ceramics occur in a context that Early (1990) dates to between ca. 1650 and 1700. The Deceiper phase occupation of the Mid-Ouachita basin apparently represents the region's terminal Caddoan occupation, which ended abruptly prior to any sustained contact with Europeans (Williams and Early 1990, 2–13).

European trade goods are not known in the Arkansas portion of the Ouachita River Valley, with the exception of a mid-seventeenth-century–style glass bead from a Deceiper phase burial at the Hardman site (Williams and Early 1990, 7–44). There is evidence of significant interregional contact between Caddoan groups along the mid-Ouachita River and Menard Complex groups along the Arkansas River. Early (1990, 13–27) indicates this began about "the same time as the De Soto expedition," and this contact appears to have been based on salt trading.

Historic period Glendora phase occupations are concentrated around the confluence of Bayou Bartholomew and the Ouachita River in northern Louisiana (see Fig. 23). The Glendora phase occupations appear to all date prior to 1730 and include Caddoan, Natchezan, and Tunican vessels in a diverse ceramic assemblage that probably evolved out of a Coles Creek, Plaquemine, to Tunica continuum (Kidder 1986; Kidder 1988, Tables 18–24; Belmont 1985; Gibson 1985b; Rolingson and Schambach 1981). Yazoo Bluffs pottery found at the Keno Site (i.e., Cracker Road Incised var. Crackerroad) also attests to additional contacts with aboriginal peoples living in that part of the lower Mississippi Valley (I. Brown 1983). A burial from the late Chakanina phase occupation at the Cedar Grove site contained a Natchitoches Engraved jar believed to be from the Keno-Glendora locality (Schambach and Miller 1984, 140–141), indicating that these occupations in the Boeuf basin may date as late as the early to mid-eighteenth century (see Table 9).

The Glendora phase used to be considered a Historic period Caddoan manifestation representative of the Ouachita Caddo because of the dominance of Keno Trailed and Natchitoches Engraved ceramic types among burial goods (Moore 1909; Williams 1964). Examination by Kidder (1988) and others of the unillustrated pottery have led them to note that these occupations also have Yazoo bluffs, Natchez, and upper Tensas basin ceramic varieties that were more likely the local domestic wares, and thus the Caddoan vessels are more likely to have been imports from the Red River and the middle Ouachita River (Hally 1972; Weinstein and Kelley 1984; Jeter 1986; Kidder 1988, 1990a, 1990b). If these settlements are those of the Historic period Tunican peoples, their location would be in general accordance with the late seventeenth- to early eighteenth-century ethnohistorical records (Swanton 1946, 13; Dickinson 1980, 7) on the respective location of Caddoan and Tunican groups in the Ouachita River basin.

Overall differences in 1687, 1700, and later ethnohistorical records in the relative geographical relationship between Cahinnio and Ouachita Caddo, and Tunica and Koroa groups show that there was a general movement south (and/or west) (Kidder 1987, 1988, 1990b) before 1730, and an eventual abandonment of the area as new salt and horse trade opportunities were developed (Brain 1979, 265). Jean Filhiol, the commander of the Post du Ouachita at the confluence of the Ouachita River and Bayou Bartholomew, noted in 1786 that "the nation which inhabited it [the Ouachita River] formerly must have been very populous. We do not know what became of it; the oldest people of the place do not remember ever having seen a single one of them" (Rickey 1937, 476).

The cemetery excavated at Gee's Landing (see Fig. 23) was apparently intrusive into a Mississippian period Gran Marais phase midden (Rolingson and Schambach 1981, 189–193) and contained vessels of the Wallace Incised, Keno Trailed, and Hudson Engraved types (see Table 14), indicating a very late seventeenth-century occupation. Cultural similarities to the Glendora phase burials at Glendora and Keno (Moore 1909, 27–80, 120–151) are evident, except that burials at Gee's Landing contained no European trade goods (White 1970). Thirty-four burials were in the Gee's Landing cemetery compared with 121 at Glendora and 255 at Keno. However, evidence of earlier Mississippian settlement at the last two sites suggests that a significant portion of the burials in the cemeteries pertain to a different, and earlier, occupation (see Moore 1909, fig. 133, 134, 139, 140, for example, and Kidder 1990b, Fig. 4). Only eighteen burials at Glendora contained European glass beads and sheet brass, whereas similar European trade materials were found in twenty-one burials at the Keno site. The lack of more specific burial contextual information prohibits the association of more aboriginal burials, containing no European trade goods, with the remainder of those that do have trade goods.

The Hodges collection from the middle Ouachita River (Webb 1959; Early 1986) further attests that eighteenth-century Caddoan peoples still lived in the middle Ouachita basin, though by 1690 they had apparently already moved a hundred kilometers downstream, primarily to the Camden, Arkansas area. The Cahinnio Village in the Camden area was described by Joutel in 1687 (Margry 1877–1886, 416): "the cabins of this village are all assembled together, to the number of 100 or thereabouts, unlike those of the Cenis [Hasinai], the Assonis [Nasoni], and others that we had formerly seen scattered out." Only one Cahinnio Caddo village was described, and ethnohistorical records do not suggest there were other villages. This one village was at least three times larger than the one upper Nasoni *ranchería* described by Terán in 1691–1692 (see Fig. 26).

If the melding of styles, technologies, and vessel forms seen in the Caney Bayou phase ceramic assemblage from the lower Ouachita River is any indication of ethnic identity (Kidder 1990a, 74–76), there was an amalgamation of diverse groups within the Ouachita River basin who then remained in the valley until ca. 1720. Ethnohistorical records suggest that the Cahinnio and Ouachita Caddo, possible ethnographic analogues to the upriver Protohistoric peoples attested to in the archaeological record, had left the area by then (Swanton 1942, 50). The Cahinnio Caddo were living with the Kadohadacho on the Red River in 1700, whereas most of the Ouachita Caddo had gone to live with the Natchitoches sometime between 1690 and 1700.[5] In 1700, in fact, Bienville and St. Denis reported that the Ouachita village had only five cabins (Swanton 1942, 50).

Recent excavations at One Cypress Point in the Felsenthal region by the Arkansas Archeological Survey have recovered what may be a distinctive Historic period Quapaw hunting camp (Hemmings 1982, 178–185). The assemblage of lithic tools—mainly scrapers and large knives—is suggested to be an early regional expression of the developing lower Mississippi Valley fur trade. No European trade goods or diagnostic aboriginal ceramics were found at the site. Instead, the assemblage is composed almost entirely of stone tools and Nodena projectile points. The most conspicuous class of stone tools present are large flake and bifacial scraping implements. This type of stone tool assemblage is not characteristic of Prehistoric or Protohistoric Caddoan occupations in the Ouachita River basin but has also been noted at Quapaw settlements on the lower Arkansas River and elsewhere in the lower Mississippi Valley at that time (Williams 1980).

By 1685 Quapaw groups had begun to move into the sparsely populated lower Ouachita River basin and into Southeast Arkansas in general (Jeter 1986) to exploit salt and other natural resources as part of their commerce with the French at Arkansas Post (Joutel [1713] 1906). If it could be determined when the Quapaw began to exploit the Ouachita River basin, it might be possible to understand the rate or tempo of the Caddoan and Tunican abandonment of the region.

Red River Basin

Historic period Caddoan occupations along the Red River cluster in several localities. The highest density of known archaeological sites is around Natchitoches and the Spanish presidio/mission established at Los Adaes in 1719 (Gregory 1983) (Fig. 28). These historic Caddoan archaeological sites are thought to be ethnically related to a number of Caddoan groups who lived around the French trading post at Natchitoches and at Spanish Los Adaes (Webb and Gregory 1978, 17–33). Attempts at archaeological identification of Caddoan tribes in Louisiana has not been very successful, however, simply because the records on tribal locations and village composition are limited to only a few areas (Kniffen, Gregory, and Stokes 1987) and the archaeological record of the Historic period is sporadic in comparison to that of the Prehistoric record.

Consider that Natchitoches Engraved, for example, is one of the most common ceramic types on all Caddoan historic sites around the Natchitoches post, whether the sites are identified as Natchitoches, Adaes, or Doustioni occupations. This type has a wide distribution throughout the Caddoan Area (Harris and Harris 1980). The same can be said for the Caddoan ceramic type Emory Punctated-Incised. The farther the tribal group from European centers such as Natchitoches or Los Adaes, the less likely such ethnic identifications become when they are based principally on subtle

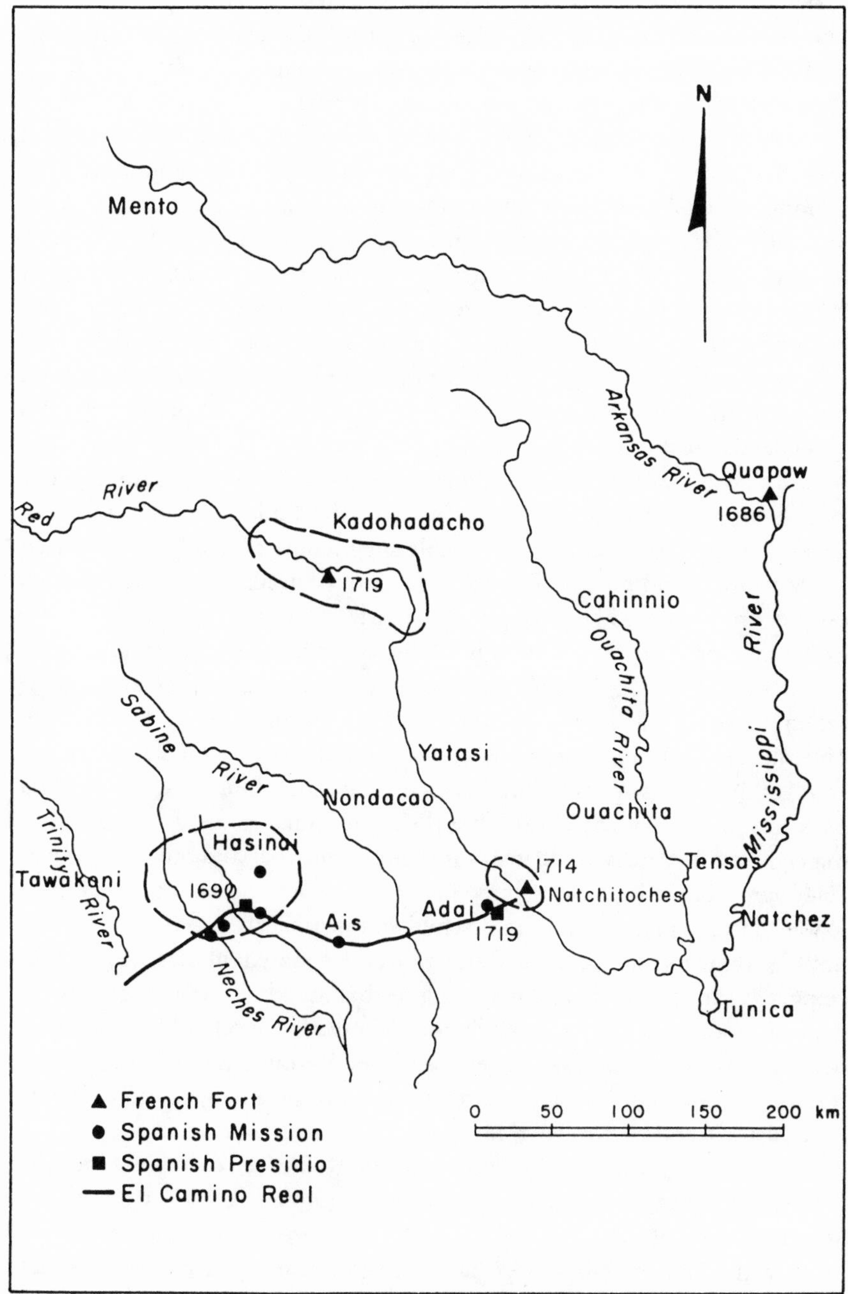

FIG. 28. Late Historic period European settlement and the location of certain ethnographically recorded aboriginal groups (after Swanton 1942).

variations in decorated ceramic assemblages. To obviate this problem, Corbin, Alex, and Karlina (1980, 210–214) proposed specific "intra-drainage ceramic traditions." These were based on associated decorated ceramics, primarily Natchitoches Engraved, and on specific types of tempered wares (i.e., bone versus grog or shell-tempered wares) that could be correlated with the Lawton, Kinsloe, and Allen phases and the areas around Mission Dolores de los Ais in the Angelina drainage (see Fig. 23). These differences in temper within the same types, however, are not only inconsistent with the use of the type-variety system as it is applied in the Caddoan Area, but may just as easily be temporal or technological rather than ethnic (Schambach and Miller 1984, 124). For instance, Schambach and Miller (1984, 124) note that "a distinction should be made within Natchitoches Engraved, not between shell or no shell, but simply between fine temper of any kind and coarse—really coarse—shell temper. It seems to us that the very latest vessels, those that turn up on full historic sites with abundant trade goods and that clearly date to the sunset years of the Caddo ceramic tradition, generally have very coarse, easily visible shell temper. Usually they are also crude in form and design. This is crude pottery in all aspects because the ceramic tradition was beginning to fall apart."

Another problem in attempting ethnic identifications utilizing ceramic types or attribute sets (Brain 1989) is the widespread exchange and importation of aboriginal ceramics by the Caddo to the Spanish and French. Not only did the Caddo peoples apparently manufacture ceramic flatwares that were influenced by Spanish and French ceramics (Corbin, Alex, and Karlina 1980, 214; Gregory 1973, 126), but their traditional ceramics were a thriving eighteenth-century trade item for the Natchitoches and other Red River Caddoan groups. Because of these factors, it is difficult to argue that, as a whole, specific material culture assemblages necessarily equate with recognizable ethnic units. That some distinctions are apparent in these eighteenth-century ceramic assemblages may suggest that an ethnic coherence existed, which is poorly defined as yet and not manifest in such other historic period occupations as the more heterogenous Caney Bayou and Glendora phases, resulting from population movements and group amalgamations in the Protohistoric and Historic periods.

Historic occupations in this section of the Red River continued into the nineteenth century until the majority of the Caddoan people left Louisiana after the treaty of 1835 (Flores 1984; Williams 1964, 558). The establishment of the French trading post at Natchitoches in 1714 prompted other Caddoan groups to settle there to better gain, manipulate, and control access to French trade. The importance of the location of the French fort at Natchitoches and the Lawton phase associated with the French settlement is that it was established outside the area where the Late Caddoan and

Protohistoric period Belcher phase people seem to have lived (see Fig. 27). Thus, Caddoan groups moved downriver, outside the "traditional" Caddoan Area, to facilitate trade relationships with Europeans and non-Caddoan peoples (Gregory 1973, 293). Based on the archaeological record from the Belcher site, which has the best record of Belcher phase settlement, this movement could have taken place any time between ca. 1600 and 1700. Even as the Natchitoches community became established around the French fort, the native population in the region continued to decline, from about eighteen hundred people in 1700 to less than seven hundred by 1720 (see Fig. 8 in Chapter 3). This decline was accompanied by direct French trade expansion on the middle Red and Arkansas rivers, which supplanted native middlemen in these regions and offset the dwindling contribution of the Natchitoches to French commerce, outside horse trading, after 1720.

Peltry from the Caddo had already been obtained from the Red River district around Natchitoches in 1716 (Archives Nationales, Colonies, Serie C-13, vol. 4, fols. 355–365). By 1725, the contribution of the Red River Caddoan tribes amounted to about 3 percent of the peltry trade in New Orleans (Surrey 1916, 346). While Caddoan participation in the fur trade may have continued to increase through the eighteenth century, the actual Caddoan contribution to the French and Spanish Louisiana economy continued to decrease relative to that of the Arkansas (or Quapaw), Osage, and Illinois groups.

As a measure of their relative importance, in 1770, we can examine the lists of Indian presents distributed by the Spanish to the Texas and Louisiana provinces (Kinnaird 1949, 148). Of the 3,755 pesos distributed to native Americans, only 378 pesos were distributed to the Caddoan tribes, 49 of which went to the Natchitoches. By comparison, over 33 percent of the presents were distributed to the lower Mississippi Valley tribes, principally the Arkansas (or Quapaw) (515 pesos) and the Tunica (122 pesos). In the Illinois province over 1,600 pesos worth of goods were distributed to the Indians.

The historic European sites located around the Bénard de la Harpe post (Fort de St. Louis), and the later Grappe trading post and military garrison probably established by St. Denis, are contemporaneous with eighteenth-century Caddoan settlements at the Hatchel-Mitchell-Moore site complex (Wedel 1978, 15; Creel 1991b). Caddoan occupations spanning the majority of the eighteenth century can be demonstrated from the Roseborough Lake site, Area B (Miroir et al. 1973), identified by Wedel as being affiliated with the Nanatsoho Caddo (Wedel 1978, 8). Prior to 1719 the Nanatsoho had apparently lived ten leagues (27.6 miles) farther upstream (Wedel 1978, 6) but had more recently moved to be closer to the upper Natchitoches, upper Nasoni, and Kadohadacho groups already congregated at the upper end of the Great Bend on the Red River. Following the establishment of the French trading post or garrison, there appears to have been a short-term local increase in population density because of the incorporation of Caddoan groups from both north and south of the Red River. The fort was maintained as a trading post until the 1770s (Gilmore 1986a), and the main Kadohadacho town remained in the vicinity of the fort, even after it was deactivated with the cession of the area to the Spanish after 1762.

The Chakanina phase (Trubowitz 1984; Schambach et al. 1983) presumably represents the archaeology of one of the two more recent Kadohadacho villages situated in the Great Bend of the Red River ca. 1700–1790. Other than the presence of Keno Trailed var. Phillips vessels in collections from the Red River midway between the Spirit Lake and the Hatchel-Mitchell-Moore complexes (Schambach and Miller 1984, 123), only in the Spirit Lake locality can post-1650 Caddoan Historic period occupations be clearly demonstrated in this part of the Great Bend.

Epidemics in 1777 and continued Osage depredations (Bailey 1973, 40; Wiegers 1988) contributed to further Kadohadacho regional population decline and to an eventual abandonment of the area about 1790. The continuing amalgamation of population remnants of different Caddoan tribal groups, as attested to in the ethnohistorical literature, is another facet of Historic period changes in these groups' size and social organization. These records indicate that in 1690 there were apparently five villages, or *rancherías,* of Caddoan peoples in the Great Bend area, three villages or *rancherías* after 1719, and only one by 1790 (Swanton 1942). That community was located in the area around Caddo Lake west of Shreveport, Louisiana (Flores 1984, 145, 168).

The Hunt phase sites had been tentatively identified as late eighteenth-century Kichai occupations by Williams (1964, 564); however, the limited number of European trade goods, particularly glass beads, and the infrequency of Natchitoches Engraved in the Hunt phase ceramic assemblages suggest that these sites must date to before the mid-eighteenth century (Gregory 1973, 154). Therefore, no specific Caddoan ethnographic descriptions can be applied to this small cluster of Historic period settlements in the Sulphur River drainage.

One of these settlements, the Atlanta State Park site (41CS37) was definitely occupied between 1700 and 1740, and it is located near the portage of the Nasoni described by de la Harpe in 1719 (Harris, Harris, and Miroir 1980). In 1719 the Nasoni lived north of the Sulphur River on the Red River. However, the approximate location of the Hunt phase is in the same general area as the Nissohone province described by de Soto (see Fig. 2 and discussions in chapter 2). Given this apparent geographical continuity between the Nissohone province and the Nasoni Caddo's early 1700s location, the Hunt phase probably represents the Historic period expression of that lower Sulphur River Caddoan group. Control of the Nasoni portage was important in the early eighteenth century because of its position at a major stream crossing on the Caddo Trace between the Hasinai and Kadohadacho confederacies. Therefore, the lack of a Caddo Historic period settlement there after about 1740 implies that the importance of the Nasoni portage decreased after that time and/or that the Nasoni were no longer able to effectively control its use.

The last group of Historic period Caddoan occupations on the Red River was between the mouth of the Blue River and the area around the mouth of the Kiamichi River. Except for the Womack site (Harris et al. 1965), those sites all date to before 1700–1720, based on associated glass bead types, the presence of Keno Trailed var. Phillips, Quapaw phase or Menard Complex trade materials, the lack of Natchitoches Engraved, and a general scarcity of European goods (Perino 1981, 1983; Skinner, Harris, and Anderson 1969).

The Kaufman-Williams site (41RR16) has a number of small Historic period household cemeteries and associated structures, and the latest occupation at the Roden site in McCurtain County, Oklahoma, was contemporary with the Caddoan settlements across the river. A colleague and I (Bruseth and Perttula 1991) have suggested that the Kaufman-Williams and Roden sites may have been part of the same community, in the sense of the upper Nasoni Caddo village described by Terán de los Ríos in 1691. Perino (1978, 75), commenting about the Williams site Historic period occupation, observed that "trade material is very sparse at the site. Collectors have found three or four burials with small numbers of blue glass beads. . . . Metal objects are rare and consist of a few pieces of sheet brass and copper. One circular item seems to have been a small coin hammered thin. Only a half dozen gunflints of the French variety have been found in the area."

The Womack site, occupied between ca. 1700 and 1729 (Harris et al. 1965), represents a Caddoan settlement or hunting camp of a group already heavily involved in the French fur trade (Gregory 1973, 247). While the period of maximum trade for deer hides between the Caddo and the French appears to be after 1740, even by 1716 some peltries were obtained from the Red River area (Surrey 1916, 335). For instance, in 1725, one thousand skins of the French Louisiana peltry trade derived from the Caddoan Red River groups (Surrey 1916, 346). This was part of the twenty-five thousand skins shipped to France in that year from Louisiana. In 1744, by contrast, one hundred thousand deerskins were shipped to France, plus buffalo skins (Archives Nationales, Colonies, Serie C-13a, vol. 28, fol. 35–36).

At sites such as Womack, the archaeological assemblage is dominated by items reasonably associated with hunting and hide preparation. This includes native-manufactured stone end and side scrapers, large knives or bifacial cutting tools, projectile points, iron knives, numerous gun parts, lead shot, and native and French gunflints (Fig. 29). These types of locations also are generally characterized by trade goods probably derived from the French as payment for skins (Gregory 1973, 242). They may have been hunting camps returned to on a regular but seasonal basis. Another candidate for a hunting camp, One Cypress Point on the Saline River in the Felsenthal region (Hemmings 1982), dates to before dependence on the horse in hunting and before implementation of the French policy of sending out resident traders to the seasonally maintained hunting camps. A lithic tool assemblage dominated by stone arrow points, end scrapers, and large bifacial knives (see tool *h* in Fig. 29) marks this distinctive, and possibly Quapaw, hunting encampment.

A similar archaeological example from the Yazoo basin of the lower Mississippi River Valley includes a distinctive lithic assemblage from the Historic period Russell phase (Brain 1978b). At the Russell site (22-N-19), large thumbnail end scrapers, bifacial scrapers, and projectile points dominate the 1682–1706 Tunica assemblage (Brain 1975a, 42). Late seventeenth-century and early eighteenth-century Natchez assemblages from the Natchez bluffs area (see tools *i* and *j* in Fig. 29) have a similar indigenous lithic technology (Brown 1985, 185). By the early to middle eighteenth century, however, iron and copper implements became available to the Natchez in sufficient quantities that their lithic technology was not maintained.

European goods at the Womack site are mainly derived from contact and trade with the French (see chapter 6 for a discussion of bead types and nationality associations). The great similarities in bead styles, for instance, between the Womack site and the Little River phase about one hundred kilometers downstream suggest that payments and traders derived from the French-controlled Fort de St. Louis.

Bolton (1915) discusses another French post located on the lower Kiamichi River in 1767 that is a probable French hunting enterprise. From these temporary quarters, French traders and trappers made their forays. Gregory (1973, 243) notes that the "French hunters operated from the Natchitoches post on a sort of share cropper basis. Men were outfitted with French firearms, flints, powder and shot, to go to the vicinity of the Wichita to hunt hides."

East Texas

The area between the Sabine River and Red River, except for the Gilbert and Pearson sites at the headwaters of Lake Fork Creek and the Sabine River, respectively (see Fig. 23), essentially has no post-1700 Caddoan archaeological record.[6] The Gilbert and Pearson sites are not strictly contemporaneous, but together they represent most of the middle to late eighteenth

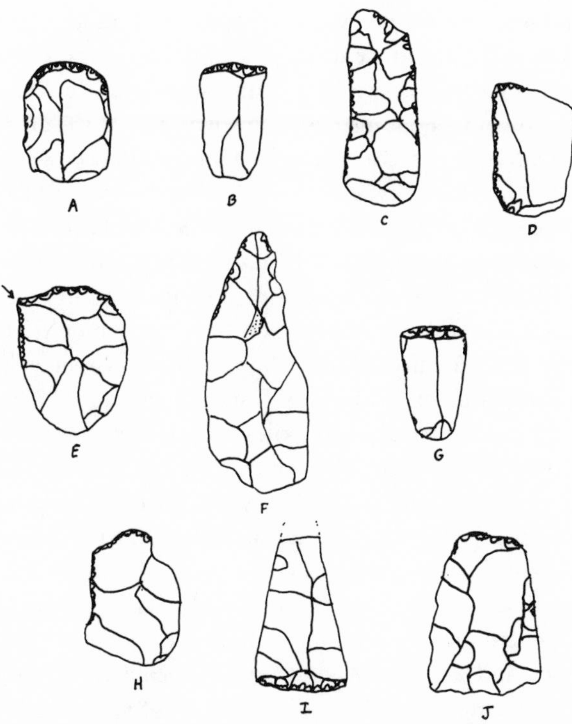

FIG. 29. Examples of eighteenth-century lithic tools, illustrated full size, from Caddo, Norteno Wichita, Tunica, Quapaw, and Natchez sites: *A,* Gilbert site end scraper (Jelks 1967, Fig. 70a), 1740–1770; *B,* Gilbert site end scraper (Jelks 1967, Fig. 71f), 1740–1770; *C,* Gilbert site knife (Jelks 1967, Fig. 72j), 1740–1770; *D,* Womack site side scraper (Harris et al. 1965, Fig. 2k), early eighteenth century; *E,* Womack site snub-nosed scraper with graver beak (Harris et al. 1965, Fig. 3a); *F,* Oliver site triangular knife (Brain 1988, Fig. 199ii), ca. 1700; *G,* Oliver site snub-nosed end scraper (Brain 1988, Fig. 199rr), ca. 1700; *H,* One Cypress Point site bifacial cutting tool (Hemmings 1982, Fig. 48g), ca. 1600–1700; *I,* Antioch site bifacial end scraper (Brown 1985, Fig. 84f), late seventeenth century; *J,* Trinity site biface (Brown 1985, Fig. 115f), early eighteenth century.

century. The presence of English Brandon flints at the Pearson site probably indicates that the site was also occupied after 1780 (Kenmotsu 1987b, 1990). The artifact assemblages from the sites appear also to be representative of Historic Caddoan hunting camps (Gregory 1973, 239–252). There is likely an association with Fort Le Dout or La Doutte (Gilmore and Foret 1988), possibly a French trading post whose date of founding and exact location are unknown, except that it was probably on an upper tributary of the Sabine River (Campbell 1976, 306; Perttula and Gilmore 1988).

This western aspect of the Caddoan Area, along the post oak Savanna and blackland prairie ecotone, was reoccupied by Caddoan hunting groups mainly in the late eighteenth century, probably as a result of their fur trade expansion into a habitat where large game animals were abundant. Before reutilization of the upper Sabine basin, this was part of the area between the Hasinai and Kadohadacho confederacies that Bolton (1908:251) described as "uninhabited territory between the upper Angelina and the Red River."

Archaeological information from the upper Sabine basin has documented that both Caddoan and southern Wichita-speaking groups lived in the area during the eighteenth century. A significant concentration of Caddoan Historic period components have been found on the Sabine River and tributaries in the general vicinity of major Sabine River crossings known in the Anglo-American period as Trammell's Trace (Jones 1968; Webb et al. 1969; Clark and Ivey 1974; Perttula and Skiles 1989). Archival information suggests that these Caddoan groups were the Nadaco or Anadarko. Scholars believe these people remained there until at least 1790 because Vial and Fragoso placed them near what is Cherokee Bayou, Rusk County, Texas, in 1788 (Nasatir and Loomis 1967, 344).

Possible Caddoan Historic period archaeological sites in the Lake Fork Creek drainage, Sabine River basin, include the Woldert site (41WD333), sites 41WD331 and 41WD206, and several localities recently discovered near the Woldert site (Perttula and Gilmore 1988; Perttula et al. 1986, 1988). The Woldert site[7] and 41WD331 are located on Mill Race Creek, about one kilometer north of the confluence of Lake Fork Creek and the Sabine River (see Fig. 20). Site 41WD331 had limited Historic European trade goods—beads and gun barrels—as well as artifacts of native Caddoan manufacture, but the Woldert site had copper and brass fragments, iron knives, iron hatchets, approximately fifteen hundred glass trade beads, lead balls, fragments of mid-eighteenth-century French flintlock musket or fusil barrels and gun parts (Hamilton 1980), an undated silver coin, and a copper cross (Woldert 1952, 484). The quantity of European-manufactured goods at the Woldert site and other nearby localities, the association with a Historic Caddoan settlement immediately downstream, and the archival information all suggest that a mid-eighteenth-century French "factory" or hunter camp was probably located near Lake Fork Creek and its tributaries (Bolton 1915; Campbell 1976; Perttula and Skiles 1989).

Norteno phase archaeological sites are present at the western end of the upper Sabine basin at the Gilbert (Jelks 1967) and Pearson (Duffield and Jelks 1961) sites. Archival and archaeological data indicate that these sites were occupied beginning in the mid- to late eighteenth century and were probably specialized hunting camps of Tawakoni, Yscani, and Caddoan peoples involved in the fur trade (Gregory 1973).

It is suspected that Norteno groups were sufficiently mobile at this time, because of the diffusion of horses across the southern plains, to carry hunting forays from the prime bison grounds into the prairie-woodland border. The presence of Womack Engraved from 41WD206 in the Lake Fork Creek basin and at the Culpepper site (Scurlock 1962) in Hopkins County, both Titus phase occupations, suggests that Norteno and Titus phase groups were partially contemporaneous and interacted to some extent. Neither 41WD206 nor the Culpepper site contains European trade goods, though, and the period when there was Norteno and Titus phase interaction has not been clearly ascertained. The suspected interactions between Caddoan and southern Wichita-speaking groups in the late seventeenth and early eighteenth centuries and possible temporal and spatial variations within the Norteno phase (Story 1985b, 90) hint that these relationships are manifestations of a complex process.

The *ranchitos* of the Kinsloe phase from the middle Sabine River basin Historic period and the household cemeteries associated with them have been described by Jones (1968). The Nondacao province mentioned by the de Soto *entrada* was in this same general locality (see Fig. 2), as were the Nondacao or Nadaco group in the eighteenth century, according to ethnographic records. Other than this territorial relationship, there is not much that can be said about the Historic period Caddoan use of the middle Sabine River because the habitation pattern is an aspect the archaeological record of this area fails to disclose. Earlier Titus phase mounds and shaft burials have been recorded (Webb et al. 1969), along with a scattering of Titus phase settlements on tributary streams (such as Potters Creek), but their regional significance and sociopolitical relationship to the remainder of the Titus phase remains unclear. Based on the archaeological data in the Cypress Creek basin immediately to the north, the Kinsloe phase may represent a spatial contraction of a Sabine River cluster that would be analogous to the Cypress Creek cluster, as defined by Thurmond (1981, 1985, 1990a).

Sometime between 1542 and 1717 Nadaco Caddo settlements were split between those on the Sabine River and the more recent settlements in the vicinity of the Nacao Caddo in the Angelina River drainage. A 1717 map by John Senex entitled "A Map of Louisiana and the Mississippi River" sets the southern Nadaco group near the Hasinai tribes. On the map is the notation: "Nadacoe destroyed by the Chicachas in 1714." The "Chicachas" may be the Chickasaw—the Chickasaw had already begun to raid the Caddo and the lower Mississippi Valley tribes by 1714 (Stubbs 1982; White 1983). Also depicted on the 1717 Senex map are two arms or forks of the Sabine River west of the Caddo Ais and Adai tribes. These arms probably represent the Sabine River and Lake Fork Creek, its largest tributary. According to the Senex map there were no aboriginal groups located on this part of the Sabine River in 1717.

In 1752 the Tebancanas, or Tawakoni, were described by the Nasoni Indians of the Hasinai confederacy as living about twenty leagues (about fifty-five miles) northwest from the upper Angelina River (Johnson and Jelks 1958, 414). This would place the Tawakoni village on the Sabine River near its confluence with Lake Fork Creek. As previously mentioned, the Tawakoni were one of the Wichita groups that had begun to move out of the Arkansas River basin south to the Red River between 1742 and 1757—because, in part, of Osage harassments—and on into the Sabine River Valley about the same time (Wedel 1982).

Visits by Fray Calahorra (1760) and de Mézières in the 1770s (Bolton 1914, 1 : 206–220) placed the Wichita groups on the Sabine River and tributaries along the prairie-woodland margins of East Texas. No historical documentation suggests that Wichita groups lived farther east in the Sabine Basin, however. Fray Calahorra is fairly specific in placing the associated Tawakoni-Yscani villages "on the other side of the other arm of the Sabinas [Sabine River]" (Johnson and Jelks 1958, 412). This "other arm" of the Sabine River was described by Fray Calahorra as a creek with "an abundance of water in pools," but it was not a permanently flowing stream in May 1760 when the journey from the Nacogdoches mission was made.

In 1770 some of the Wichita groups had moved to the Trinity and Brazos rivers north and west of the Camino Real, but it is likely that the upper Sabine River basin was still occupied by some of these Nortenos even though their main villages were twenty-five to thirty leagues (sixty-nine to eighty-three miles) to the south-southwest. This supposition is based on the archaeological evidence from the Gilbert and Pearson sites near the headwaters of Lake Fork Creek and the Sabine River, respectively (Jelks 1967; Duffield and Jelks 1961), since the types of European trade goods present there indicate some occupation after ca. 1780.

When Pedro Vial traversed the upper Sabine River basin in August 1788 he apparently followed the Tawakoni-Taovayas trail from the Red River to the Sabine River crossing (see Bolton 1915) in East Texas. He did not note any aboriginal settlements along the route once he left the Taovayas village near present-day Spanish Fort, Texas (Bell, Jelks, and Newcomb 1967) until he reached a Nadaco Caddo village near, but west of, the Sabine River (Nasatir and Loomis 1967, 342–345). Apparently this group of Nadaco Caddo had not been destroyed by the "Chicachas" in 1714.

From the Sabine River crossing southeast to the Nadaco village was a distance of 25.5 leagues, approximately seventy miles (Nasatir and Loomis 1967, 344–345). The village had thirteen to fifteen houses scattered over a distance of three leagues, but the houses were evidently distributed along tributaries of the Sabine River because the second Sabine River crossing by Vial was five to six leagues to the east of the village (Nasatir and Loomis 1967, 346). The presumed location of the Nadaco Caddo village in 1788 is in the same general locality as the Nondacao province mentioned by the de Soto *entrada* (see Perttula et al. 1986).

European trade goods recovered from such sites as Ware Acres (41GG1), Millsey Williamson (41RK3), and Taylor (41RK36) (on tributaries of the Sabine River, including Rabbit Creek and Martin Creek) are associated with post-1760 Nadaco settlements in the vicinity of the second Sabine River crossing by Vial (Jones 1968). The occurrence of a special bell (var. Flush-loop) (Brown 1979a, 201) and black English Brandon gunflints suggests that the Nadaco continued to live on the Sabine through the first quarter of the nineteenth century (see Ewers 1969, 138).

In the Neches River drainage the archaeological data evidence a territorial continuity between Protohistoric and post-1680 Caddoan occupations (see Figs. 27 and 28). This is exemplified by the Frankston and Allen phases in the upper reaches of the Neches and Angelina drainages in East Texas (Story and Creel 1982, 30–34). As previously mentioned, the Allen phase represents the archaeological remains of at least some of the Hasinai tribes, whose prehistoric Caddoan ancestors are identifiable as part of the Frankston phase. This particular phase extends back to ca. 1400 (Kleinschmidt 1982).

In comparing the ethnographically recorded locations of the Hasinai groups to the locations of post-1685 Caddoan archaeological sites in the Neches and Angelina River drainages, two points are apparent: first, that fairly specific Caddoan ethnic affiliations may be feasible for the Allen phase components in proximity to El Caminos Reales (Corbin 1991) and, second, that Allen phase components in the upper Neches River basin cannot be presently affiliated with any known Caddoan group, "band," or tribe. It is suspected that the Allen phase components in the upper Neches River basin primarily date to before 1730.

In this area beginning in 1690 the Spanish established a series of missions and presidios among the native Caddoan groups as part of the settlement of East Texas and as a buffer against French exploration and colonization of the region (see Fig. 22). The province of Tejas was abandoned, however, in 1693 by the Spanish because of a host of difficulties, most notably ill-will and a lack of cooperation from the Caddoan inhabitants in the area (Swanton 1942, 47–50).

The *conna,* or shaman, of the Hasinai tribes "had convinced the Indians that the waters of baptism were fatal to them, because most of those who were baptized in articulo mortis died. . . . Father Massanet deplored deeply that the Indians refused to believe that there was but one God. He explained that the Indians declared there were two: one who gave the Spaniards clothing, knives, hatchets, and all the other things they had; another who gave the Indians corn, beans, nuts, acorns, and rain for their crops. They had lost all respect for the priests and had on various occasions threatened to kill them" (Castañeda 1936, 1:373).

As part of the Spanish colonial policy in the Provincias Internas, mission establishments were located where aboriginal populations were the largest, and then the missionaries attempted to force the native American converts of Christianity to live in nucleated mission settlements (Bolton 1917; Thomas 1988). This early attempt at Caddoan resettlement and conversion had failed, as did subsequent Spanish attempts at controlling the East Texas Indian tribes. Because the effects of the missions in East Texas were not overtly socioeconomic or socioreligious in nature (Bolton 1915, 100–101), they were not the inducement to population resettlement that the French system of trade and presents was (Sabo 1987, 37–38). As Fray Benito Hernández de Santa Anna noted in 1731, "as each family of the Texas Nation lives separately in its own ranchito—they left them [the missionaries] alone, or came and went without settling down. They [the Texas Indians] often come to have the padres cure their deer-skins" (Pichardo in Hackett 1931–1946, 3:para. 421).

The Texas governor de Barrios y Jáurequi (1751–1759) had said about the success of the Spanish mission versus French trade policies that "no Cadohadacho, Nacogdoches, San Pedro (Nabedache) or Texas Indian is to be seen who does not wear his mirror, epaulets, and breech clout—all French goods. And now, for the winter, they are giving them blankets, breech clouts, powder, and shot. Hence these nations say: The Spaniards offer fair words; the French fair words and presents" (Pichardo in Hackett 1931–1946, 3:para. 402).

Spanish frontier policy was explicitly based on a restriction in trade among the Hasinai tribes in an attempt to force native dependence upon the missions for supplies (Bolton 1914, vol. 1). Poor and unreliable means of supply transport to frontier provinces and the proximity of the French at Natchitoches and New Orleans, however, all helped to economically insulate the Hasinai Caddo from any measure of Spanish mission control. They continued to maintain communities or *rancherías* of dispersed farmsteads into the nineteenth century[8] and later under the Republic of Texas government (see chapter 2).

Following the initial Spanish abandonment of the missions, the French colony of Louisiana initiated a concerted exploration of the Hasinai Caddo country in an attempt to develop strong trade with them. Le Moyne d'Iberville explored the Red River area in 1700, and Bienville and Louis Juchereau de St. Denis did the same in 1700 (Swanton 1942, 50–51). The establishment of the Compagnie des Indies in 1712 systemized the commercial ventures of the French in the lower Mississippi River Valley and resulted in "the expansion of the French frontier toward the valley of the Red River" (Giraud 1974a, 333). In 1714 St. Denis established the Natchitoches post at the abandoned 1702 Natchitoches village and commenced the French involvement in the profitable trade of salt, pelts, and horses that the Hasinai, Kadohadacho, and Tunica (most notably) had already established (Swanton 1946, 737–738).

The presence of French traders in this frontier area further compelled the Spanish to reassert sovereignty in the Tejas province. A second phase of presidio and/or mission construction began in earnest in 1716 with the establishment of Mission Nuestra Padre San Francisco de Tejas and the Presidio Nuestra Señora de los Dolores de los Tejas near the Neches River and El Caminos Real (Corbin 1991). Further missions were constructed between 1716 and 1721 for the Nacogdoche, Nasoni, Ais, and Adaes Caddo groups with the Presidio Nuestra Señora del Pilar de los Adaes chosen as the capitol of Tejas province in 1731 (see Fig. 22 and 28). The isolated frontier outpost, the difficulty in coercing the Hasinai tribes to settle at the missions, and the unreliable supply network and excessive transportation costs along the frontier of Nueva España all contributed to the development of contraband and later officially sanctioned trading between the French at Natchitoches and Spanish settlers in East Texas (Griffith 1954). This allowed for the uninterrupted, if still illegal, interaction and trade between the French and the Hasinai groups, who continued to maintain residence in the same territory as before.

Within the Hasinai confederacy that developed in the Spanish mission area "the tribes . . . did not live in groups which maintained the same constituent elements unchanged from generation to generation" (Swanton 1942, 8). Rather, there was continued fragmentation, there were changes in location and intergroup alliance, or there were possibly some groups that simply disappeared from the ethnohistorical and historical records. The relatively independent Caddoan alliance of probable "kin and/or dialectical groupings" (Gregory 1973, 15–16) assured that a flexible approach by European colonists would be ultimately more successful than a narrow and restricted one in furthering European goals and ultimately drawing the Hasinai and Kadohadacho into the eighteenth-century market economy (Bolton 1914, 1:28–61).

By 1750 individual French traders could be found in each of the Hasinai and Kadohadacho villages (Morfi 1935, 91), and Caddoan groups were firmly established as middlemen to groups on the southern plains who also participated in the French trade. Increased trade opportunities brought by the expansion of the fur trade made traditional agricultural pursuits of the Caddoan peoples increasingly more marginal and also caused their hunting and trapping territories to shift and expand.

SUMMARY AND CONCLUSIONS

Beginning ca. 1685 the nature of European contact with the Caddoan peoples changed from indirect and intermittent to sustained, direct, and face-to-face (Perttula and Ramenofsky 1982). This culture contact was accompanied by permanent European settlement in the Red River Valley and in parts of East Texas. The different French and Spanish colonial policies were to increasingly involve the Caddoan peoples in the rapidly changing, politically and economically motivated European frontier of the Spanish Borderlands West. Caddoan peoples played pivotal roles in the Spanish-French and American colonization of the Red and Arkansas River valleys. Their importance is certainly well documented in the archival and ethnohistorical records of the colonial powers and American states.

Contact during the Historic period meant acculturation for both the European and Caddoan inhabitants of the Caddoan Area. That acculturative process was predicated on economic exchange, in which the local Caddoan communities supplied food products, material items, and marketable goods (e.g., horses, pelts, and bear grease) in return for European goods. This relationship between European and Caddoan groups was initially symbiotic, but as it developed, it eventually incorporated Caddoan economic strategies into the European-dominated trade and economic network.

Both archaeological and ethnographic data are relevant sources of information for studying Caddoan lifeways after the mid–sixteenth century. The ethnographic record, however, does not report processes of historical causation, but they can be inferred by (*a*) carefully controlling the context in which ethnographic data are used in the study of native history (Trigger 1974, 1986b) and (*b*) by relating the data to aspects of the history in French and Spanish archival materials. Quantitative information on trends in the French and Spanish colonial economies, the contribution of the aboriginal peoples to those economies, and changes in colonial policies on trade and exchange with the aborigines are critical aspects of the Historic period record in the Caddoan Area. As such, they provide parameters and temporal baselines from which to infer changes in the ethnohistorical record, changes that have archaeological implications. In this sense, while the archaeological and historical data bases are different, they can complement each other in relatively specific terms.

The Historic archaeological record of the Caddoan Area indicates that only certain communities or *rancherías* continued to be maintained into the ethnographically recorded Historic period. Although these communities existed within the same general areas of territorial continuity carried over from ca. 1520–1685, the areas of settlement were greatly contracted. Local amalgamation of groups and communities, along with patterns of valley abandonment initiated during earlier episodes of European contact and interaction, were already more or less established by the time of direct European contact and colonization.

These localities of Historic period settlement by Caddoan peoples, as documented in the ethnohistorical records, were strong inducements to planned European colonization and settlement efforts. This colonization and settlement helped to extend Caddoan trade relationships by including Europeans as part of the trade network. In these settings the symbiosis between Europeans and the Caddoan peoples developed. Here the intensity of European contact was high, and the economic situation, trade opportunities, and the access to European goods all mitigated to some extent the negative impact of European contact (i.e., the introduction of acute epidemic diseases) and contributed to the short-term success of the expanded trade among partially resettled Caddoan populations. The adaptive value of this type of interaction was realized by the Caddoan peoples primarily in their dealings with the French out of Natchitoches, inasmuch as the French mercantilistic trade policy was based on using gifts and trade goods to encourage and maintain strong Indian trade alliances. The Spanish, on the other hand, tried to restrict commercial interaction with Caddoan groups in an attempt to bring the East Texas Caddoan populations into the foundering mission system.

Out of the differences in French and Spanish colonial policy developed patterns of contact and interaction less related to mutual accommodation than to European manipulation. In general, this relationship pattern can be traced to the development and participation of the Caddoan people in the fur trade. Some aspects of the traditional economic strategies were abandoned as the Caddoan economy became more dependent on European manufactured goods and forms of payment (credit) that could not be integrated into existing modes of subsistence and trade.

With the development of the Caddoan fur trade in the early eighteenth century, certain hinterland areas that had been depopulated or abandoned before ca. 1700 were reoccupied and utilized, at least on a seasonal basis, by other Caddoan peoples. The headwater areas of the Sabine and Cypress Creek basins are two such areas; occupations there in the Historic period date after ca. 1740 (see Duffield and Jelks 1961; Jelks 1967; Perttula et al. 1988). In these hinterland areas no permanent or sustained European settlements existed, although seasonally established French trading posts were known in the 1760s, 1770s, and 1780s in the upper Sabine and Kiamichi river basins in the Western Caddoan subarea (Bolton 1915).

It is probably no coincidence that the Caddoan Area Historic period confederacies are in the three locales where direct and permanent European settlements existed throughout much of the eighteenth century. Whereas the use of the term *confederacy* may not be appropriate to describe Historic period Caddoan sociopolitical integration (Gregory 1973, 277; Story 1978, 51; Wyckoff and Baugh 1980, 231), the abandonment of major portions of the Caddoan Area is clearly related to the timing and development of these local population aggregates. Being amidst European settlements, agglomeration provided an adaptive advantage to those Caddoan groups forming or maintaining population clusters from different remnant Caddoan groups.

This was only a short-term adjustment in regional population density, however, which was changed by the increasing importance of the French fur trade and a continuing population decline due to the effects of recurrent European acute epidemic diseases (Ewers 1973). With the increasing availability of French guns, fur trading became a more common way for Caddoan peoples to interact with the Europeans and also make improvements in means of subsistence. Continued population dispersion not only favored the success of the fur trade since uninhabited but exploitable territory was available, but also may well have contributed to the increased survival of more intensive fur trading groups relative to other more sedentary Caddoan agriculturists because dispersion minimized direct European contact during some seasons of the year. Thus, agglomeration continued even as more Caddoan peoples moved away from the European settlements and their involvement in the fur trade expanded.

6 / Special Aspects of the Eighteenth-Century Caddoan Archaeological Record

Before the coming of the Spanish missionaries they [the Hasinai] had obtained indirectly from the Spaniards or other nations such things as hawk-bells, shells, etc. These they suspended with their native gew-gaws round the neck or sewed them to their buckskin garments in such a way as to make the most noise. This love for ornament was the key to much of the hold acquired by the Spaniards and French over the Hasinai natives.

—*Herbert E. Bolton, 1987*

European colonists influenced patterns of mortuary variability, material culture, and sociopolitical organization in Caddoan populations. Although a systematically collected data base on post-1685 Caddoan mortuary practices is not available, information on known sites indicates the absence of vertical differentiation or hierarchical ranking. French and Spanish archival and ethnohistorical records also provide detailed temporal and quantifiable measures of the importance of the Indian trade to the transplanted European economy in the New World. Patterns of trade have specific implications for the nature of the Historic period Caddoan archaeological record. Symbiotic economic European-Caddoan interaction affected intertribal relationships and the stability and maintenance of Caddoan territoriality.

MORTUARY VARIABILITY

Although a number of Caddoan archaeological sites with burials presumed to postdate 1685 have been excavated since the late 1920s, these sites have been, in general, unsystematically investigated, often disturbed by pothunters, or found, unfortunately, lacking in critical contextual detail. Consequently, while valuable comparative information on types of Caddoan burial treatments and grave good assemblages have been obtained on an areal basis (see Cole 1975 and Gregory 1973, 223–231), findings of local and regional social differentiation reflected in mortuary practices, in the periods following direct European contact with the Caddoan peoples, have been mostly fortuitous.

Ideally, for the study of mortuary remains (i.e., the skeletal remains and associated grave goods) to contribute to the analysis of cultural change it is

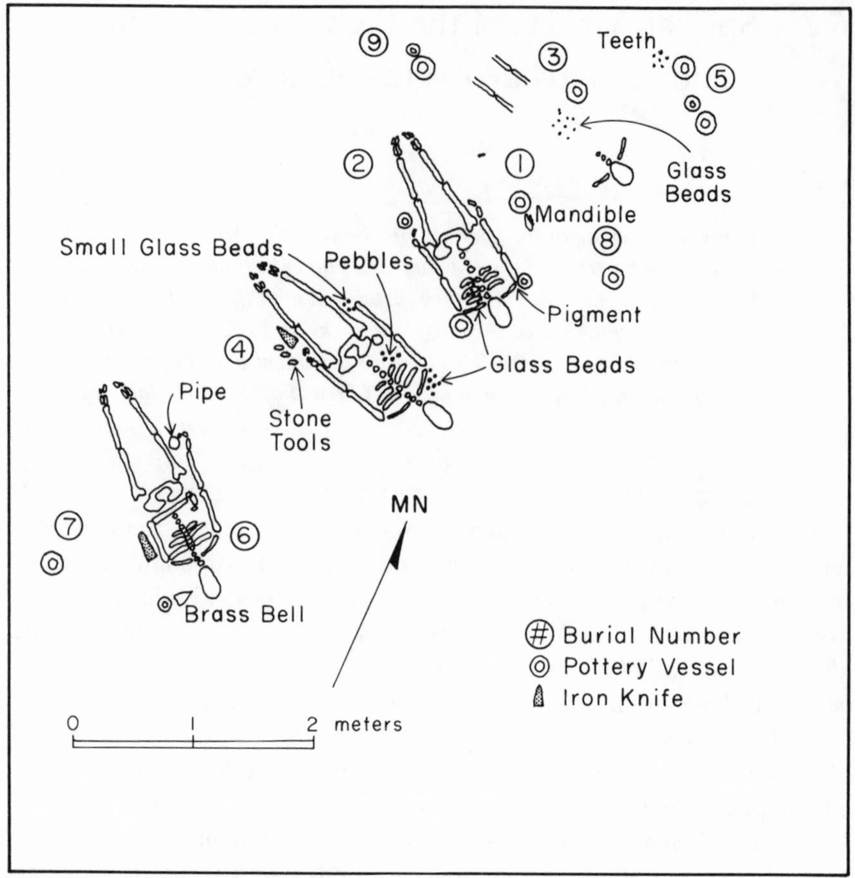

FIG. 30. Deshazo site cemetery plan (*MN*, magnetic north) (from Good 1982, Fig. 28).

necessary that (*a*) cemeteries be comprehensively excavated, ensuring that the range and spatial component of burial practices be systematically documented for both adults and children (Burnett 1990b, 1990c), and (*b*) that close-order or fine-scale chronological control be documented in the cemetery collection (see O'Shea 1984; Mainfort 1985; Voorrips and O'Shea 1987). Seldom are these types of conditions met in even optimal archaeological situations (and the grave assemblages to be discussed herein are no exception), but useful information on Historic period Caddoan mortuary variability can be obtained from those few sites where fairly detailed investigations have been conducted.

The cemetery at the Deshazo site (41NA27), which dates from the late seventeenth to the early eighteenth century, is located fifty-five meters south of an Allen phase hamlet or small village on an alluvial fan overlooking Bayou Loco, a tributary of the Angelina River (see Figs. 23 and 24 and Table 14). Excavations in the 1930s by avocational archaeologists at the site recovered Burials 1–9 (Fig. 30), and one other extended burial (Burial 10) is reported to have come from the same cemetery (Good 1982, 80). Another three burials in the hamlet or village are of children interred in pits dug through the floor of two structures in Area D at the site (see Fig. 24). A limited number and variety of artifacts were recovered from the Deshazo site burials, including sixteen aboriginally manufactured ceramic vessels, a ceramic pipe, stone tools, an assortment of European manufactured glass beads (Creel 1982a, 120–125), and a small number of European metal trade goods (Table 15).The burials at the Deshazo site are readily separable into those containing aboriginal artifacts and those containing both aboriginal and European trade goods. The latter burials, which are better preserved, appear to represent a later burial episode than those containing strictly aboriginal artifacts as grave goods (Good 1982, 84, 86). The burials with European goods are, however, not suspected to be more than a generation younger than the earlier group (Story n.d.).

All of the adults were buried in an extended position. The low diversity of grave offerings and the overall similarity in the number of grave goods between both burial groups suggest that the mortuary patterning is the product of a society with only limited internal differentiation or gradation in rank between individuals (O'Shea 1984, Table 4.3). However, that the greatest number and variety of goods, one indication of wealth (see Mainfort 1985), occurs in those burials with European trade goods may indicate that a Caddoan individual's access to these goods enhanced social importance. This seems likely inasmuch as trade goods appeared to be extremely scarce items at the time the site was occupied (Story n.d., 538). If such were the case, then it follows that either the relative wealth of the Deshazo inhabitants increased after European contact or that a system of vertical differentiation or special status might have been present. The former appears to be more probable, given the frequency and quality of the grave goods included with the burials with European goods.

The European trade goods obtained from the Deshazo site include both tools (iron knives) and nonutilitarian (glass beads and a bell) items, commodities that bespeak different interpretations of value in both the economic and ceremonial/ideological spheres (Miller and Hamell 1986, 315–326). Even so, European goods had not replaced those of native manufacture because aboriginal Caddoan ceramics and lithic artifacts were abundant. Given the estimated date of the Allen phase component at the Deshazo site (ca. 1700–1730) and the European presence at that time in the Caddoan Area (see chapter 2), it is most likely that the European goods found in the

TABLE 15. Grave Goods Associations at the Deshazo Site, Nacogdoches County, Texas

Burial No.	Total Specimens	Ceramic Vessels	Trade Goods: Beads	Trade Goods: Other	Miscellaneous
1	1	1			
2	155	3	151		Pigment
3	1	1	—[a]		
4	485	1	479	1	Rattle?
5	3	3			
6	4	1		2	
7	1	1			
8	1	1			
9	1	1			
10[b]	?		—[a]		
11[c]	1	1			
12[c]	1	1			
13[d]	1	1			

Source: Adapted from Good 1982.

Note: Burial 4 also had three native stone implements, and Burial 6 had one ceramic pipe.

[a]Not quantified (Creel 1982b).

[b]Exact location unknown.

[c]Area D, unit 1 (structure 3).

[d]Area D, unit 9 (structure 9).

graves were native exchange goods that were then treated as exotic items marking some individual's special status, but not indicating a hereditary ranking system.

The early to mid-eighteenth-century cemetery at the Cedar Grove site in the Great Bend area of the Red River includes nine individuals—two infants, two juveniles, and five adults (four males and one female) (Table 16). The infants were buried within structure 3, and the remainder were interred in two groups a short distance north of the house (see Fig. 25). With the exception of European trade goods, which are virtually totally lacking (Trubowitz 1984, 264 and Figs. 13–18), a wider variety and greater number of grave goods accompanied the burials at the Cedar Grove site than accompanied those at Deshazo. The number of native ornaments, implements, and ceramic vessels at the Cedar Grove site are more similar to the Period 3, subphases a–c, typical Titus phase burials (see chapter 4) than they are to the Allen phase component at the Deshazo site.

The Gulf Coast conch shell pendants and beads from Burials 4–7, 9, and

TABLE 16. Grave Goods Associations at the Cedar Grove Site, Lafayette County, Arkansas

Burial No.	Total Specimens	Ceramic Vessels	Native Ornaments			Native Implements	Miscellaneous	Age (yrs.)/Sex
			Beads	Disc	Other[a]	Bone/ Shell		
Late A								
1	3	2					Mussel shell	Infant, 1–1.5
2	5	3					Drilled turtle shell/eagle[b]	Infant
3	117	1	113				Mussel shell/bald eagle	45–49/Female
5	14	5	8				Mussel shell	35–39/Male
6	2				2			8/?
7	11	5			1	2	Mussel shell/pigment/clay	20–24/Male
Late B								
4	21	6	12	1		1	Mussel shell	20–24/Male
9	19	11		2[c]	2		Pigment/fish/mussel shell	50/Male
10	18	10			5	1	Fish/mussel shell	12–15/?

Source: From Trubowitz 1984.

Note: Burial 8 belongs to earlier occupation. No ceramic pipes, no stone native implements, and no trade goods were found in this burial.

[a] Pendant/gorget.

[b] Bald eagle skeleton.

[c] Bone (presumed to be buttons).

10 have their counterparts in the Protohistoric period mound shaft burial grave assemblages from the Belcher site in that most burials are associated with these items of exotic origin (see Webb 1959, 1984). Given the context of the Belcher site shaft burials, inclusion of these exotic goods with burials of all ages was evidence of certified rank or vertical differentiation among that Red River Belcher phase Caddoan population (Webb 1984).

At the Cedar Grove site, however, status is more ambiguous because the burials were recovered in a nonmound context and grave assemblages and their treatment do not vary significantly one to another (Trubowitz 1984; M. Kay 1984, 204). Thus, instead of interpreting the Chakanina phase cemetery at the Cedar Grove site as representing a ranked mortuary community, one may alternatively explain the cemetery assemblage character by hypothesizing that through time (i.e., from ca. 1670 to 1730) this group as a whole acquired more access to goods of exotic origin. In such situations, therefore, these items must be considered to have been less restricted or controlled by rank prerogatives than they had been during the preceding Belcher phase, when they were employed as part of the warfare/cosmogony complex (see Knight 1986, 677), and consequently were more widely distributed in the community. In this sense, the fact that the use of Gulf Coast conch shell was pervasive in the youngest Chakanina phase mortuary program (100 percent, or 3/3 burials), compared with a moderate use in the older Chakanina phase mortuary program (50 percent, or 3/6 burials), suggests an increasing "communalization" (Knight 1986, 682–684) of these types of artifactual remains over a relatively short time (Sabo 1987:39).

Other Historic period cemeteries illustrative of Caddoan mortuary practices include several sites in Northeast Texas. The Clements site (41CS25) is located on a small tributary near the headwaters to Black Cypress Bayou, not far from the divide between the Cypress Creek and Sulphur River basins in Northeast Texas. The Goode Hunt Site (41CS23) (see below) is about eight kilometers to the west in a similar geographic setting[1] (see Fig. 23).

The Clements Site cemetery was excavated by the University of Texas in 1932, and twenty-two burials were exposed over a 600-square-meter area adjacent to a habitation locale whose trash midden was its only extensively examined aspect (Lewis 1987; Jackson n.d.a). Twenty of the burials were apparently single, primary extended inhumations, but a semi-flexed burial (Burial 2) was also recorded along with a multiple burial (Burial 11) containing three individuals. According to Jackson (n.d.a) the three individuals are from three superimposed primary extended burials rather than the product of one burial event as was recorded, for instance, from the double burials noted in the Titus phase cemeteries (see Thurmond 1990a; Turner 1978).

The site had been disturbed prior to the University of Texas excavations. Some skeletal remains had been rearranged, and, likely, some artifacts from

Burials 3, 9, 10, 13, and 17 removed (Table 17). Therefore, discussions and summary quantification of the grave goods recovered are presented for the site as a whole and then separately for the graves that were the least disturbed by pothunting. The Clements site dates from ca. 1680 to 1720.

A relatively diverse grave good assemblage was recovered from the site. Conch shell grave goods were the most common inclusion, including probable bead necklaces from at least two burials (Burials 8 and 15), ear discs, and portions of pendant necklaces. The zoomorphic style of the conch shell pendants from the associated midden at the Clements site is very similar to ones recovered at both the Belcher (Webb 1959, 172–173) and Cedar Grove (M. Kay 1984, Figs. 13–22) sites, as well as from Belcher phase components at the Foster, Friday, and Battle sites along the Red River in Southwest Arkansas. Half of the Clements burials had conch shell ornaments, certainly indicative of a ready access to these materials of exotic origin; a similar relationship was demonstrated in the Chakanina phase burials at the Cedar Grove site. Along with the shell ornaments were European glass beads (one to twenty-six per burial) from five separate interments. In two instances, shell beads or other shell ornaments were found together in the same burial with the European glass beads (see Table 17).

Trubowitz (1984, 270) argues from the Cedar Grove burial data that conch shell objects are replaced by European trade goods as status markers in Kadohadacho society, thus in essence gradually devaluating the symbolic designation of the shell ornaments and making them available to the broader population. The Clements site cemetery as a Caddoan mortuary component may be an intermediate example of this hypothesized replacement process.

Given the fact that the Clements site and the Chakanina phase burials at the Cedar Grove site are broadly contemporaneous but probably representative of distinct ethnic and social groupings, it can be further suggested that the changes in the mortuary program in these two regions reflect a broader pattern of change in the "communalization" of hereditary social rank markers. For with the exception of Burial 15 (see Table 17) at the Clements site, there are no distinct differences in grave good assemblages or in the type of burial treatment (O'Shea 1984) that would denote the existence at that time (ca. 1680–1720) of vertical differentiation in this local population. The other burials at the site with European trade goods are not different in number and variety of goods (aboriginal and/or European in origin) than those burials containing only aboriginal grave goods as assemblages.

European trade goods' presence, albeit limited, at the Clements site and their absence from the contemporaneous Chakanina phase settlement at Cedar Grove are in accord with certain aspects of the Great Bend Contact era model proposed by Trubowitz (1984, 39–40). The infrequency of European

TABLE 17. Grave Goods Associations at the Clements Site, Cass County, Texas

Burial No.	Total Specimens	Ceramic Vessels	Ceramic Pipes	Native Ornaments		
				Beads	Disc	Other[a]
1	14	2				
2	8	1		2		
3	4	2				
4	8	5		1	1	
5	6	2		1		
6	5	3				
7	6	3				
8	22	2		12		
9				No artifacts remained		
10				No artifacts remained		
11	10	9				
12	4	3				
13				No artifacts remained		
14	12	5				1
15	69	6		36		
16	6		1	5		
17				No artifacts remained		
18	12	3		5		2
19	4	1	1	1		
20	2				1	
21	6	3		1		
22	6	2				

Source: From Jackson, n.d.a.
[a]Pendant/gorget.

trade goods in late seventeenth to mid-eighteenth-century Caddoan sites in the Great Bend area of the Red River is seen primarily as a consequence of three factors: (*a*) geographic position combined with (*b*) the filtering of the flow of European products by other Caddoan (and non-Caddoan) groups and (*c*) the retention of these trade goods by the social elite, when acquired, even as deposits in graves with other burial goods. It is unlikely that before 1730 European goods would have been accessible to the broader Caddoan population or found in village contexts (see the discussion below in the

Native Implements		Trade Goods	
Stone	Bone/Shell	Beads	Miscellaneous
		9	Pigment/mussel
			Shell/deer
1	1		Mussel shell
1			Pigment
			Pigment
3			
1		1	
		3	Pigment
4	2		Turtle shell/ pigment
			Pigment
1			Mussel shell/ deer mandible
		6	Pigment
		26	Pigment
			Canine tooth
	1		Mussel shell
			Mussel shell
			Mussel shell
2			Pigment
3			Mussel shell/ pigment

section "French and Spanish Colonial Policy and Implications for the Distribution of Trade Goods to the Caddoan Indians"). The Clements site, however, is near to the Nasoni portage on the Sulphur River that was used by early eighteenth-century French explorers such as Louis Juchereau de St. Denis and Bénard de la Harpe (Wedel 1974, 1978). This portage was used instead of navigating through the Great Raft (Tyson 1981) on the Red River to reach Kadohadacho groups living at that time on the middle Red River (see Fig. 25).

Another hypothesis proposed to explain the few European trade goods on early eighteenth-century Kadohadacho sites and their more common presence at contemporaneous sites (Clements and Deshazo in Northeast Texas) is Ray's (1978) theory of the role of the native American middleman in using and trading European goods. Ray proposes that in native American retrading of European goods, many of the goods originally obtained were not worn out and discarded at their first exchange locality. Instead they were exchanged with other groups for other types of goods, presumably mainly of aboriginal manufacture. Orser (1984) suggests, therefore, that if certain natives were middlemen in the exchange of European trade goods, sites occupied by their group should contain fewer European goods than were actually traded to them. Moreover, those goods retained would be likely to be deposited as grave goods. An adequate evaluation of Ray's (1978) "middleman hypothesis" requires both a regional Historic period archaeological data base and fine-scale chronological control and, further, it assumes a representative investigation of Caddoan habitation and mortuary contexts at a sample of appropriate sites. All these types of data sets are unfortunately lacking in the investigated Caddoan sites representing the archaeological record for the period following 1685. It is a hypothesis well worth further examination as the scale of investigations on Historic period Caddoan settlements expands in the future (Williams and Early 1990).

Other similarities between the Clements and Cedar Grove mortuary programs include the common use of aboriginal pottery vessels as grave goods and the common presence of red and green pigments in mussel shell containers. Fifteen of the burials at the Clements site had pigment and/or mussel shell offerings (see Table 17); ten burials with European goods had pigments, particularly a green pigment (Jackson n.d.a).

Vermillion traded by the French was used as a red pigment by early eighteenth-century Caddoan groups in East Texas (Jones 1968; Harris, Harris, and Miroir 1980), but the different colored pigments at the Cedar Grove site proved to be of indigenous origin (Ericson and Coughlin 1984, Table 12-4). Since the pigments from the Clements site occur in burials with European trade goods, a pigment analysis could be conducted on any remaining samples to determine their origin. Jackson (n.d.a) also noted that the amount of green pigment placed in graves at the Clements site was similar to the Titus phase J. M. Riley site in Upshur County, Texas (see chapter 4). This site dates presumably to the late seventeenth century, late in the Turner (1978) proposed temporal arrangement (see the appendix), but did not contain obvious European materials in the cemetery offerings. The green pigments, however, may be of some significance in documenting the existence of early European-Caddoan interaction in East Texas (Thurmond 1985, 198).

The Goode Hunt site was also excavated by the University of Texas in the summer of 1932 (Jackson n.d.b). An area roughly 500 square meters was excavated to expose a cemetery with seventeen human burials, an isolated ceramic vessel, and a single dog burial (Fig. 31). The Caddoan burials were single, primary, extended inhumations for adult individuals; only three subadults (Burials 5, 11, and 17) were recorded (Jackson n.d.b). Unlike the Clements, Cedar Grove (Trubowitz 1984, Fig. 10-2 to 10-16), and Deshazo (Good 1982) sites, the Goode Hunt site had grave pit orientations that were not consistent or uniform in direction (see Fig. 31). One group—Burials 1, 8, 12, and 13—is oriented with the head to the south and feet to the north, while the remainder are oriented with the head to the northeast and the feet to the southwest. Differences in the types of decorated ceramic vessels present in the two groups suggests that they represent two sequent burial episodes.

The first, which we refer to as group 1 (Burials 1, 8, 12, and 13), is contemporaneous with the Belcher III component at the Belcher site, estimated to date from ca. 1550 to 1650 (see chapter 4). The presence of a Belcher Engraved var. Soda Lake bottle (Schambach and Miller 1984, 120) in Burial 1 (see Jackson n.d.b, 5) is an excellent marker for the earlier part of the Belcher phase on the Red River (Schambach and Miller 1984, 120, 167). Group 2 burials at the Goode Hunt site are estimated to date between 1700 and 1730 on the basis of a ceramic assemblage quite comparable to the Late A and Late B, or Chakanina phase, mortuary ceramics from the Cedar Grove site (see Table 9). Ceramic types and varieties identified from the group 2 burials include Hodges Engraved var. Candler (Burial 2), Hodges Engraved var. Kelley's Lake (Burial 7), Hodges Engraved var. Armour (Burial 14), Keno Trailed var. Phillips (Burial 3), and possibly Natchitoches Engraved from Burial 6 (Jackson n.d.b, 7, 10, 19, 22, 34).

There are significant differences between the two burial groups in the amount and variety of grave goods associations (Table 18). Group 1 burials contain few grave goods, predominantly aboriginal ceramic vessels, with minimal differentiation between individuals. Group 2 burials have a greater number and variety of grave goods, with any intragroup variability in social differentiation being accountable primarily as a function of age and/or sex. (In table below, SD is standard deviation, and CV is coefficient of variation.)

	MEAN	SD	CV
Group 1	2.0	0.5	25.0
Group 2	7.1	4.6	64.8

The two juveniles or subadults (Burials 11 and 17), which were interred at the margins of the cemetery (see Fig. 28), had a mean of only 3.5 grave

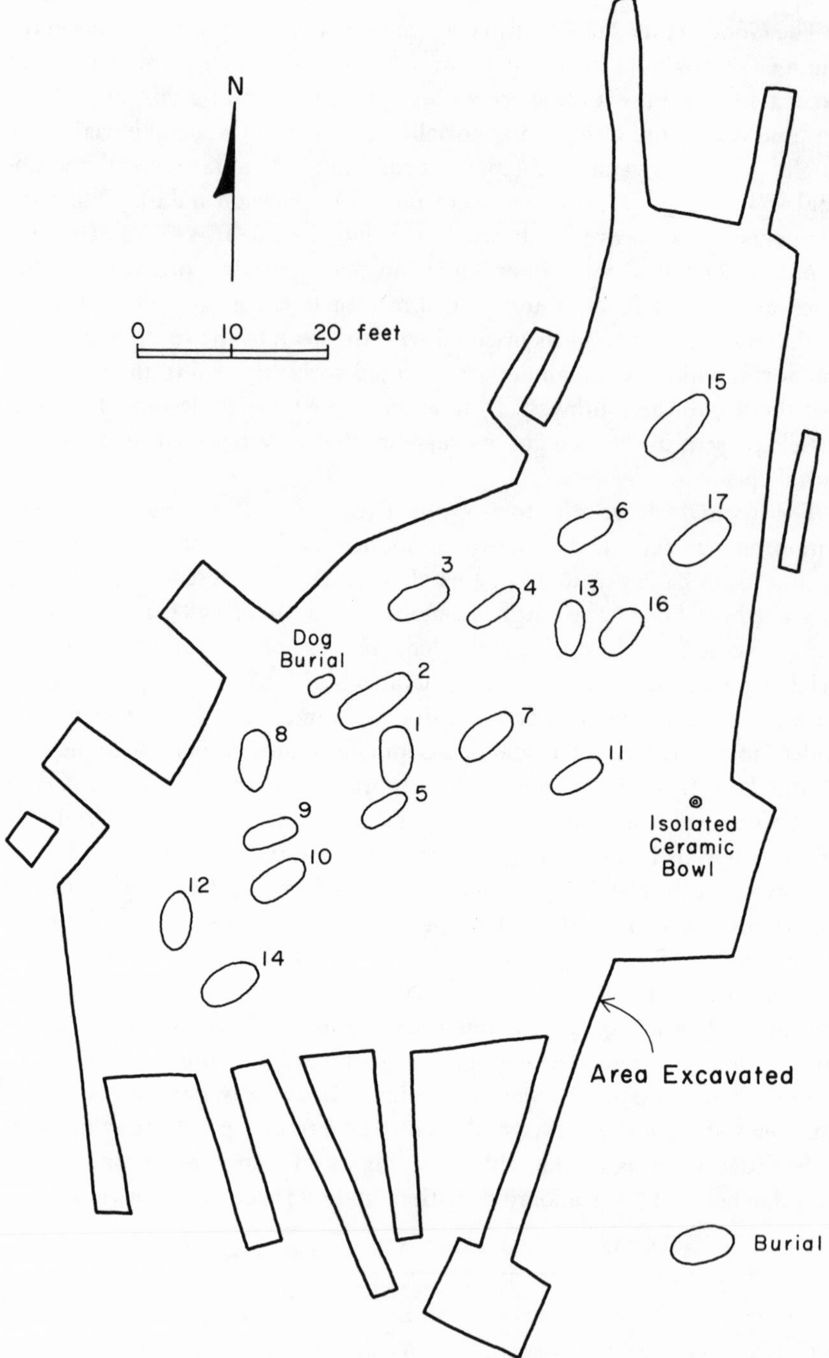

FIG. 31. Cemetery plan at Goode Hunt farm, Cass County, Texas (from Jackson n.d.b.).

goods per burial. The burial of the six- to eight-year-old child near the center of the cemetery, (Burial 5), however, contained eight pottery vessels and two offerings of pigment (see Table 18).

Group 2 burials are also characterized by associations of aboriginal stone and shell implements, including manos, pitted stones, an abrader, and several hafted mussel shells likely to have been used as hoes. Burials with these sorts of implements are uniformly distributed in the cemetery. Green, red, and gray pigments were placed in about 40 percent of the group 2 burials, comparable to their frequency at the Clements site (see Table 17). The burials containing pigments occur near the center or along the margins of the cemetery. Whether the pigments are of local aboriginal or European origin has not been established (see above). A single thin sheet of metal was found behind the skull of Burial 7 (Jackson n.d.b, 21). The unidentifiable piece may be a fragment of European sheet brass such as those found in the contemporaneous Glendora, Keno, and Kaufman-Williams sites of the post-1685 Historic Caddoan period.

The grave assemblage at the Goode Hunt site suggests again that social differences within the groups are based primarily on age distinctions, a characteristic of egalitarian, simple societies with horizontal differentiation (see Table 6). There is no clear evidence in the grave goods or in methods of burial treatment that distinctions exist, elevating certain individuals above others in the social system. The only evidence possibly contradicting the absence of social ranking is the character, internal location, and placement of a child (Burial 5). Not only does this burial contain many grave goods, but its position near the center of the cemetery is very much consistent with the general spatial distribution of ranked individuals noted in certain Titus phase cemeteries (see chapter 4).

Intersite Comparisons

The mortuary variability in post-1685 Caddoan Historic period sites is little known, but analyses of the few sites that have undergone the more comprehensive investigations provide useful information about internal patterning in grave assemblages and the possible character of social distinctions during two to three generations following initial direct European contact. In Table 19, I summarize statistics on the four different cemeteries considered in detail in the previous section and data for two burials from the Roseborough Lake site (see Fig. 23), which was the probable location of the 1731–1778 Caddo post, Fort St. Louis de Kadohadacho, and was also an upper Nasoni *ranchería* (Miroir et al. 1973; Gilmore 1986a).

Social ranking or vertical differentiation as a hypothesis is not consistent with the observed mortuary variability of the Deshazo, Cedar Grove, Clements, and Goode Hunt cemeteries. Items considered indicative of high

TABLE 18. Grave Goods Associations at the Goode Hunt Site, Cass County, Texas

Burial No.	Total Specimens	Ceramic Vessels	Native Implements		Miscellaneous
			Stone	Bone/Shell	
1	3	1	1		
2	7	6	1		
3	8	6	1	1	
4	6	5			Pigment
5	10	8			Pigments
6	7	3	3	1	
7	6	5			Pigment
8	2	2			
9	6	5		1	
10	2	2			
11	3	3			
12	2	2			
13	1	1			
14	11	9		1	Pigment/mussel shell
15	11	9	1		Pigment deer mandible
16	12	8	3	1	
17	4	3	1		

Source: From Jackson n.d.b.

Note: Only Burial 1 had a ceramic pipe; no burial had native ornaments; and only Burial 7 had one trade good artifact, a piece of thin sheet metal, which was possibly intrusive.

rank or status—sociotechnic artifacts (Binford 1962)—(e.g., the conch shell ornaments) occur in Red River basin Caddoan mound shaft burials dating to the fifteenth and sixteenth centuries, but seemingly occur in post-1685 cemeteries in a habitation context. This change in context is consistent with a "communalization" of once symbol-laden goods (Knight 1986). The greater access of conch, still an overall indication of wealth (as measured by the number and variety of goods included as grave offerings), may also indicate a relationship between the social enhancement of a much broader proportion of Caddoan society and the initiation of sustained European interaction and trade. Trubowitz (1984) argues that the overall greater access to items and paraphernalia previously considered of ritual significance is accompanied by a substitution or replacement of their role by European trade goods that are retained as before by members of the society with high rank. This proposed relationship was not clearly demonstrated at the Cedar Grove site, however (Trubowitz 1984, 270), and the frequency of conch shell at the Roseborough Lake and Clements sites indicates that the general argument is unlikely to be the case.

In this set of sites, only at the Clements and Roseborough Lake sites do conch ornaments and European goods occur together in the same burials. At the Roseborough Lake site conch shell in necklaces was probably in the process of being replaced by glass beads; conch shell bracelets were still in use (Miroir et al. 1973, Figs. 3, 4). In another case, an iron disk from a late seventeenth- or early eighteenth-century burial at the Bob Williams site (see Fig. 23) apparently was used as an ear ornament, again replacing shell ear disks (Perino 1983, 67). In general, however, these cemeteries date to before the time when one would reasonably expect that Caddoan groups were saturated with European goods. A consideration of French, English, and Spanish colonial policy (see below) supports the inference that trade goods were not abundant or readily distributed to the various allied Caddoan groups until after ca. 1770. Computer simulations of European trade good flow among the Arikara, who lived on the Northern Great Plains, by Orser and Zimmerman (1984, 199–210) imply that where European goods are abundant and dependable aboriginal-European trade relationships are established, the saturation point (i.e., when the frequency of European goods reaches a level that makes them easily accessible to all members of aboriginal societies) may be reached within a generation's time.

Summary

Historic period Caddoan adults and juveniles generally received similar treatment at the time of death. They were placed in cemeteries in proximity to their community's settlements and were commonly accompanied by ceramic vessels and other domestic items (including implements of various sorts) as grave goods. Children, however, were more likely to be placed in pits below house floors than in the cemeteries used for the adults and juveniles.

With a few exceptions, adults and juveniles received comparable amounts and kinds of grave offerings, but children seem to have been buried with only a few grave goods. The exceptions include a number of Caddoan adult burials dating after ca. 1750 who were accompanied by considerable amounts of European trade goods, particularly glass beads used as ornaments, which had become accessible to much of the Caddoan population. The use of red and green pigments in mussel shell containers as additional offerings was of particular importance in the Cedar Grove and Clements burial programs. In no case were Historic Caddoan burials documented that suggested a causal relationship between social rank, the trade of European goods, or

TABLE 19. Mean Number of Grave Goods in Selected Post-1685 Caddoan Cemeteries

Site	No. of Burials	Specimens	Ceramic Vessels	Native Ornaments	Native Implements	Trade Goods
Deshazo	13	50.8	1.2	0.0	0.2	49.4
Roseborough Lake	2	561.5	6.0	15.5	3.0	537.0
Cedar Grove						
A	6	25.0	2.7	20.5	0.5	0.0
B	3	21.1	9.0	7.7	0.7	?
Clements	22	9.3	2.4	3.1	0.9	2.0
	[18]	[11.3]	[2.9]	[3.8]	[1.1]	[2.5]
Hunt	17	5.8	4.6	0.0	1.1	?

participation in the fur trade, which is unlike burials of the Tunica, Natchez, and Arikara during the same time period (Brain 1979:279; Neitzei 1965, 1983; O'Shea 1984:279–283).

CHANGES IN MATERIAL CULTURE

In the study of Caddoan material culture changes, Historic period Indian archaeological assemblages can reflect the many and varied effects adoption and trade of European items—fabrics, glass beads, and glass bottles—had on native American aboriginal societies (Brain 1979, 1989; Brown 1979b, 1979c; Hester 1989b; Waselkov 1989). Just as important, however, to this study is an appreciation of context when interpreting how these changes are expressions of aboriginal behavioral change (see Miller and Hammell 1986; Hamell 1983). That is, European items were obtained and used in ways by native Americans that had no relationship to their intended European use. The use of European items can thus be informative not only about the demise of certain native crafts relative to new ones dependent upon European goods and technologies, but also as a measure of sociocultural change (Brown 1979b, 148). As an example, the presence of brass kettle scraps on Historic period Caddoan sites could indicate that kettles were used for cooking activities as a replacement for native ceramic vessels. However, in certain instances these kettles appear to have been used only as sources of raw material for making arrow points and other metal artifacts (Gregory 1973, 250).

As Brain (1979, 271) has noted, useful distinctions to make in studying the material culture of Protohistoric and Historic Indian groups are first between those European artifacts used in a context and manner similar to those seen in pre-European times (before 1540) versus those items used strictly in a nontraditional, European manner, and second, changes in the frequency of European artifacts in aboriginal assemblages, ranging from being absent to being all of European derivation. Examples of the former would be the use of an iron knife, instead of a stone knife, to cut and slice bone or wood, the use of bottle glass to cut and scrape objects, or the use of flattened kettles or barrel staves for metal arrow points. One of the better examples of the use of European items in a nontraditional manner is the adoption and considerable importance of flintlock muskets for hunting; another is the use of horses for travel and moving equipment. These examples of change in material culture and technology certainly had long-lasting consequences for the Caddoan peoples and the retention of traditional technologies and lifeways (see Kniffen, Gregory, and Stokes 1987, 210–213).

That Caddoan peoples ultimately adopted and became dependent upon European tools and trade goods (usually of a nonutilitarian nature) need not imply that the aboriginal adoption of European goods can be directly equated with systemic behavioral changes. Rather, the fundamental meaning and importance these goods had in changing aboriginal life in the Historic period necessitated different means of interaction, technological change, and changes in perceptions of exchange between the Caddoan peoples and Europeans, and among the various Indian groups living in the region, such as the Tunica, Wichita, and Cherokee. It is not surprising, therefore, that at the same time mass-produced European goods were introduced among the native Americans in the Caddoan Area there should arise evidence in the archaeological record for increasing pan-tribal stylistic and cultural homogeneity in ceramics, dress, and personal adornments (Gregory 1978, 161).

Perhaps the most important European product to have been introduced to North America was the horse. Not only did it facilitate rapid movement and transportation of all native and European goods, but the increased mobility it brought was the prime mechanism for development of Plains-oriented economic strategies in North America (Osborn 1983). Ethnohistorical records show that by 1680 horses were the prime exchangeable commodity for Caddoan societies south of the Red River. Horses were commonly equated with guns as a basic standard of value (Ewers 1955), and the transactions involving these two goods formed a mutually profitable trade for those aboriginal groups best supplied with each resource (Schilz and Worcester 1987).

Apaches were probably one of the first groups to have horses in the Southern Plains (Worcester 1944), from which they were exchanged in trade north and east from the peripheries of the Spanish settlements in the Santa Fe area. Sometime after 1664 Juan de Archuleta from the New Mexico province mentioned Apache horse trading at El Cuartelejo, identified now as the Scott County pueblo in western Kansas, and the presence there of metal artifacts from French sources that must have come originally from the Great Lakes area (Thomas 1935; Witty 1983).

The Jumano middleman Juan Sabetea described well-fed horses in the as yet little-known "Kingdom of the Tejas" in a deposition made to Spanish authorities in Santa Fe in 1683. During La Salle's ill-fated expedition from Fort St. Louis on Matagorda Bay in 1687, he was able to set out toward the Mississippi River on horses previously purchased from the Caddoan Hasinai tribes in Northeast Texas (Joutel [1713] 1906, 113). Father Anastasius Douay, accompanying La Salle, said that horses were common property among the Hasinai and could be purchased from them for a single iron hatchet (Pichardo in Hackett 1931–1946, 1: para. 361–363). According to Griffith (1954, 144–145), "When the French first appeared in the area, the Red River seems to have marked the approximate eastern limit of the horse frontier. The Hasinai were the last Native group to possess the animals in anything like numbers and were, through trade, becoming the agents through whom the horse frontier advanced to the north and east. Henri de Tonty noted, in 1690, that the Cadodoquis [Kadohadacho] Nation on Red River had a total of only about 30 horses, while the Naovidiche [Nabedache] possessed them in such numbers that there were four or five about each house."

The Caddoan peoples living in East Texas apparently first began acquiring horses by trading with the Jumano and by conducting western raids on such groups as the Canohatinno who had plentiful supplies of horses (Joutel [1713] 1906). The livestock brought by the Spanish to East Texas became part of the Hasinai herd after the missions were initially abandoned in 1693. It was from this stock that the Hasinai tribes were able not only to meet their own needs, but were also able to eventually help supply the French Louisiana and Illinois colonies' demand for horses and mules. In exchange for horses sold in the French post of Natchitoches, the Hasinai received firearms, powder and lead balls, hatchets, knives, hoes, glass beads, mirrors, cloth, garments, and alcohol, while to a Frenchman horses would bring more than thirty livres in New Orleans (Surrey 1916, 282).

Horses were cheaply purchased by the French from the native American groups that had a ready supply. Compare the thirty-livre price of a horse in New Orleans with the price of a Pawnee slave (three hundred to twelve hundred livres) in Sainte Genevieve, Illinois province (Surrey 1916, 172–179). Even though currencies fluctuated in value throughout the period of the French Louisiana colony, thirty livres was equivalent to six dollars or six pesos at 1769 prices. Since goods supplied to the Indians in return were typically of poor quality but expensive to purchase, the trade from the French perspective was assuredly a profitable one. As an illustration, consider that the annual presents given out from Natchitoches in 1770 to Red River Caddoan groups amounted to about 310 pesos, as follows (Kinnaird 1949:148): Great Cado (Kadohadacho), 127 pesos and 6 reales; Little Cado (Petit Caddo), 91 pesos and 7 reales; Natchitoches, 49 pesos and 5 reales; Yatasse (Yatasi), 42 pesos and 4 reales.

This is equivalent to 1,555 livres, or roughly 50 horses. Fifteen hundred fifty-five livres was also about the price of one hundred guns. A flintlock musket could be purchased by the Caddoan hunter in exchange for ten large deerskins per gun if the price of the gun had not been excessively marked up by the French trader or by someone at the post. Mark-ups of 50 percent above cost were common, however, in French Louisiana trading posts (Surrey 1916). Therefore, only about one thousand deerskins supplied by the Red River Caddoan groups to the French traders were necessary each year to offset the cost of the annual French presents to the Caddoan groups along the Red River. Considering that horse trading in New Orleans and Natchitoches commonly involved transactions of several hundred horses at a time, the cost of annual presents was certainly not prohibitive to the French. Presumably horses were cheaper to purchase from Indians for merchandise than to have to buy them from Spanish sources directly; in any event, for much of the eighteenth and early nineteenth centuries trade in livestock and horses between the French in Louisiana and the Spanish in Texas was outlawed by the Spanish authorities (Jackson 1986). From the point of view of European economic strategies and profit-making ventures, the horse trading was inexpensive, profitable, and helped to develop the cattle trade in French Louisiana (Gregory 1973).

Brain (1979, 280–282) has pointed out that it was the ability of the Tunica to control the horse and salt trade with the Europeans that ensured their economic success and "wealth." The Tunica "were in a position to oversee all trade up the Red River and its tributaries . . . when a new item of trade became available through European introduction, the Tunica managed to assume the role of middlemen in its distribution."

The Tunica treasure from the Tunica Trudeau site (Brain 1979, 1989), located opposite the Red River confluence with the Mississippi River, dates from as early as 1731. In its artifactual diversity, including both aboriginal and European goods, it gives ample testimony in mortuary goods of Tunican accumulation of European items collected in active trading and commerce with the French. Presumably their commercial interest in the horse trade dates, if not earlier, from the establishment of Natchitoches in 1714 and New Orleans in 1719. Kidder (1990a, 76) suggests that the Tunica had usurped the overland trade routes in salt and maize by ca. 1706–1707 from the Caddoan and other lower Mississippi Valley aboriginal societies.

The case can be made that certain Caddoan groups were in a similar economic position with respect to the horse trade because most of the horses purchased by the French came from Natchitoches and were supplied by western Caddoan groups. Pichardo (in Hackett 1931–1946, 3:para. 653) commented in his early nineteenth century historical study of Texas that "the Frenchmen of Natchitoches, with double-dealing and dissimulation, likewise solicit them [horses] in Texas . . . in order to supply those Frenchmen who were settled among the Ylinoes [Illinois] and at New Orleans."

As direct suppliers to the French at Natchitoches, Caddoan groups involved in the trade could not be easily supplanted as middlemen by other Indian groups; consequently, the merchandise they obtained in selling horses was more than the merchandise and goods that were eventually passed on indirectly to other aboriginal groups in the trading network. This was particularly the case, of course, when horses could be obtained in raids.

It was only after the establishment of New Orleans that the Tunica were able to effectively and opportunely set themselves up as better placed entrepreneurs than the horse-dealing Caddoan tribes because of their relocation at a series of key trade portages (Brain 1979, 257–268), especially at the confluence of the Red and Mississippi rivers. Aboriginal changes in location and trade position continually reoriented the nature of the horse trade in the Caddoan Area. Increased competition raised the risks involved in obtaining horses and thus directly affected one of the key bases of Hasinai and Kadohadacho wealth. Intertribal relationships also changed or fluctuated because of the escalated rivalry between aboriginal groups trying to capture or maintain the position as preeminent supplier of horses to the French. Attempts to supplant one another, which threatened their livelihood, led the Caddoans and Tunicans to mutual enmity. In 1687 Joutel ([1713] 1906) listed the Tunica, Kichai, and Apache as Caddoan allies, but a hundred years later the same groups, by then all heavily involved in the horse trade, were considered enemies by the Caddoan peoples (Pichardo in Hackett 1931–1946, 2:para. 745).

Within the Caddoan Area itself there were differences in the patterns of trade, and investigating the material acquisitions noted in the ethnohistorical documents may help us understand Historic period Caddoan archaeological assemblages with European goods. Griffith (1954, 148), for instance, thinks that "Espinosa's account of the disparity in the number of guns possessed by the Hasinai in comparison with the Cadohadachos, and the inverse disproportion in ownership of horses which was evident when the two groups visited each other, indicates that, as of about 1716, the Hasinai and the Cadohadachos marked, respectively, the saturated frontier of horses moving eastward, and of muskets moving westward in trade. The tendency of the commerce with the French and their Indian allies was to establish an approximate equilibrium in the supply of each commodity on both sides of the frontier."

This disproportional accessibility to guns and horses affected how different Caddoan groups participated in trade with Europeans and other non-Caddoan groups. The competitive advantage of having an abundance of European guns could be offset by not having the mobility to expand hunting and trapping territory when it was necessary, to conduct raids to acquire slaves, or to pursue bison on the prairies. Furthermore, any competitive advantage the Caddoan peoples may have had because of having relatively more guns and/or horses than other groups in the immediate area would change when dealing with such native American groups as the Osage who were well supplied with both products.

Of the horticultural tribes in North America, the Osage were probably the best supplied in horses (Ewers 1955, 13 and Table 2). They were also able to obtain guns from both the French and English throughout the eighteenth century (Hamilton 1960a). A gunsmith's cache found at the Osage Plattner site in southwestern Missouri, occupied ca. 1730–1780, indicates that a gunsmith was present on the site during its occupation and that he was available to the Osage customers to repair their guns (Bray 1978, 30); the guns in this case were of English manufacture (Hamilton 1960b).

The combination of adequate numbers of guns and horses allowed the Osage to extend their hunting trips and forays closer to other unprotected Indian settlements and hunting camps, where they were able to successfully procure slaves and harass Wichita and Caddoan groups (Wiegers 1988). The main source of Indian slaves gathered by the Osage were Wichita and Caddoan peoples who were living near the Arkansas and Red rivers (Bailey 1973). The Wichita groups were seemingly little match for the Osage in this regard because of the chronic shortage of guns at the time (Wedel 1981, 41–43). Osage harassment of the Wichita groups was one factor responsible for the Wichitas' movement between 1742 and 1757 out of the Arkansas River basin southward to the Red River Valley. Osage depredations against the Kadohadacho tribes were primarily a late 1770s phenomenon brought about by a change in the "nature of war . . . from a raiding type [to acquire slaves] to a war of conquest, as the Osage expanded their hunting and trapping territory" (Bailey 1973, 40). The Kadohadacho on the Red River could not cope with the more mobile Osage, who were also equal to if not superior to the Kadohadacho groups in firepower; consequently, from the 1770s to 1790 the Kadohadacho consolidated their population into two larger villages, and then after 1790 they relocated south, around Caddo Lake and closer to Natchitoches (Williams 1964).

Gun parts are found most frequently in the Historic Caddoan period sites

TABLE 20. Comparative Inventory of Gun Parts from Eighteenth-Century Indian Sites

	Osage			Caddo
Gun Parts	Plattner 1730–1780[a]	Gilbert 1740–1770[b]	Pearson 1775–1830[c]	Womack 1700–1730
Locks	1	3	1	
Lock plates	10	2		
Cocks	3	10		1
Frizzen springs		6		
Frizzens	5	8	1	1
Buttplates	12	20		13
Triggerguard	14	29	7	17
Side plates	4	9	2	15
Rampipes	4	16		3
Mainsprings	4	2		1
Triggers	2	1		1
Triggerplate	1	1		
Flint screw	1	13		
Tumblers		2		
Tumbler briddle	1	1		
Barrel fragments	33	23	5	9
Bullets/lead ball	16	10	7	8
Breech plugs	5	6		
Gunflints				
Native	95	69	10	23
French		43	1	4
English				4
Flash pans		2		1

[a] Hamilton 1960a, 1960b. Does not include Osage gunsmith cache.
[b] Jelks 1967.
[c] Duffield and Jelks 1961.
[d] Harris et al. 1965.
[e] Corbin, Alex, and Karlina 1980.
[f] Miroir et al 1973.
[g] Brain 1979.
[h] Hartley and Miller 1977.

		Tunica	Wichita
e los Ais 22–1773[e]	Roseborough 1719–1778[f]	Trudeau 1731–1746[g]	Bryson 1700–1740[h]
		20	
	1		1
			1
	1		2
	4	13	1
	6	13	
	2	7	4
	6	9	
2	1		1
			2
			1
	1		1
			2
1	3	20	
	56	110	1
	2		
	84	1	9
12		11	
1			

on the Red River and in the upper Sabine River basin (Table 20). Inventories of trade materials from eighteenth-century Hasinai sites do contain trade guns or parts (Cole 1975), but they do not occur in the frequency noted elsewhere in the region or at the frequency that might be expected based on the Caddoan ethnographic record (see Schilz and Worcester 1987). At the Allen phase Deshazo site (dated between ca. 1680 and 1750), perhaps the most thoroughly excavated Historic Period Caddoan archaeological site known, a gun worm and four lead balls from Area C and units 1 and 2 in Area D constituted the only evidence for the use of guns (Story 1982, 126–129). Other gun parts are known from the Kinsloe phase settlements on the middle Sabine River, but they are not common apparently in burials (Jones 1968). At least one large cache of mid-eighteenth-century French flintlock muskets, or fusils, has been reported from the Woldert site (41WD333) and vicinity in the upper Sabine River basin (Perttula and Skiles 1989), but in this case it is unclear if the associational context is aboriginal or French (Gilmore and Foret 1988, 91–99).

The ethnographic evidence reviewed above alone suggests that guns and gun parts might be common in the eighteenth-century archaeological record. In 1718 when Alarcon reentered the Hasinai country he "was received with shots from more muskets than the said governor had on his side" (Morfi 1935, 77), and Fray Espinosa counted ninety-two guns among the Hasinai (or Hainai) at the Mission de la Purísima Concepción on the Angelina River (Morfi 1935, 106). If these are accurate accounts, what happened that explains their absence at contemporaneous Caddoan archaeological sites in Northeast Texas? Hypotheses include:

1. Gun parts were rarely burial accompaniments in Historic period Caddoan graves.
2. The context of gun disposal (e.g., in caches or storage pits) may not be closely associated with habitation/burial areas, so any unsystematic excavations in these areas will produce little evidence of guns.
3. Gun parts were scavenged, reworked, or traded when they were no longer in good repair and could not be fixed by a gunsmith.

Nevertheless, if and when comparable excavations can be carried out in habitation and burial contexts on Hasinai, Kadohadacho, and other Caddoan Historic period settlements, proportionally more guns and gun parts should be expected in the archaeological deposits associated with the Kadohadacho settlements. Just the inverse relationship can be proposed in the representation of horse gear (predominantly of Spanish manufacture), including saddlery, bridle chains, stirrups, saddle ornaments, and *ficas* (these are medallions with a clasped hand symbol on them, and they were used by the Spanish to ward off the evil eye). Proportionally more items of horse gear should be present among the Historic Hasinai settlements.

Another important factor to consider is the relationship between the types of Historic period aboriginal settlements and the nature of the trade good assemblages found in different contexts. The Caddoan occupations[2] of such hunting camps as the Womack and Gilbert sites (see Table 20) contain the highest number of guns, gun parts, and related artifacts in eighteenth-century settings in the area. Caddoan peoples who were actively involved in the fur trade must have been the highest consumers of trade guns. Not only were the flintlock muskets an effective hunting tool, eventually replacing the bow and arrow, but also Caddoan groups, which seemingly did not have the technological means of repairing damaged guns, continually had to turn to the French traders to replace their stock. Thus, the life of an individual gun as a Caddoan hunting tool probably was not long relative to the gun's use as a recycled product.

Comparisons of gun inventories between contemporaneous Wichita,[3] Tunica, and Osage settlements show some overall differences in quantity that support the ethnographic record on the relative number of guns among different groups (see Table 20). At least among the Tunica and Natchez, certain high-status individuals were buried with guns and gun parts (Brain 1979, 278; Gregory 1978, 153; Neitzel 1965, 43).

French and Spanish Colonial Policy and Implications for the Distribution of Trade Goods to the Caddoan Indians

The quantity of European trade goods made available to the Caddoan peoples by the French and/or Spanish governments varied from year to year for a number of reasons. Shipping problems, war between the colonial powers, and changes in Indian policies all caused occasional shortages or the lack of trade goods in colonial trade centers in French Louisiana. In Spanish Texas prior to 1762, however, colonial Indian policy was not founded on a commercial basis. Trade was permitted only under strict regulations (Bolton 1915, 32–39). Weapons and ammunition were strictly prohibited as trade items in the province of Nueva España, but were by necessity an essential part of the French and British encouragement of the fur trade. Grain shipments between Spanish Los Adaes and French Natchitoches, however, were apparently one of the covers used for contraband trading of such items from Spanish military and government employees with the French and Hasinai tribes. Bolton (1915, 418) commented that "the Spanish colonists who engaged in hunting took advantage of the market for their peltries, exchanging them for the goods in which the French dealt." As a result, during the 1751–1759 Spanish Texas administration of governor de Barrios y Jáuregui, the

Spanish trade of merchandise secured by them at Natchitoches was authorized. The Spanish used this merchandise in exchange for Hasinai maize, hides, and horses, which were eventually conveyed back to Natchitoches as payment (Bolton 1915, 65–66). Therefore, the fact that from 1751 to 1759 the Spanish actively and legally participated with the French in trade with Caddoan peoples is quite significant when it is considered that this period correlates closely with the fur trade boom in French Louisiana (Surrey 1916).

Between 1739 and 1756 the yearly contribution of the peltry trade increased 750 percent, from 16,000 to 120,000 livres a year (Table 21). The peltries acquired from the fur trade constituted more than 10 percent of the yearly total exports from French Louisiana until 1758, when they began to decrease rapidly until Louisiana was ceded to Spain in 1762. It was not that the absolute value of pelts decreased during that time, but rather that the relative contributions of indigo, tobacco, and other goods increased that much more rapidly (Surrey 1916). Therefore, from the French-Spanish economic point of view, the peak period in the fur trade appears to have been between ca. 1740 and 1758 in Louisiana.

For the native inhabitants of Louisiana, including the various Caddoan groups, the importance of the fur trade continued into the American period (after 1803) and the establishment of the United States factory system (Prucha 1984, 115–134). The Sulphur Fork Factory, at the confluence of the Red and Sulphur rivers in southwest Arkansas, did over five thousand dollars' worth of fur trade business in one year with the Indians living in the district (Magnaghi 1978), which included some Red River Caddoan peoples along with such immigrant Indians as the Cherokee, Delaware, Shawnee, and Coushatta (see chapter 2).

What is important about these fur trade data with respect to the availability of trade goods to the different Caddoan groups is that they signify an ever-increasing amount of merchandise was being traded by the French to Caddoan peoples during the eighteenth century. Given this information, there is thus no point in time one can specify when aboriginally manufactured items begin to be replaced or supplanted by the increasingly more accessible European goods. Pottery vessels were produced until at least 1805 among the Red River Caddoan groups (Gregory 1973, 267), and even as late as the 1770s Caddoan ceramics outnumbered European imports by a wide margin at such mission sites as Mission Dolores de los Ais (Corbin, Alex, and Karlina 1980; Corbin et al. 1990). Similar patterns are apparent in the stone tool industry and production of native bone and shell ornaments, whose use declined during the period of French administration in Louisiana. Consequently, Caddoan adoption of European merchandise for

TABLE 21. Fur Trading in Louisiana as an Aspect of Commerce, 1718–1762

Year	Value of Pelts (Livres)	Value of Combined Exports	Contribution of Pelts to Total Exports (%)
1718	3,000[a]	NA	NA
1725	8,000	NA	NA
1731	10,000	NA	NA
1744	32,000	203,000[b]	15.8
1750–1754	250,000	2,056,000	12.2
1756	120,000	859,900	14.0
1757	150,000	1,258,000	11.9
1758	180,000	1,868,000	9.7
1759	240,000	2,886,000	8.3
1760	240,000	4,440,000	5.4
1761	NA	5,611,000	NA
1762	250,000	6,662,000	3.8

Source: Adapted from Surrey 1916.
Note: NA, not available.
[a] One thousand pelts at thirty sols/pelt.
[b] Yearly average of 812,250 livres combined exports from 1743–1746.

cooking, hunting, butchering, and ornamentation is expected to have increased only after ca. 1730 and then particularly after 1770 when new Spanish policies in Indian relations were established in both Louisiana and Texas (Bolton 1914, 1:66–79).

The ceding of Louisiana to Spain in 1762 (though the cession was not completed until 1769), following France's loss to the British in the French and Indian War, led to a reevaluation of Spain's Indian trade policy. The initial reaction of the new Spanish governors of Louisiana was to maintain the French practices of giving annual presents to the friendly tribes and keeping European traders in each village (Kinnaird 1949, xxii–xxiii). This policy was temporarily rejected, however, in 1772 by the first viceroy of the Provincias Internas because "he objected to fixed annual gifts to buy peace and wanted presents given only as reward on occasions when Indians had demonstrated their loyalty and devotion to the King" (Bolton 1914, 1:271). In an effort to maintain control of the Indians who were already dealing with the traders of Louisiana (including Caddoan and Wichita groups), the Baron de Ripperdá, governor from 1770 to 1778 in Texas, was able to overcome these objections and put into effect, along with the Louisiana authorities, this new Indian policy more successfully in the province of Texas. The key points of the revamped Spanish trade policy were the following:

1. Annual distribution of presents was to be reestablished with those tribes considered loyal to the king of Spain.
2. Traders in each village were to purchase furs and other items in exchange for supplies. Every village headman or chief was to be provided with a table of prices to ensure that fixed prices could be maintained.

The implementation of these two points of policy was to ensure good economic and political relations with the Indians of Louisiana and Texas. This was necessary in Spain's eyes because these groups served as buffers against the English on the east side of the Mississippi River; moreover, the policy would negate the trade influences of the English in the two provinces.

Annual presents to the native Americans in the Provincias Internas were distributed in Louisiana even as the cession to Spain took place, with distribution points at Natchitoches, Arkansas Post, New Orleans, and St. Louis. The Kadohadacho and other Caddoan groups living on the Red River received their presents at Natchitoches. Approximately 360 pesos worth of goods were distributed to them in 1770; based on Kinnaird (1949) this is probably a typical amount up to 1776. In 1770, the 127 pesos' worth of goods given to the Gran Cado (the Kadohadacho) as an annual present included:

A hat trimmed with galloons	24 large knives
An ornamented shirt	40 small knives
Two fusils	48 awls
Two blankets of 2½ points	48 worm-screws
Three ells of cloth	200 flints
Two ordinary shirts	24 steels
A copper kettle	48 hawksbells
20 lb. powder	200 needles
40 lb. balls	90 ells of tape
1 lb. vermillion	10 rolls of tobacco
2 lb. glass beads	Two jugs of brandy
1 lb. thread	Six mirrors
One axe	2 lb. wire
Two adzes	One flag
Half a piece of cord	Two hatchets
25 lb. of salt	One ell of ribbon for the medal

The amount of goods necessary to annually supply the Gran Cado (the Kadohadacho) in trade and exchange for furs, horses, and bear oil was twenty to thirty times larger than the annual presents. This suggests that 7,200–11,000 pesos was an amount sufficient to stock the Natchitoches post for the Kadohadacho, Natchitoches, and Yatasi needs (Bolton 1914, 1:132–134, 143–146).

Following the formal establishment of the Provincias Internas in 1776, annual gifts began to increase significantly (Table 22). Before 1776 annual gifts or "friendship" to the Indian populations in Louisiana accounted for five percent or less of the total yearly annual expenses of the province. Afterward, they accounted for between 10 percent and 40 percent of yearly expenses.

In Spanish Texas the administration tried to follow the trade and gift patterns reestablished in Louisiana and already promised to the Texas Indians by de Mézières in 1779, but it was constrained by the scarcity and cost of trade goods (John 1975, 622). In October 1780 the supply of trade goods ran out at both Natchitoches and Nacogdoches, the new distribution center in Spanish Texas (John 1975). Nevertheless, during this period European goods were available at an unprecedented level and began to dominate the character of aboriginal assemblages. Particularly common were those items having new forms, such as steel axes, hoes, glass bottles, and kettles, and materials requiring new methods for their use (Brain 1979, 273–274), for example skillets, scissors, strike-a-lights (metal bars used to strike a light), drawknives, and nails.

For the Spaniards, the development of new means of trade and Indian relations after 1780 raised serious questions concerning what goods should go to which Indian groups, which groups should be excluded from trade, how much should be given, under whose jurisdiction should it be given, and from what site should the goods be distributed (Kinnaird 1949, 2:80). Tribes and headmen (*caciques*) friendly to the Spanish were rewarded by annual gifts, but those groups considered to be hostile were excluded from receiving annual presents. These judgments naturally varied year to year, depending on the Spanish desire to maintain a balance of power in the area within and beyond their control. Essentially, the gifts could be used in a manipulative sense to cause changes in tribal alliances, particularly those changes in alliances considered necessary to offset further English trade and economic influences. Generally speaking, those Indian groups who dealt with the English or directly threatened Spanish settlers (first the Apache and then the Comanche) were considered to be hostile by the Spanish authorities.

Recommendations circulated in 1783 by the Spanish government concerning annual presents to be given to the different friendly tribes in Texas provide an idea of the kinds and amounts of trade goods to be found on post-1780 Historic period sites (Table 23). Additionally, friendly chiefs, appointed

TABLE 22. Expenses of the Province of Louisiana by Fiscal Categories, 1766–1785 (in *Reales de Plata*)

	Allotment		Extraordinary		Marine		Friendship to Indian Populations		
Year	(No.)	(%)	(No.)	(%)	(No.)	(%)	(No.)	(%)	Total
1766	227,992	83.1	28,688	10.5	17,633	6.4	NA		274,323
1767	961,052	82.4	61,464	5.3	84,292	7.2	60,242	5.1	1,167,050
1768	918,202	69.1	268,636	20.2	118,268	8.9	23,072	1.8	1,328,178
1769	1,444,243	69.3	423,472	20.3	194,952	9.4	19,864	1.0	2,082,531
1770	969,768	75.2	208,040	16.2	86,706	6.7	24,304	1.9	1,288,818
1771	801,854	93.2	25,804	3.0	NA		32,599	3.8	859,257
1772	876,960	93.5	15,785	1.7	NA		45,387	4.8	938,132
1773	806,890	95.5	7,018	0.8	NA		31,253	3.7	845,161
1774	802,887	91.0	43,076	4.9	NA		36,212	4.1	882,175
1775	810,451	92.9	23,614	2.7	NA		38,052	4.4	872,117
1776	808,018	92.0	49,024	5.6	NA		21,085	2.4	878,127
1777	790,833	78.1	114,953	11.2	NA		109,453	10.7	1,016,239
1778	848,221	64.5	266,174	20.3	NA		198,066	15.2	1,312,461
1779	1,517,934	32.7	2,094,424	45.1	NA		1,028,544	22.2	4,640,902
1780	1,897,547	40.7	2,098,131	45.2	NA		653,050	14.1	4,648,728
1781	2,487,272	37.0	3,389,166	50.3	NA		857,969	12.7	6,734,407
1782	1,788,907	32.9	1,463,345	26.9	NA		2,186,902	40.2	5,439,154
1783	1,784,328	42.7	1,425,227	34.1	NA		968,241	23.2	4,177,797
1784	1,707,814	40.2	951,065	22.4	NA		1,586,917	37.4	4,245,796
1785	2,341,752	44.8	1,986,352	39.2	NA		762,852	15.0	5,090,856

Source: Data from Archivo General de Indios, Legajos 597.

Note: Expenses are measured in *reales de plata* (Treasury silver) and related percentages.

capitánes or *gobernadores* by the Spanish and then presented with medals to signify their position (see Ewers 1974; Sabo 1988), were to receive:

One axe	One pair of knitted stockings
One hatchet	One pair of shoes
One mattock	One pair of buckles of common metal
One gun	
4 lb. gunpowder	1/2 lb. vermillion
8 lb. bullets	Six large heavy knives
One pair trousers	1 lb. beads
One fine trimmed shirt	One tobacco bundle

One pound of beads was probably sufficient to make one beaded shirt (Gregory 1973, 156) using the seed beads common in post-1750 Historic period sites in the Caddoan Area.

Even as the Spanish government began to finally develop a commercially oriented Indian policy in Texas and Louisiana, it faced stiff competition first from the English trading houses east of the Mississippi River and then equally stiff competition from the Americans. The English were able to well supply such groups as the Osage or Pawnee who lived in Spanish Louisiana but who had never been consistently favored or considered to be friendly by Spanish authorities. Furthermore, English merchants sent trade expeditions along the Texas Gulf Coast and up some of the major streams, and they also illegally maintained traders among some of the Caddoan groups in East Texas after 1780 (Pichardo in Hackett 1931–1946, 2:para. 709). The firm of St. Maxent and Ranson had been appointed commissioners of Indian affairs for Louisiana in 1769, and all goods distributed there were supposed to be purchased only through them. The British, working out of Pensacola, Florida, however, had a major controlling interest in the St. Maxent and Ranson firm (Clark 1970) and were able to use that control to unload their trade goods at a suitable profit (Kinnaird 1949, 1:104). Thereby, they negated some of the Spanish efforts to maintain a socially and economically viable trade venture.

Consequently, after ca. 1770, trade goods of English derivation became available legally and illegally in the French and Spanish markets. Traders living among the Caddoan groups in Louisiana especially but also in Spanish Texas began to distribute English trade goods to them, taking into account the preferences of the different Indian groups with which they dealt.

Glass Beads

Glass beads found on Caddoan sites occupied during the eighteenth and early nineteenth centuries demonstrate changes in the nature of European-Indian contact and trade good supply that support a real "clustering of cer-

TABLE 23. Recommendations Concerning 1783 Annual Presents to Friendly Tribes in the Province of Texas

Present	Tawakoni	Taovayas	Tonkawa	Texas	Bidai	Arkokisas/ Cocos/ Mayeyes	Kichais
Axe	12	24	12	6	6	3	3
Hatchet	6	12	6	3	3	2	2
Mattock	6	12	6	3	3	2	2
Gun	6	12	6	3	3	2	2
Gunpowder (lbs.)	36	72	36	18	18	9	9
Ball (lbs.)	72	144	72	36	36	18	18
Ells cloth	16	32	16	8	8	4	4
Shirts	14	28	14	7	7	4	4
Vermillion (lbs.)	6	12	6	3	3	2	2
Knives (dozen)	7	14	7	3.5	3.5	2	2
Beads (lbs.)	14	28	14	7	7	4	4
Combs (dozen)	8	16	8	4	4	2	2
Tobacco (bundles)	16	40	16	8	8	4	4

Source: From Kinnaird 1949, 2:80.

tain varieties with a particular European nationality at a particular time" (Brain 1979, 116). Brain's 1979 analysis of the temporal-spatial relationships of bead varieties from Eastern North America shows that certain bead types have a restricted spatial distribution that can be reasonably interpreted as being the result of specific national areas of contact and/or supply (i.e., French, Spanish, or English). This temporal-spatial relationship seems to be the case regardless of the fact that most glass beads of the eighteenth century were made in Venice and Amsterdam (Karklins 1985, 114), and each European country operating in Eastern North America had the same general range of bead types to distribute. It does appear likely that, all things being considered equal, distinctive bead assemblages found in different aboriginal locales might also be evidence for particular Indian color and size preferences (see Hamell 1983), which were accommodated by the different Europeans for a considerable time.

Brain's categorization of nationalities of European contact in the examination of bead types, the median age of the beads, and their distribution on Historic Caddoan period sites supports some changes in Indian-European relationships in the mid– to late eighteenth century that were expected based on the archival and documentary records. Bead assemblages from the Norteno phase sites on the Red River (ca. 1700–1750+), the Norteno phase sites on the upper Sabine River (ca. 1740–1780+), the Lawton phase (ca. 1714–1803), and the Little River phase (ca. 1719–1780) were examined to ascertain changes in patterns of contact and trade within certain parts of the Caddoan Area (Table 24).

French contact dominates the bead assemblages across the entire eighteenth century, its origin being primarily from the lower Mississippi River and its distribution centers at New Orleans and Natchitoches. Evidence of French contact from outside the lower Mississippi Valley is most common at Caddoan sites along the middle Red River, the area of the Kadohadacho and ethnically related groups, in an early, pre-1740, context. It is probable that this contact relates to interaction with the French Illinois colony that was known by 1710 to have obtained horses in trade with Caddoan groups on the Red River (Giraud 1974a:343) and to have had interaction and exchange relationships with the Osage. In the Little River phase, contemporaneous with the establishment of adjacent Fort de St. Louis by de la Harpe in 1719 (Wedel 1978), bead types signaling French contact from the lower Mississippi Valley account for 94 percent of the glass beads present. Of greater significance is that no bead type present is indicative of primary Spanish contact. The Little River phase beads were likely obtained directly from the French traders at Fort de St. Louis. The other localities evidence some Spanish (or Spanish-English) contact. Based on the archaeological context these glass beads were derived from Spanish annual gift distribu-

TABLE 24. Bead Assemblages on Eighteenth-Century Caddoan Phase Sites: Median Bead Dates by Sources

	Median Dates and other Data on Bead Types					
	French[a]	French[b]	English	Spanish/ English	French/ Spanish/ English	French/ English
Norteno phase (Red River)	1735	1740	1763	1748	1742	1739
Norteno phase (Sabine River)	1745	1743	1763	1752	1742	1755
Lawton phase	1745	1739	1788	1752	1742	1749
Little River phase	1741	1739	1797	—	1739	—
Bead types (mean)	3	9	2	1	5	2.5
Seed bead types (%)	0	9	29	0	21	20
Wire-bound bead types (%)	8	17	62	0	0	80

Source: Adapted from Brain 1979, 117–133.
[a]But not lower Mississippi Valley sources.
[b]Louisiana sources.

tions after 1769. The highest frequency of bead types of English or English-French nationality (see Table 24) are found in certain Lawton phase bead assemblages and in a post-1780 Pascagoula-Biloxi cemetery on the Red River below Natchitoches (Gregory and Webb 1965).[4] The Lawton phase assemblages span a considerable length of time, but the high percentage of seed beads and wire-bound beads denote significant Caddoan occupations after ca. 1760 (Brain 1979; Deagan 1987). (*Seed beads* were drawn beads generally less than four millimeters in diameter.)

Trends in bead sizes in the eighteenth century, particularly the high frequency of seed beads in certain assemblages, correlate well temporally with the overall shift in Spanish Indian trade policy, annual presents, and the increasing percentage of the yearly budget spent on Indian gifts. Gregory (1973, 154–155) further notes that the introduction of seed beads is associated not only with the increasing use of beads by Caddoan groups, but also with a shift about 1750 in the style of clothing. Beaded shirts, which were shirts having borders of seed beads or beads as bands crossing the waist, came into vogue.

Archaeological examples of this type of bead use in Caddoan clothing is represented in the Pearson site assemblage from the upper Sabine River Norteno phase (Duffield and Jelks 1961, 51) and from the Kinsloe phase on the middle Sabine River (Jones 1968). This type of clothing apparently became even more popular in the 1800s after the introduction of special small needles (Gregory 1973; Berlandier 1969). Seed beads do not necessarily represent only the late eighteenth-century Caddoan use of beaded clothing styles, for burials in many areas demonstrate seed beads were distributed before 1750. Rather, the patterned arrangements of bands of seed beads on clothing is most indicative of this Historic development in Caddoan adornment. Earlier in the eighteenth century, in fact, beads were generally larger and were primarily worn as necklaces and bracelets rather than sewn onto articles of clothing. Other items of European use, especially silver, may also reflect the same kind of stylistic change that accompanied the wide-scale adoption of European dress provided in the annual gifts to the Caddoan peoples. These European clothes were distinctly altered to conform to native concepts of dress, however (Gregory 1978; Perttula 1991).

This type of aboriginal use of European manufactured items is closely related to the reorganized Indian trade post-dating the French cession of Louisiana to Spain. Pre- and post-1760 Caddoan archaeological sites thus manifest distinctly different patterns of contact as seen from a general accessibility of trade goods, material culture changes, and changes in ways of life. Since there are specific observable differences in the archaeological record generally, single-component Historic period Caddoan sites should provide an even better opportunity to relate specific occupations to particular systems of contact, trade relationships, and means of interaction.

CHANGES IN THE COMPLEXITY OF CADDOAN SOCIOPOLITICAL ORGANIZATION

The confederacies among the Hasinai, Kadohadacho, and Natchitoches Caddo are distinct entities in the ethnographic and ethnohistorical record (Swanton 1942, 7–16). But how well does the term *confederacy* reflect Caddoan sociopolitical organizations that existed in the Contact record? Are the notions of tribal confederacies and complex sociopolitical order appropriate concepts (Woodall 1980) to apply to the southern Caddoan-speaking polities of the seventeenth and eighteenth centuries?

Direct ethnographic evidence demonstrates that the Natchitoches Caddo confederacy was not formed until after 1700. Its formation seems to have been a result of French exploration and settlement of the Red River. Before forming the confederacy, most of the Natchitoches had abandoned their main village on the Red River and followed St. Denis to the French fort at the mouth of the Mississippi River, while the remainder moved up the river toward the Kadohadacho, where they maintained a separate *ranchería* through the first half of the eighteenth century (Clark 1902; Wedel 1978). The "lower" Natchitoches followed St. Denis to Lake Pontchartrain, where they lived until 1714, when St. Denis took them back with him to their old village when he built the post of Fort de le St. Baptiste at Natchitoches as a trading depot (Swanton 1942, 53).

The Ouachita Caddo group had already begun to join with the Natchitoches on the Red River by 1690; they had only five cabins left on the Ouachita River in 1700 (Dickinson 1980). The Yatasi and the Doustioni then joined with the Natchitoches and Ouachita after the establishment of the Natchitoches trading depot. The Yatasi had previously lived on Red River between the Natchitoches and Kadohadacho in the vicinity of present-day Shreveport, Louisiana, but segments of the Yatasi were eventually absorbed by the two larger groups (Swanton 1942, 13). Webb and Gregory (1978) consider the Yatasi to be a kin-linked band lumped into a category comprising only small, scattered groups in the late seventeenth century, and in all likelihood, these bands were remnants of the much larger Caddoan populations known to have been present in that part of the Red River Valley in the sixteenth and possibly early seventeenth centuries. The Kadohadacho term *Yatasi* means only "those other people" (Webb and Gregory 1978 : 29).

The Kadohadacho confederacy was composed of two separate Kadohadacho villages, or *rancherías,* as well as the Nanatsoho, Nasoni, and "upper" Natchitoches groups. It represents the same sort of kin and linguistic grouping of once-separate entities and remnants of populations already noted to be characteristic of the Natchitoches confederacy.

Both the Nasoni and Natchitoches were remnants of larger groups who lived elsewhere in the Caddoan Area in the sixteenth and early seventeenth centuries. The Nasoni apparently lived in the lower Sulphur River basin ca. 1540 (see Fig. 2). When they fragmented, one remnant became affiliated with the Kadohadacho (Wedel 1978); the other, with the Nadaco of the Hasinai confederacy (see Fig. 22). The Nanatsoho in 1690 lived on the Red River upstream from the other Kadohadacho groups, but between 1690 and 1719 they moved ten leagues (twenty-eight miles) downstream to establish a *ranchería* in the midst of the larger Kadohadacho community (Wedel 1978, 8). Documentary evidence also indicates that other Caddoan groups in the late seventeenth century lived twenty leagues (fifty-five miles) or more upstream of the Kadohadacho community, but they are not recorded in post-1727 documents (Table 25).

It is clear that the Kadohadacho confederacy was in existence prior to the onset of sustained European contact, since its constituent members were already in association at the time they were first described by French and Spanish explorers in 1690. The confederacy was also an enclave for scat-

TABLE 25. Archival Documentation of Caddoan Groups in East Texas

Native Groups	Late Seventeenth Century—ca. 1727	Post-1727
Anadarko (Nadaco)	X	X
Anao	X	
Cachae (Cataye or Caxo)	X	
Cantey[a]	X	
Dotchetonne	X	X
Hacanac	X	
Hainai		X
Haqui[b]	X	
Lacane	X	
Naansi[b]	X	
Nabedache		X
Nabeyxa[b]	X	
Nabiri (Nabiti)	X	X
Nacachau	X	
Nacaniche[c]		X
Nacau	X	X
Nacogdoche	X	X
Nacono	X	X
Nakanawan	X	
Nanatsoho	X	X
Nasayaha	X	
Nasoni	X	X
Nechaui		X
Sassory	X	
Sico	X	
Tadiva	X	
Vinta	X	
Neche	X	X

Source: From Campbell 1976; Swanton 1942.

Note: X indicates presence.

[a] Seventy miles west of the Kadohadacho on the Red River.

[b] In the Sabine/Sulphur river basins.

[c] Later form of *Lacane*.

tered Caddoan populations from other areas outside of the Red River. The Cahinnio Caddo community on the Ouachita River in Southwest Arkansas was abandoned shortly after 1687. Remnant groups moved to the Red River among the Kadohadacho, others moved near to the Quapaw on the lower Arkansas River, and still others moved to the upper Arkansas River to merge with the Mento Wichita band (Dickinson 1980).

Eleven bands or tribes have traditionally constituted the Hasinai Caddo confederacy (Swanton 1942, 7–14); however, documentary evidence published by Campbell (1976) suggests that there were at least twelve additional bands or groups in the East Texas area during the late seventeenth century, and most of them appear to have been territorially independent units or entities at that time. Ethnographic information is extremely limited for these other bands, and thus they are known primarily from pre-1727 documentary materials where their names are recorded on tribal lists compiled by the Spanish and French authorities (see Table 25).

They were probably absorbed by other Hasinai groups or became extinct during the eighteenth century. Specifying locations for these groups is also difficult, but many seem to have lived north of the Hasinai confederacy (see Fig. 22) in the area described by Bolton (1908, 251) as uninhabited territory in the mid-eighteenth century. Even some recognized members of the Hasinai confederacy, such as the Nacao, Nacachau, Nacono, and Nechaui bands, were mentioned only infrequently after ca. 1716 in the archival documents. By that time, they had apparently lost their separate ethnic and band identity through such processes of fragmentation and ethnic absorption because the Hasinai confederacy consolidated around the Hainai and Neche bands after that date (Griffith 1954).

At one time all Caddoan-speaking groups in the Caddoan Area appear to have spoken separate dialects (Lesser and Weltfish 1932). The available linguistic evidence parallels the sociopolitical changes noted above in that it documents a progressive between-group homogeneity and the subsequent disappearance of most of the Caddoan dialects.[5] The confederacies existed at the time of sustained European contact, and while they were referred to as confederacies throughout the eighteenth century, overall control of Caddoan society was already based more on individual kin group than the confederacies by around the middle of the eighteenth century (Wyckoff and Baugh 1980; Gregory 1973). The confederacies are best considered short-lived products of intragroup fragmentation and intergroup agglomeration in a few select and traditional locales. Groups changed alliances and relationships from generation to generation and were often divided between the confederacies. The confederacies were probably also a response to regional depopulation (see chapter 3) and Osage depredations, but the ensuing local settlement aggregation had an important effect on how diverse kin and/or dialect groups could be integrated into a newly created and functioning Caddoan society.

SUMMARY

Archaeological evidence from the Red and Ouachita river valleys suggests early Caddoan and Tunican participation in the fur trade pre-dated 1700, and the temporal setting and isolated nature of early fur trading sites indicate that the trade was independent of direct European participation or supervision. In these situations, access to European goods, particularly guns, was variable and unreliable. By 1740–1750, however, European goods were being distributed by European traders who lived as semipermanent residents in most Caddoan villages, and the importance of the fur trade grew for Caddoan peoples with the economic incentive.

In terms of the French Louisiana colonial economy, the years between 1739 and 1757 were the most important years for the development of the fur trade. Even so, the fur trade never contributed more than 15 percent of the total annual exports from French Louisiana. For the Caddoan groups, fur trading was to become a dominant economic activity, particularly with respect to conditioning the nature and extent of European interaction, at about the same time the relative influence of the fur trade within the colonial economy was declining. The continuation of Caddoan participation in the fur trade in the American and Texas Republic periods is owed at least in part to its being the activity best suited to maintaining stable trade alliances between European, Anglo-American, and Caddoan peoples.

When the Spanish were ceded the Louisiana colony, they kept this trade policy in force. They buttressed the policy by spending between 10 percent and 40 percent of their total expenses in the province of Louisiana from 1766 to 1785 on annual trade presents and other gifts to the Indians. As access to European goods became more dependable, Caddoan groups in East Texas and the Red River Valley were able to extend their influence south and west among non-Caddoan groups who were not capable of directly contacting the French or Spanish in Natchitoches or New Orleans or who had no French traders in villages.

Trade goods in abundance in Historic Caddoan settlements date primarily to the years after 1730 and after the establishment of reliable fur trade relationships. European goods are not common on Historic period Caddoan habitation sites or cemeteries dating to before that time (Cole 1975; Story 1982, n.d.; Trubowitz 1984). The European trade goods found in pre-1730 contexts are restricted to ornamental artifacts, reworked metal scraps, and other nonutilitarian objects primarily found in mortuary contexts as grave goods. Guns, axes, knives, powder and shot, and clothing items are also much more common on trade good inventories after 1740.

Differences in the types and amounts of annual presents distributed by the Spanish to native Americans after 1760 in the region had their basis in variable aboriginal populations and to perceived relationships of power between native groups and the Spanish. A comparison of the annual presents given to each tribe imparts some idea of the nature of intertribal and Spanish interaction in the late eighteenth century. In the province of Texas, the most important tribe, the Taovayas Wichita, received four times as many trade goods as did the Hasinai Caddo or Tejas tribes.

Coincident with the establishment of the Spanish Louisiana administration and the continuation of the French policy of annual presents and permanent resident traders was the introduction of trade goods by the English from their Gulf Coast and Atlantic Coast colonies. Most of the Spanish trade goods distributed in the late eighteenth century were purchased from the British, and the British had also begun to send traders directly to the Caddoan *rancherías*. British trade goods at Caddoan sites are, therefore, reliable markers for post-1760 Caddoan occupations from the Arkansas River to East Texas (Brain 1979).

PART 3

Summary

Conclusions and Future Prospects

Archaeology [is] essential to understanding better the nature of human beings and their place in the world. —*Bruce Trigger, 1990*

In this summary I take stock of our study of the Caddoan archaeological and ethnohistorical record for 1520–1800, reviewing these records and what they tell us about the Caddoan peoples of the Trans-Mississippi South. This study is essentially a first-order approximation of the character of the contact and acculturative process between the Caddoan peoples and Europeans and as such stays close to the available data most of the time. Nevertheless, from time to time the archaeological and ethnohistorical records were sufficiently robust to prompt me to more broadly generalize, hypothesize, and speculate than previously about the Caddoan Contact era. Future work and collaborative research efforts will be necessary to evaluate more thoroughly these generalizations and to corroborate them or propose more comprehensive and/or alternative understandings.

That being the case, I also discuss in this concluding chapter future prospects for study of Caddoan archaeology and ethnohistory. These future prospects include what I consider to be the key research goals, methods, and data needs that must be further assessed and developed for there to be positive and substantive increases in our understanding of the cultural heritage of the Caddoan peoples. They include the comprehensive study of (*a*) Spanish, French, and American archival and documentary records, (*b*) the archaeological record of the fur trade, (*c*) the archaeology and ethnohistory of the post-Removal period, and (*d*) the paleodemographic and bioarchaeological data.

THE ARCHAEOLOGY OF THE PROTOHISTORIC PERIOD

The Protohistoric period, 1520–1685, precedes any sustained contact between Europeans and Caddoan peoples of the Trans-Mississippi South. Any systemic change in aboriginal adaptations that would have occurred during this time, the Protohistoric "Dark Ages" (Dye 1986), are not retrievable from archival records or ethnographic observations of the Spanish or French colonists, missionaries, or traders, but must be documented and studied in the Caddoan archaeological record. That record was explored in this study to detect systemic cultural change from precontact to Historic times among Caddoan peoples and, knowing that, determine later how such changes might be manifestations of any more comprehensive reorientation in Caddoan lifeways arising after interaction with Europeans.

The lack of regionally based representative samples of Protohistoric period settlements in any locality or region of the Caddoan Area prohibits accurate archaeological estimates of population changes during these times. Instead, qualitative differences in various sociopolitical and community-wide aspects of Caddoan lifeways must be examined, first, as one means to characterize 1520–1685 Caddoan peoples and their cultures and, second, to assess apparent group or phase differences over time and their relationship to any impact and population loss from European diseases, settlement movements, and changes or disruptions in social and political organization.

By the time of sustained European contact after ca. 1685, large portions of the Caddoan Area had been abandoned by Caddoan peoples. Consequently, spatial continuity between the late Caddoan period (ca. 1400–1520) occupations, early Historic or Protohistoric Caddoan cultural phases, and historically recorded Caddoan groups is fragmentary, producing a disjunctive Historic archaeological and ethnographic record.

Particularly along the major streams such as the Arkansas, Red, and Ouachita rivers, most of the abandonment by Caddoan peoples seems to have occurred between ca. 1600 and the first substantial episodes of face-to-face European contact. This abandonment did not take place at the same time from region to region, but did have two common features: (*a*) the substantial movement of groups in the late sixteenth and seventeenth centuries and (*b*) a coalescence of local Caddoan groups with other groups only in major riverine settlements on the Red River or on the lower Ouachita River.

In the Arkansas River basin of eastern Oklahoma, Caddoan settlement ends ca. 1550–1600. Indications of more mobile settlement systems becoming successful about this time on the southern plains appear to correlate with a northern Caddoan reorientation of subsistence patterns (brought about in large measure by the adoption of the horse and the pursuit of bison) and with such differences in sociopolitical complexity as becoming more egalitarian (Peterson 1989, 119). The archaeological record suggests a rapid movement out of the basin by the remaining Caddoan populations during the seventeenth century. That movement, toward the Red River or west up the Arkansas River and out onto the southern plains, was accompanied by intensification of a plains-oriented subsistence system based on seasonal bison hunting using horses (R. E. Bell 1981, 1984b; Baugh 1982) and trading bison hides and other goods (Vehik 1990).

In the Ouachita River Valley some Caddoan groups may have moved downriver through the sixteenth and seventeenth centuries into areas that had been vacant since about 1400 (Gibson 1985b, 328–331). In certain respects, they were probably made up of a diminished but diverse number of groups in the region who had formerly been separate sociopolitical entities. The Caddoan occupation of the Ouachita River Valley ended rather abruptly in the late seventeenth to early eighteenth century, prior to sustained contact with Europeans.

Up until the time of abandonment, there appears to have been a relatively dense population in the valley, with mound use in some form continuing until approximately 1650 (Early 1990). The bioarchaeological evidence from the Ouachita River basin, which is relatively comprehensive compared with that of most other regional sequences in the Caddoan Area (Burnett 1990a, 1990b), suggests that despite an epidemic of smallpox between 1500 and 1650, in general the Caddoan populations of the region had adapted well and experienced no diminishment in adaptive efficiency during the Protohistoric period. There does appear to have been a lower population density after ca. 1650 and an overall decrease in maize consumption.

The Red River Valley in the central Caddoan subarea is one of the better known archaeological regions of the Early Historic or Protohistoric period. Excavations at the Belcher and Cedar Grove sites (Webb 1959; Trubowitz 1984; Jeter et al. 1989) have provided substantial evidence on diachronic patterns of mound use, mortuary practices, and community sociopolitical complexity between ca. 1500 and 1740. Periods of mound use and/or mound pit burials on the Red River for the McCurtain, Texarkana, and Belcher phase regions generally predate ca. 1650. Their discontinuation coincides with evidence of decreased social differentiation and/or complexity and with less extensive settlement within the Red River Valley. Settlements are widely separated in the Protohistoric period, and they appear to be made up of clusters of farmsteads and family communities. These localities are maintained, however, up to about 1730 on the middle Red River, and perhaps as late as 1790 in the Great Bend locality, and were the focus of whatever regional processes of Caddoan population amalgamation and settlement that took place. This kind of regional settlement density is consistent with local population amalgamation and regional population decline. The amalgamations, however, did not bring Caddoan populations within these locales up to the densities probably characteristic of the region during Late Caddoan or Protohistoric times.

In the western Caddoan subareas of East Texas and the Ouachita Mountains, the archaeological record for the Caddoan rural communities is broadly indicative of changes in sociopolitical complexity accompanied by a localization of community systems. Both these processes share similarities with the archaeological record in the Red River Valley. In the Ouachita Mountains, moreover, it is likely the case that much of the mountains were not permanently inhabited after 1600.

Relatively specific changes in the nature of Caddoan settlement and community organization during the Protohistoric and Historic periods were noted in the Cypress Creek and upper Sabine River archaeological sequences. Examples of nonmound shaft burials and isolated community cemeteries associated with distinct spatial groups (referred to as *clusters* or *subclusters* by Thurmond [1985]) were readily identified as manifestations of a form of sociopolitical integration that replaced mound centers. The mound centers were replaced by the formation and use of community-wide cemeteries ca. 1550–1600, and these cemeteries were used by relatively egalitarian Caddoan societies. However, both the community cemeteries and the nonmound shaft burials were short-lived phenomena, apparently being maintained (as evidenced by the archaeological record) only until ca. 1650–1670.

Therefore, while processes of regional abandonment and possible depopulation affected East Texas and western Caddoan populations in the Protohistoric period, evidence that community reintegration did take place may mean that cultural disruptions and depopulation were not as severe initially among these rural Caddoan communities as it was for some of the Caddoan populations in the major river valleys. That the Sabine, Neches, and Angelina river basins in East Texas appear to have had a higher density of Protohistoric and post-1685 Historic Caddoan settlements than is evidently the case on the major rivers (with the possible exception of the Ouachita River basin up until 1650) within the Caddoan Area also points to the possibility that there was a greater depopulation in town communities than in rural communities following the initiation of European contact and interaction.

Nevertheless, even in these regions of East Texas the occupations are more scattered than they were ca. 1520, with many of the minor river valleys being unoccupied or having a much smaller overall population in the Protohistoric and Historic periods than previously was the case. Even ca. 1700, the Caddoan populations in East Texas were larger than the Kadohadacho and the Natchitoches groups on Red River. The East Texas Caddoan groups maintained that numerical superiority throughout the eighteenth century, even as the total Caddoan population decreased from about 7,000 to 1,400 individuals (Swanton 1942).

THE HISTORIC PERIOD ARCHAEOLOGICAL RECORD

The archaeological record in the Caddoan Area dating after ca. 1685 is unfortunately not based primarily on comprehensive investigations in habitation contexts, but on a record—albeit extensive—obtained from excavating associated household cemeteries. This bias in archaeological investigations severely constrains the examination of systemic changes in Caddoan lifeways that are associated with sustained contact with Europeans.

We may first note that community cemeteries are not part of the archaeological record at this time. Settlement data from more intensively surveyed locales within the overall Caddoan Area indicate no change in the dispersed pattern of farmsteads and hamlets (referred to in the ethnographic record as *rancherías*) noted from the 1520–1685 period. There is ethnohistorical evidence that may indicate that *rancherías* were larger among the Kadohadacho and aggregated Caddoan tribes on the Red River and that there were more separate but smaller *rancherías* among the Hasinai tribes in East Texas. Except for a single nucleated community of Cahinnio Caddo on the Ouachita River and some archaeological evidence indicative of small *rancherías* on the Sabine, Sulphur, and middle Ouachita rivers, the Hasinai and Kadohadacho Caddo *rancherías* represent only widely separated groups between abandoned areas devoid of settlement until after ca. 1740, when possible fur trade or hunting campsites may have been present.

Another cluster of Caddoan settlements was located around the French trading post at Natchitoches and the Spanish presidio/mission established at Los Adaes. These settlements comprised a number of once ethnically distinct but recently affiliated Caddoan groups who moved there together in attempts to better manipulate and control access to the French trading effort and also to increase their chances of obtaining available trade goods—glass beads, guns, and metal implements. The Caddoan community around Natchitoches declined 61 percent in the first two decades of French settlement in the early eighteenth century.

At the Kadohadacho–Upper Natchitoches–upper Nasoni communities located in the vicinity of Fort de St. Louis, at the upper end of the Great Bend on Red River, there are a number of sites with post-1685 components. The relative density in this locality suggests a short-term and limited increase in population that was probably the result of the incorporation of Caddoan groups from both north and south of the Red River. This Caddoan *ranchería* was maintained at this place on the Red River until about 1790, when it was reestablished around Caddo Lake about seventy miles to the south. By the 1830s the *ranchería* was located along tributaries of Cypress Bayou and the Red River in Northeast Texas (Perttula 1991). An epidemic in 1777 was a contributing factor in the abandonment of the Red River locality.

In most of the other places within the Caddoan Area where Caddoan occupations postdating 1685 have been investigated, with the exception of the Sabine River Nadaco groups, there is no solid evidence to indicate that settlements lasted much beyond 1740. Sites such as those on the Sulphur River (which are considered to be part of the Hunt phase) or on the middle Red River (the Bob Williams–Sam Kaufman–Roden sites) cannot be ascribed with any confidence to any known ethnographic entities in the Caddoan Area.

Mortuary variability in post-1685 Caddoan sites indicates that differences within Caddoan groups in social status cannot be ascribed to rank distinctions or vertical differentiation. Such items previously associated with Caddoan status positions as conch shell ornaments may be found in these sites in a nonrestricted context. This change in associational context and location suggests a communalization of previously symbol-laden goods and a substantial reorganization of the status system (Knight 1986; Smith 1987).

THE ETHNOHISTORICAL RECORD

The processes of amalgamation and patterns of mobility initiated during the earlier phases of European contact were more or less already established by the time major European explorations were undertaken and the Caddoan peoples were described. The nature of contact 1685–1800 can be best described as one of acculturation for both the European and Caddoan inhabitants of the Trans-Mississippi South (Gregory 1973, 1983). By *acculturation* I mean "culture change as it is generated by culture contact . . . [and] initiated by the conjunction of two or more autonomous cultural systems" (Social Science Research Council 1954, 974). As McEwan and Mitchem (1984, 279) point out, for the Europeans key processes of acculturation involved both realms of the diet and techniques of food preparation: "because supplies to these relatively isolated regions were limited and irregular, items which were rapidly depleted or perishable (such as food), or goods which were easily damaged, would logically require the most immediate alternative solutions for replacement or supplementation."

In this type of scenario European settlements relied upon the local aboriginal communities for supplying necessary food items such as salt, bison, venison, vegetables, cultivated crops, and bear oil. In return, European goods and products were supplied to the aboriginal communities as payment. Thus, the relationship between European and Caddoan groups when permanent settlement began was one of symbiosis: the exchange of ornamental and utilitarian European-manufactured goods for subsistence-related items supplied by the Caddoan groups. This symbiosis characterized French settlements from Natchitoches to Fort de St. Louis.

As a process, the establishment of permanent settlements and economic exchange by the Europeans was an opportunity for Caddoan groups to extend already extant trade relationships to include newcomers in their midst.

These new economic opportunities led, however, over the long term to the eventual incorporation of Caddoan peoples and lifeways into a European-dominated trade and economic network (Brown 1975; Usner 1989). This change from a traditional Caddoan economic strategy that was basically independent of the European world economy to one that was inextricably intertwined and dependent upon it seems to follow the same trends as Murphy and Steward (1956) noted in their classic study of aboriginal acculturation and its relationship to capitalistic trade. They concluded that

> outside commercial influence led to reduction of the local level of integration from the band or village to the individual family and in the way in which the family became reintegrated as a marginal part of the much larger nation. The local culture core contained the all-important factor of almost complete economic dependence upon trade goods.... These products did not achieve importance until the native populations became parts of larger sociocultural systems and began to produce for outside markets in a mercantilist pattern.... The culmination point may be said to have been reached when the amount of activity devoted to production for trade grows to such an extent that it interferes with the aboriginal subsistence cycle and associated social organization and makes their continuance impossible.

Trade and interaction strategies developed and successfully used by Caddoan groups in dealing with other aboriginal groups were extended to include the Europeans who could supply them with unique goods in exchange for their products. The Caddoan peoples dealt mainly in trade with the French and only rarely with the Spanish, because of the latter's prohibitions against trade with the Caddo. Consequently, Caddoan groups living near the Spanish continued to deal directly with the French on the Red River who were their source of European goods. Illegal trading activities between the French and Spanish became common by the mid-eighteenth century as some Spanish colonists tried to establish profitable trading partnerships with the East Texas Caddoan groups utilizing the methods of the French (Bolton 1915).

One other aspect of the extension of trade strategies to include Europeans can be noted in the Caddoan Area. This was the movement of groups to new geographical locations that were better in regard to middlemen, subsistence systems (traders), and ready access to goods. This usually meant, in practice, a movement of Caddoan groups closer toward European settlements (Gregory 1973). This particular strategy of trade was only briefly followed for the basic reason that more efficient transportation systems were continually being developed by the European settlers. These changes in trade systems thus brought desired goods to native American groups directly and (at least in theory) controlled the quantity and flow of goods without participation of Caddoan or other native American middlemen;

nevertheless, the archaeological record for the Historic period suggests that native American middlemen continued to operate in Louisiana and Spanish Texas through the latter part of the eighteenth century.

As a means of obtaining European tools and weapons, which were of considerable economic and military value, Caddoan fur trading established dependable supply networks with the French. Because the quantity and quality of such trade items were variable before aboriginal groups began to play a larger role in the colonial aspect of the European world economy, domination of the fur trade could only follow establishment of dependable supplies and trade good shipments (Lehmer 1977). Caddoan tribal locations relative to European supply points on the Red (Fort de St. Louis and Fort St. Jean de Baptiste aux Natchitoches), Arkansas (Arkansas Post), and Mississippi (New Orleans) rivers were of primary importance, therefore, in exerting power in developing and maintaining fur trade in the Trans-Mississippi South. Documentary evidence on the proportion of the French and Spanish Louisiana budget spent on Indian gifts and trade goods and the value of pelts in the combined exports from the colonies indicate that it was not until ca. 1740–1750 that such dependability was firmly established (Surrey 1916) among the native American groups of the Caddoan Area and French Louisiana.

FUTURE PROSPECTS

Through the study of archaeology and ethnohistory, we have learned a great deal about the native history of the Caddoan peoples of the Trans-Mississippi South. We have learned from the Caddoan peoples themselves about their cultural heritage (Newkumet and Meredith 1988), and professional archaeologists and ethnohistorians have finally come to appreciate that Caddoan peoples today, like many other native American tribes, have a strong and abiding interest in retaining, preserving, and enhancing their cultural heritage (Parker 1990, 167; Perttula in press). Certainly it is true that "Indian tribes and their individual members are generally more concerned with heritage preservation than even preservation minded non-Indians. Native Americans recognize that it is their culture that sets them apart. It makes them distinct and unique, and preserving these qualities is essential to their unique status as dependent sovereigns. . . . Native Americans generally realize that it is their heritage, both in its physical and intangible manifestations, that makes them unique. This recognition leads directly to a heightened concern for the protection and preservation of heritage resources" (Downer 1990, 89).

We can learn a lot more about the Caddoan peoples, and in doing so we can learn more about ourselves and our place in the world. Tremendous opportunities exist today for archaeologists, ethnohistorians, historians, and Caddoan peoples to begin working together to better understand the long and short-term courses of cultural change in Caddoan native history and to comprehend "that culture change undergone by Native American peoples was neither one-sided nor solely governed by European intentions and strategies" (Wilson and Rogers 1992, 1). The discussion below outlines a course of research that represents a step in that direction.

A first step toward expanding the archaeological and ethnohistorical study of Caddoan lifeways in the period after 1520 must include the following: (*a*) developing a solid knowledge of the context of Prehistoric Caddoan settlement and subsistence strategies in the Caddoan Area (Story 1990; Jeter et al. 1989) and (*b*) determining at least relative population sizes within each of the regions and river basins inhabited by Caddoan peoples. It is reasonable to suppose that existing cultural patterns of Caddoan groups at the time of first contact would certainly condition how they responded to the new circumstances created by the arrival of the Europeans. Any disruption or reorientation of aboriginal cultures that occurred as a result of contact and interaction with European groups is, in part, a product of that record, as is the success of adaptation methods developed by these native groups that proved effective in ensuring cultural survival in a changed world. During the Historic period, Caddoan groups found themselves in a new setting, a setting defined by the intermeshing of European and aboriginal cultural systems, behaviors, objectives, and motivations (Gregory 1973, 294).

Depending upon pre–Contact era Caddoan population sizes in particular regions, patterns of settlement size and nature, and the position of dense population clusters (or town communities) relative to trails or axes of communication, each region within the Caddoan Area would be affected differently by the Europeans. Therefore, settlement relocation, abandonment, and aggregation may not all take place within each of the regions and river valleys, and it is not to be expected that population declines and their impact would be regionally uniform. To ascertain why some regions were abandoned and never reoccupied while others served as focus sites for reintegration of disparate groups, we must also know more about Prehistoric settlement sizes, the minimum number of people necessary to maintain an integrated and coherent entity given existing subsistence and settlement strategies, and the means available for the agglomeration of independent cultural groups.

Ordinal scale measurements of Caddoan populations are also important to obtain in particular regions and temporal intervals in the Late Caddoan, Protohistoric, and Historic Caddoan period archaeological record. The dispersed character of Caddoan settlements during all the time periods under consideration will necessitate comprehensive site survey programs within critical regions of the Caddoan Area, given comparable levels of survey intensity (see Fish and Kowalewski 1990), designed specifically to locate evidence of historic Caddoan occupations (Perttula and Gilmore 1988; Perttula et al. 1988). Only in this way is it possible to obtain quantifiable estimates of site and population density within specific research parameters.

Another critical research requirement that can certainly aid the study of the Protohistoric and Historic archaeological record in the Caddoan Area is the development of a reliable, fine-scale chronological framework for post-1520 Caddoan sites. Certainly sites are known within the Caddoan Area where quite detailed chronological frameworks can be constructed (Schambach and Miller 1984; Williams and Early 1990; Creel 1991b; Perino 1983) for the Protohistoric and Historic periods, but these are typically cemetery assemblages. It is important that the existing chronological framework be extended to contemporaneous habitation sites and midden mounds. This is particularly the case for the Historic Caddoan archaeological record since only a handful of habitation locales have been thoroughly examined (see Story 1990, n.d.; Trubowitz 1984). Improvements and refinements in measurements of chronology for individual components and phases in the Protohistoric and Historic Caddoan periods, and thus improvements in the definition and recognition of archaeological phases, should provide the temporal framework necessary to consider important and new information that addresses the effects of European contact.

Smith (1987, 23) noted that "to measure culture change in situations where historic documentation is lacking, it is necessary to establish chronologies based on stylistic changes in categories of archaeologically recovered materials." Smith (1987, 23–53) utilized European-introduced trade goods as horizon markers (Willey and Phillips 1958, 33) to define four periods spanning the Early Historic period (1525–1670) in the Southeast interior. Each of the periods lasts only between thirty and forty years. His method of dating and chronology construction, though potentially of some considerable utility in deriving calendrical ranges on Caddoan sites containing European trade goods, must be considered to be of only minor utility in work concerning the Caddoan Area before ca. 1700 because European trade goods are uniformly scarce and regionally variable. It is doubtful, therefore, that most Caddoan sites post-1520 can be chronologically arranged by "comparing the frequency of occurrence of European trade items with that of items of native manufacture" (Smith 1987, 24).

Using thermoluminescence dating of ceramic sherds, daub, fired clay from hearths, or even burned rocks, which are abundant on all Caddoan habitations and many contemporaneous French and Spanish settlements (see chapter 5), is recommended for discrete single-component assemblages to culturally stratified occupations. Testing these types of samples may provide the absolute dates on all ceramic-bearing Historic period Caddoan occupations, inasmuch as radiocarbon dating on Protohistoric Caddoan sites has been unprofitable. It is important that any absolute dates obtained by thermoluminescence on ceramic sherds have small (<10 percent) standard deviations, otherwise the dates will not be useful for specific discussions of temporal questions because the probable date range will be too broad. A suite of dates from a range of contexts and a range of Caddoan ceramic styles and wares will provide perhaps the most dependable results for dating occupations.

No one questions that absolute dating of discrete single-component Protohistoric and Historic period Caddoan occupations is a critical research need. It will permit recovery of relatively comprehensive contextual information on the structure and occupational history of the sites from one finite period, rather than the total Caddoan Area Historic period. Until radiocarbon and thermoluminescence samples are systematically retrieved and processed from a series of post-1520 sites within different regions of the Caddoan Area, the analytical framework and research perspective will not permit researchers to address basic questions of settlement and sociopolitical change in anything less than 100- to 150-year blocks of time.

The study of Caddoan mortuary remains (burial goods and skeletal remains) has been a crucial component in all aspects of Caddoan archaeological research since the early 1900s, the post–Contact era archaeological record being no exception. These studies have contributed a wealth of information, not only concerning changes in Caddoan lifeways and health conditions, but also by providing unique data particularly useful for further studies of such topics as aboriginal social organization, the development of chiefdoms, and the existence of interregional exchange networks (Hoffman 1987). Cemeteries and burial assemblages provide the type of discrete, closed contexts discussed above that are most appropriate for obtaining information to address issues relating to rapid cultural change.

With the passage of the Native American Graves Protection and Repatriation Act (P.L. 101-601) the issue of reburial (McW. Quick 1986) and repatriation along with its implications for Caddoan archaeology needs to be squarely addressed by Caddoan tribal representatives, federal and state agencies, and archaeologists. It is important to outline how and in what respects this vital source of information about the Caddoan peoples and their cultural heritage is to be used by all concerned parties (Perttula 1989b, in press). Resolution of this issue is particularly needed now for the current and future development of paleodemographic and bioarchaeological studies about Caddoan peoples because this discipline promises to especially contribute new understandings of Caddoan lifeways and overall health status during all time periods (see Rose, Harcourt, and Burnett 1988; Burnett 1988, 1990a, 1990b; Harmon and Rose 1989).

Research Needs

Other aspects of the Caddoan Historic archaeological and ethnohistorical record important to consider to tell a better native history of the Caddoan peoples include four different but complementary themes and data sets:

1. Spanish, French, and American archival and documentary records
2. The archaeological record of the fur trade
3. The Caddoan archaeology and ethnohistory of the post-Removal period, after ca. 1840
4. Paleodemographic and bioarchaeological investigations

Each one is integral to fostering a broader perspective of the Caddoan cultural heritage, but taken together they should help us understand the intricate relationships between the European newcomers and the native Americans.

Ethnohistorical Research Ethnohistorical research is the study of changes "that have occurred in native societies from earliest recorded European contact until the present" (Trigger 1985, 166). Ethnohistory uses archival and documentary sources and oral tradition to obtain and contribute information about and evidence for changes in native American cultures following European contact (see Trigger 1982, 1986a; Brown 1990).

My colleagues and I (Perttula et al. 1986, 179–196) have discussed some of the problems and constraints involved in an objective assessment of the Protohistoric (1520–1685) and Historic (1685–1800) periods in the Caddoan Area utilizing historical documents. The main constraint has been that pertinent primary documents from French, Spanish, and American archival sources are predominantly limited to Kadohadacho groups living north on the Red River or south among the Hasinai Caddo in the Neches and Angelina drainages of East Texas. Unfortunately, no substantive archival and documentary records exist for groups occupying the areas between these two Caddoan locales.

French, Spanish, and American archival documents have certainly proved to be of considerable significance in (*a*) studying Caddoan ethnography and ethnohistory (Griffith 1954; Swanton 1942); (*b*) understanding European-Indian relationships in the Spanish and French colonies (Wedel 1978, 1982; Usner 1985, 1987); and (*c*) characterizing relationships between the Caddo, the Anglo-Americans, and the immigrant Indians in Texas and Louisiana (Kniffen, Gregory, and Stokes 1987; McLean 1988, 1989; Anderson 1990). Nevertheless, it seems evident that primary records, often still untranslated or poorly organized and indexed, are an untapped resource for the archaeologist and ethnohistorian interested in native history during European contact (Story 1984, 280). Information on aspects of military and economic policy originating in the French and Spanish ministries in New Orleans, Natchitoches, San Antonio, and other settlements may well be located that would provide a more detailed and quantitative assessment of such Caddoan archaeological and ethnohistorical topics as the development of the fur trade; religion, ideology, and ceremony; and ethnicity and territoriality (Story et al. 1990, 433; Perttula 1991).

The main sources pertinent to the continuing study of Caddoan ethnohistory and Historic period archaeology are Spanish and French archives for the colonies of Spanish Texas (1717–1836), Spanish Louisiana (1763–1803), and French Louisiana (1699–1763). These colonial records are not restricted to Spanish or French colonial capitol archives because vast archival material has been photocopied and/or microfilmed and is available at designated archives in the United States, Mexico, and Europe (see Barnes, Naylor, and Polzer 1981; Beers 1979; Rowland, Sanders, and Galloway 1984).

The Natchitoches Archives, at the Natchitoches Parish courthouse in Natchitoches, Louisiana, is potentially a valuable source of ethnohistorical information because it is known to contain records from the Natchitoches post Fort St. Jean Baptiste aux Natchitoches. This was the first tradepost maintained among Caddoan groups on the Red River and the main trade depot for them and the Spanish occupants of the East Texas missions 1716–1780 (Bolton 1914, vol. 1). French merchants and traders working among different Caddoan groups during the Spanish administration in Natchitoches were required to have a license or permit from the authorities before trading. Information contained in these permits or contracts have already yielded significant data on trade good distributions and annual presents among the Kadohadacho, Petit Caddo, Yatasi, Natchitoches, and the Taovayas-Wichita (Bolton 1914, 1:143–145). The records of the Superior Council and Spanish Cabildo also contain useful fur trade information—contracts, details on prices, and agreements on deliverable goods drawn between Natchitoches traders and New Orleans merchants (Usner 1985, 82, 90).

Another important source of documentary material that needs to be systematically assessed for Caddoan ethnohistoric, site-specific, and linguistic primary data is the Béxar Archives (1717–1836), 250,000 pages of archival materials from the colonial archives of Texas produced during the Spanish (1717–1821) and Mexican (1821–1836) periods. The Béxar Archives, which are housed at the Barker Texas History Center (BTHC) at the University of Texas at Austin, contain records relating to all aspects of military, ecclesiastical, and civil life in Spanish and Mexican Texas (Benavides 1989).

Important for ethnohistorical research on Caddoan peoples are documents referring to the establishment of the East Texas presidios, missions, and civil settlements; control measures against the Indians; commerce; slavery; and transportation (Kielman 1967). The Archivo San Francisco el Grande (1673–1800) in the BTHC has records concerned with the establishment and operation of the East Texas missions between 1690 and 1773. Transcribed documents include mission reports detailing supply requests, Indian relations, and military and political developments in the area. Of particular significance are documents involving Athanase de Mézières, the commandant at Natchitoches between 1768 and 1780, who was a major figure in developing strong European-Indian economic and political relationships during this period (Bolton 1914). Besides Caddoan groups living on the Red River in the vicinity of Natchitoches, Indian groups such as the Taovayas, Kichai, Tawakoni, and Yscani, living on the upper Sabine and Red rivers in the 1760s and 1770s, received special attention by de Mézières, and Baron de Ripperdá (Spanish commandant at Los Adaes) (Bolton 1914, 1:206–220).

The Nacogdoches Archives, also located in the Texas State Archives and the BTHC, is another archival source that must be considered in a comprehensive ethnohistorical study of aboriginal Caddoan groups. Included there are official documents of correspondence between government officials and commandants and proceedings of the Alcades and Cabildo of Nacogdoches and adjacent areas (Kielman 1967, 256–257). Because of its strategic military and economic position in East Texas, Nacogdoches is analogous to Natchitoches as a European colonial center in the eighteenth and early nineteenth centuries. Mission Nuestra Señora de Guadalupe de los Nacogdoches was established in 1716 at the Nacogdoche Caddo Indian village (see Swanton 1942) and became the main Zacatecan mission 1731–1772 (Leutenegger 1973). The Spanish town of Nacogdoches was established in 1779 and also became the major Indian trade center and distribution point in East Texas until the Texas revolution in 1836.

Other archival and documentary sources that need to be studied are the annuities and purchases of the Caddoan tribes listed in the ledgers of the Natchitoches, Sulphur Fork, and Caddo Prairie agencies or factories established among these groups 1806–1835 by the U.S. government (see Baerreis 1983 for an ethnohistoric study of the Delaware Indians utilizing such ledger records). Ledger entries, invoices, and lists of goods received for the different factories contain information on nineteenth-century Caddoan hunting and trading activities for the general region on the Red River.

Finally, the Bureau of Indian Affairs at the National Archives contains correspondence of the Caddo Prairie agencies near Shreveport (Hill 1965). Special files, dating from 1825, of the Bureau of Indian Affairs include claims brought by fur traders for individual Indian debts, which were paid out of tribal funds supplied by the U.S. government (see Clayton 1967, 68). Also in the National Archives are the Records of the Office of Indian Affairs (War Department), 1825–1848, and Reports of the Commissioner of Indian Affairs (Department of the Interior), 1849–1939 (see U.S. Congress, House, 1847). These records may be significant sources on Caddoan lifeways following the statehood of Texas.

Archaeological Research: The Fur Trade and the Removal Period The study of Caddoan Historic period archaeology and ethnohistory is in large measure a study of the fur trade (Usner 1985, 1987). While it is argued in this study that the importance of the fur trade to the French and Spanish economies in the Trans-Mississippi South probably lasted only a relatively short time (ca. 1720–1763), it had lasting consequences for the aboriginal inhabitants of Texas and Louisiana (Usner 1985, 86). (During the American period the fur trade represented only 1 percent of total U.S. exports [Clayton 1967, 68].)

Certainly the implications for Caddoan archaeology of aboriginal participation in the fur trade seem fairly clear and include (*a*) development of a distinctive lithic assemblage for processing hides, (*b*) group movements into unoccupied hinterlands and abandoned river valleys for the direct exploitation of the hide resources or a relocation and movement to the European supply and trade depots established within the Caddoan Area, and (*c*) the accumulation of trade goods by successful traders and middlemen that were deposited as grave goods at their death. Ray (1974, 1978) has pointed out that these kinds of specific native American relationships assume a general patterned character when the role of the North American fur trade, whether it be under French, English, or American direction, is considered. He concluded (1974, 228) that "the fur trade favoured economic specialization. While conditions permitted, some groups emerged as trade specialists or middlemen, some became skilled trappers, while others devoted all of their attention to the hunting of large game animals in order to supply the provision needs generated by the fur companies."

A realistic, synthetic appreciation of the significance of the fur trade in the Caddoan Area, for both the aboriginal and European inhabitants, must be a product of both archival and archaeological research studies. Tantalizing glimpses of requisite data sets exist in French, Spanish, and American archival economic records, including volumes on specific furs traded—for example, deer, beaver, raccoon, bear—and the total contribution of the fur trade to the economy. However, these need to be systematically developed in both temporal and regional dimensions to erect a quantitative framework for the fur trade that can be usefully applied to interpreting the Historic Caddoan archaeological record. Moreover, aspects of aboriginal cultural change that are engendered in the Historic period because of a full-scale participation in the fur trade need to be considered in a manner congruent with temporal, ethnic, ecological (White and Cronon 1989), and economic evidence gathered in the archaeological record (Witthoft 1967), not simply as pieces to a larger puzzle. The fur trade is only one facet of how Caddoan subsistence and economic systems changed through time and of how these changes are an expression of the ways Caddoan groups were affected by European contact.

Although a wealth of historic archival and documentary information is available on the Caddoan peoples who lived in Texas between ca. 1836 and 1859, very little specific archaeological evidence has been uncovered for their settlements (Bell, Jelks, and Newcomb 1967; Tanner 1974). By the late 1830s, most of the Caddoan groups had been removed from Northeast Texas, their lands settled by Anglo-American farmers and planters, and they had taken up residence with other affiliated groups (such as the Cherokee and the Tawakoni) on the Brazos River in North-central Texas. There they apparently continued to farm and hunt bison, even after they had been placed on the Brazos Indian Reservation in 1854.

It is unfortunate that there is a near absence of archaeological data for the Caddoan Indian settlements of the 1840s and 1850s in the North-central Texas region. These types of sites, though they may be difficult to identify because they may not contain aboriginal artifacts and they were only occupied for short periods of time, represent a very significant and unique period of increased acculturation and material culture changes among the Caddo tribes living on the Brazos River. Their study would provide an excellent opportunity to integrate Caddoan archaeological, ethnohistorical, and linguistic research to determine in economic, technological, political, social, and cultural terms how Caddoan lifeways were maintained under such acculturative and paternalistic conditions.

Paleodemographic and Bioarchaeological Research Paleodemographic and bioarchaeological data from Late Caddoan (ca. 1400–1520), Protohistoric, and Historic period skeletal assemblages are vital to assessing the impact of European epidemics, native population decline, ethnic amalgamation, and changes in birth rates and demographic profiles. They are important as well for documenting the overall survival of kin-related groups in the face of European contact and interaction (see Rose 1984; Harmon and Rose 1989). Evidence of chronic demographic stress (Piper, Hardin, and Piper 1983), modifications in traditional burial programs, and other biocultural indicators in human skeletal remains of cultural disruptions are the types of data critically needed to evaluate the consequences of long-term demographic decline and changing health conditions (Burnett 1988, 1990a).

Other than the few and recent paleodemographic and bioarchaeological studies from Caddoan sites on the Red and Ouachita rivers that date after 1520 (Rose 1984; Burnett 1986, 1990b; Loveland 1987), the comprehensive profile is incomplete in regional and temporal changes in population structure, fertility, persistence of infections, and other indications of overall health conditions under phases of enhanced social and disease interaction.

Particularly important to the study of the effects of European contact and interaction with Caddoan groups will be comparative regional assessments of bone chemistry; pathology and disease load; demography; morphology; and population changes 1520–1685, 1685–1800, and post-1800. Bone chemistry, the analysis of stable carbon and nitrogen isotopes, can be utilized to document specific dietary changes (Schoeninger, Hiebert, and van der Merwe 1987), including a decrease or increase in maize consumption, through the Contact era. This has been nicely illustrated by Burnett (1990b) with the Mid-Ouachita, Social Hill, and Deceiper phase skeletal samples from the Ouachita River basin. Analyses of enamel defects (hypoplasias) may contribute information on growth disruptions (Larsen 1987a; Hutchinson and Larsen 1988) and are thus key to understanding the periodicity and pervasiveness of stress episodes in Caddoan populations at specific times. It is important to determine which population classes or individuals were more susceptible to stress and how this condition affected their ability to survive and reproduce (Larsen 1987a, 9).

Study of structural and functional changes induced by infectious diseases may provide direct evidence for European epidemics (see Burnett 1986, Blakely and Detweiler-Blakely 1989) as well as contribute more general information on health conditions when comparative frequency data on the number of nonspecific periosteal reactions can be obtained. Rarely, however, will the types of diseases mentioned in the ethnohistorical record leave identifiable lesions directly indicating that death resulted from an acute European-introduced disease. Therefore, other approaches that help to detect the cause of death and that might reflect increased mortality levels from an epidemic or an episode of violence (Blakely and Matthews 1990) need to be taken. Possible factors to study include (*a*) the length of time between death and burial (e.g., using animal teeth marks), (*b*) the structure or configuration of the remains (e.g., mass burials in pits), (*c*) the age and sex of the mortuary population, and (*d*) the identification of cuts and punctures produced by iron weapons such as swords. In general, the investigation of subadult mortality, mean age of death, and the percentage of young versus old in the mortuary assemblage holds the most promise at present for producing the type of region-wide, diachronically based demographic data sets needed to evaluate changes in Caddoan peoples' health and adaptive efficiency during the Contact period (Burnett 1990b, 11–49).

Demographic data on survivorship and life expectancy are influenced by diet and health considerations (see Buikstra and Mielke 1985). Differences through time in survivorship profiles after European–native American contact may reflect both a depression in demographic status and a decrease in life expectancy as well as the effects of diseases introduced by Europeans (Palkovich 1981).

Such bioarchaeological data will provide a more complete assessment of how native American populations were affected by the arrival of Europeans in the Caddoan Area. It is in the direct measurement of health conditions, diet, and stress parameters in Caddoan skeletal series in combination with Historic archaeological and ethnohistorical investigations that bioarchaeology and paleodemographic studies may truly contribute to a better understanding of how Caddoan peoples lived after 1520.

APPENDIX

The Chronological Sequence in the Titus Phase of Northeast Texas

Chapter 4 reviews the archaeological record of the Caddoan Area between ca. 1520 and 1685 to ascertain changes in settlement density and location and sociopolitical organization during this period of intermittent contact between Caddoan peoples and Europeans. One task essential to the discussion has been the review and assessment of the chronological and classificatory frameworks for each of the subareas of the Caddoan Area, namely the western, northern, and central Caddo subareas (Schambach 1983).

In the western Caddo subarea is the Cypress Creek basin and Titus phase of East Texas. Its chronological and classificatory framework is examined in more detail here to critically evaluate the competing chronology theories of Turner (1978) and Thurmond (1985, 1990a). Their positions are summarized in chapter 4. Evaluating the chronological framework for this region is necessary because the highly significant Protohistoric archaeological record and the record of change preserved here (Thurmond 1990a; Perttula 1991) are crucial to evaluating the effects of European contact. Without a robust and uniform chronological framework, the significance of any changes in community cemetery organization, mortuary ritual, social organization, and periods of mound construction would be unduly obscured.

To examine the Titus phase chronological sequence, I compiled data on the cooccurrence of decorated Caddoan pottery types, design motifs on Ripley Engraved (the most common decorated type in the Titus phase and Cypress cluster), and arrow point caches in Titus phase burials from the twelve best reported cemetery assemblages: Russell (41TT7), Tuck Carpenter (41CP5), Mattie Gandy (41FK4), Joe Justis (41MX2), Richard Watson (41MX6), Thomas Caldwell (41TT6), J. E. Galt (41FK2), A. P. Williams (41TT4), J. M. Riley (41UR2), McKinney (41MR12), H. R. Taylor (41HS3), and P. S. Cash (41CP2). Changes in the frequency and occurrence of pottery types, design motifs, and arrow point caches were used to assign specific burial

TABLE A-1. Association of Pottery Types with Burials Containing Discrete Suites of Arrow Point Types

Pottery Vessels	Projectile Point Type (%)							
	Perdiz 1a	Perdiz/Bassett 1b	Bassett 2a	Maud/Bassett 2b	Maud 3a	Talco/Maud 3b	Talco 3c	All Burials
Engraved								
Ripley	60.8	76.9	60.6	56.1	30.4	47.2	55.4	54.7
Taylor					4.3	12.2	8.0	6.1
Wilder	1.3		3.0	14.6	13.0	3.8	4.4	4.7
Bailey						1.9	4.0	2.2
Belcher					4.3	1.9	0.8	0.9
Glassell				2.4		0.9	0.4	0.6
Hodges						1.9	2.0	1.3
Avery	1.3							0.2
Simms							1.2	0.6
Bowie							0.4	0.2
Brushed/Incised								
Maydelle	4.1	3.9		4.9	4.3		1.2	1.8
Bullard	2.7	3.8		4.9	17.4	5.7	3.2	4.2
Karnack					4.3	5.7	2.8	2.5
Pease	4.1					0.9		0.8

Neck-Banded								
Larue	1.3		3.0		4.3	3.7	1.2	1.8
Applique								
Harleton	1.3		9.0	2.4	4.3	6.6	7.2	5.6
Cass							2.4	1.1
Ridged								
Belcher						0.9		0.2
Pinched								
Killough			3.0					0.2
Stamped								
Cowhide							0.4	0.2
Trailed								
Keno						0.9		0.2
Noded utility jar	14.9	15.4	12.1	12.2	4.3	5.7	3.5	7.2
Plain bowl	4.1		3.0		8.7		1.2	1.6
Effigy bowl	4.1		6.1	2.4			0.4	1.3
No. of Vessels	74	26	33	41	23	106	251	554

lots to a relative temporal position through seriation methods (see Renfrew and Bahn 1991, 106–108 for a general discussion of the seriation method).

The arrow point caches were divided into seven groups: Perdiz, Perdiz/Bassett, Bassett, Maud/Bassett, Maud, Talco/Maud, and Talco (Table A-1). Definitions of these arrow point types are provided by Suhm and Jelks (1962) and Perino (1985). The Perdiz and Bassett types are notched, stemmed points with a contracting or tanged stem (Turner 1978, Fig. 17d, 17e, and 17f). The Maud and Talco arrow points are triangular in shape with concave bifurcate bases (Suhm and Jelks 1962, 281, 289). The most common ceramic types (as defined by Suhm and Jelks [1962]) associated with the different arrow point burial lots can be summarized as follows (see Table A-1):

Perdiz	Ripley Engraved, utility jars, Pease Brushed-Incised, Maydelle Incised
Perdiz / Bassett	Ripley Engraved, utility jars, Maydelle Incised, Bullard Brushed
Bassett	Ripley Engraved, utility jars, Harleton Applique, effigy bowls
Maud / Bassett	Ripley Engraved, Wilder Engraved, utility jars, Maydelle Incised, Bullard Brushed
Maud	Ripley Engraved, Bullard Brushed, Wilder Engraved, plain carinated bowls
Talco / Maud	Ripley Engraved, Taylor Engraved, Harleton Applique, Bullard Brushed, Karnack Brushed / Incised
Talco	Ripley Engraved, Taylor Engraved, Harleton Applique, Wilder Engraved

First, note that there is a qualitative similarity in the range of ceramic types represented between the seven arrow point burial lots. This denotes a basic temporal-spatial contiguity in material culture associations within the Titus phase and, moreover, consistent quantitative trends in the relative popularity of the different types across arrow point lots (see Table A-1).

The relative frequencies of the different ceramic types primarily change monotonically (i.e., consistently increase or decrease in number or relative value) from the Perdiz arrow point burial lots through the Talco arrow point burial lots. Where percentage changes do not conform to a monotonic distribution or where frequencies are not continuous in nature, variations can, in most cases, be readily accounted for by small sample sizes (especially in the Bassett and Maud arrow point burial lots). Another consideration is that these anomolous relative differences in percentage across arrow point lots are not very significant given the overall low frequency of the ceramic types in question (e.g., Harleton Applique, plain carinated bowls). Only Ripley Engraved does not have a monotonic distribution (see Table A-1).

At a minimal level, therefore, the arrow point burial lots from the twelve best reported sites (see Fig. 14) in the Cypress Creek basin are useful as ordering criteria because they satisfy an important precept of artifact seriation. That is, the general changes in frequency of ceramic types in burials with distinct arrow point lots has a consistent bell or battleship shape and monotonic pattern.

Rim decoration motifs on Ripley Engraved carinated bowls and compound bowls (Fig. A-1, after Turner 1978, Fig. 33; Thurmond 1981, 1990a, Fig. 6) were then examined, using the same site data set, for their association with Perdiz, Bassett, Maud, and Talco arrow point burial lots. This was done to ascertain if a more definitive and consistent pattern of change in motif frequencies could be isolated within these burial lots, thus negating potential ordering errors in the more comprehensive arrow point burial lot/ ceramic type association discussed above (see Table A-1). Changes in these small-scale decorative motifs within one common, broadly distributed pottery type appear to be the most appropriate ones to employ for further construction of a temporal sequence, regardless of the design's symbolic or social context (Braun 1985, 513–514; Dunnell 1978; Plog 1980).

Table A-2 presents relative frequency data on the association of the Ripley Engraved primary motifs with the arrow point burial lots (Thurmond's pendant triangle is the same as Turner's design motif 2; the scroll, as 4 and 9; continuous scroll, as design motif 3; and scroll and circle, as 1 [Thurmond 1981; Turner 1978, Fig. 33]) (see Fig. 16). The same relative ordering and monotonic distribution of arrow point burial lots is obtained with this sample of vessels (N = 131) as was in the original vessel set of all Titus phase ceramic types (N = 554). Burials containing only Perdiz arrow points as a grave offering are dominated by Ripley Engraved bowls with the continuous scroll motif (see Fig. A-1); Bassett arrow points occur with the scroll and continuous scroll motifs; Maud arrow points are found primarily with the scroll and circle and the scroll motifs on the Ripley Engraved bowls; and the pendant triangle and scroll motifs are most popular in burials that only have Talco arrow points (see Table A-2).

Both data sets can be employed to construct a proposed temporal ordering or seriation model for the Cypress Creek cluster. Available radiocarbon dates from the region (Thurmond 1981, Table 60; Story 1990, Table 81), in combination with changes in arrow point form elsewhere in the Caddoan Area and the southern plains (Brown 1976; Prewitt 1981; Prikryl 1987, 1990; Baugh 1986), indicate that the Perdiz arrow point burial lots are placed as offerings in the earliest Cypress Creek cluster burials, followed in time by the Bassett, Maud, and Talco arrow point types. Burial lots containing combinations of two arrow point types are of intermediate age (see Table A-1).

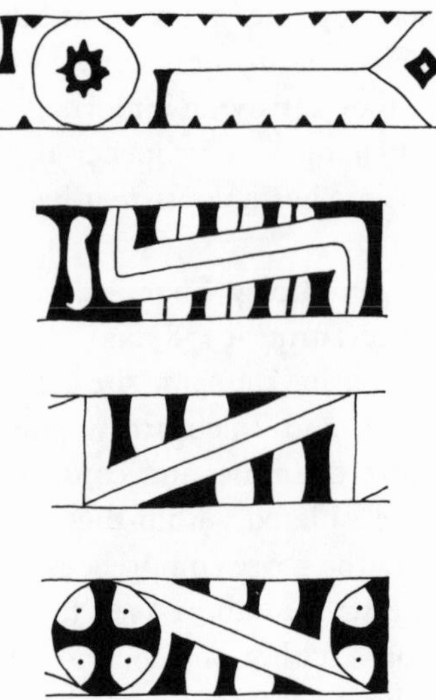

FIG. A-1. Ripley Engraved primary decorative motifs (*top to bottom*): pendant triangle, scroll, continuous scroll, and scroll and circle (from Thurmond 1990a, Fig. 6).

Based on these sets of information, three temporal periods within the Cypress cluster are proposed, with a number of subphases (see Johnson 1987, 19). The subphases are equivalent to each of the seven arrow point burial lots as outlined in Table A-1. Period 1, subphases a and b, is the same as the Whelan phase as described by Thurmond (1985, 189). It is estimated to date 1350–1450. Early period 1 occupations have calibrated radiocarbon date ranges of 1355 to 1413 (see chapter 4). The period is characterized by Perdiz and Bassett arrow points, Ripley Engraved ceramics with the continuous scroll motif, and high frequencies of Pease Brushed-Incised. Relatively high proportions of utility jars, effigy bowls, and plain bowls are also characteristic of period 1, especially in subphase a. Only the Avery Engraved type, a major Red River McCurtain and Texarkana phase fine ware (Schambach 1983, 9), represents trade ware in the Cypress cluster at this time.

Period 2, subphases a and b, is part of the Titus phase and may date ca. 1450–1600. Calibrated date ranges of 1440–1640, 1476–1648, and 1520–1580 from Tuck Carpenter and Roberts substantiate this estimate. Ceramic chalices from the Tuck Carpenter site, possibly modeled on Spanish glassware forms (see chapter 2), may also date to this period (Turner 1978; Thurmond 1990b). Bassett and Maud arrow points are the major arrow point types. The major pottery types are Ripley Engraved, with the scroll and continuous scroll motifs (see Fig. A-1); Wilder Engraved; Maydelle Incised; Bullard Brushed; Harleton Applique; and utility jars, effigy

TABLE A-2. Association of Primary Motifs on Ripley Engraved Bowls with Burials Containing Projectile Point Types Perdiz, Bassett, Maud, and Talco (Percentage Motifs Per Type)

	Motifs—Carinated and Compound Bowls				
Projectile Point	Pendant	Scroll	Continuous Scroll	Scroll/ Circle	No. of Vessels
Perdiz	7.7	19.2	69.2	3.8	26
Bassett	7.7	53.8	38.5	0	13
Maud	14.3	28.7	0	57.1	7
Talco	48.2	30.6	4.7	16.5	85

bowls, or plain carinated bowls. Glassell Engraved, a Belcher phase type (Schambach 1983, 9), is a significant item of ceramic trade ware.

Period 3, subphases a–c, is the "classic" Titus phase, as defined by Thurmond (1985, 189–190), and dates after ca. 1600. Thurmond (1990a, 1990b) suggests that the Titus phase may not date much past the early 1600s and certainly ends by the early 1700s. Period 3 is a time of more rapid ceramic decorative variation in the locally produced fine wares and a period when nonlocal, Red River ceramic wares become more common than before in East Texas. Belcher phase trade wares, which represent between 3.2 percent and 6.5 percent of the ceramic vessels in the period 3 sample (see Table A-1), include Belcher Engraved, Glassell Engraved, Hodges Engraved, Belcher Ridged, and Cowhide Stamped (Webb 1959; Schambach 1983). Types Cass Applique, Simms Engraved, and Bowie Engraved, restricted to subphase c, are Texarkana phase trade wares. Keno Trailed occurs in a number of Early and Late Historic period Caddoan phases, but it is also of Red River affiliation. Trade wares of both phases are most common in period 3, subphase c, of the Cypress cluster, amounting to 7.6 percent of the ceramic vessel assemblage. Talco and Maud arrow points are characteristic of period 3, especially the Talco type (see Table A-1).

The most common locally produced ceramic type in the Cypress, Sulphur, and Sabine River basins in periods 1–3, Ripley Engraved, was no longer made after ca. 1700. A few components of this later period contain limited amounts of European goods, and ceramic assemblages comprise the pan-regional Caddo V period types Keno Trailed (Schambach and Miller 1984, 123), Clements Brushed (Dickinson 1941), Simms Engraved, and Taylor Engraved. Locally manufactured ceramics no longer dominate the ceramic assemblages of these East Texas groups. The lack of Natchitoches Engraved and the presence of Keno Trailed var. Phillips (Schambach and Miller 1984, 123) is evidence that Caddoans occupied these locales only to ca. 1730.

Notes

1. Introduction

1. Linguistically, the Caddoan family may be divided into a northern Caddoan-speaking group, which includes the Pawnee, Arikara, and Wichita groups who lived on the Great Plains of North America (Wedel 1988), and a southern Caddoan-speaking group. This group includes the Caddo proper, sometimes referred to as the Kadohadacho; the Hasinai, who lived in Northeast Texas; and possibly the Adai, who lived in the vicinity of the Spanish mission and presidio at Los Adaes in western Louisiana (Chafe 1983; Lesser and Weltfish 1932). It is the southern Caddoan-speaking groups who are the subject of this book.

2. Discussions by Schambach (1988, 1990b) question aspects of the Caddoan affiliation of much of the northern Caddoan Area. The opposing viewpoints of Rogers (1991) and Brown (1991) reiterate that the long-term cultural and geographical continuity evident in the region's archaeological record seems more consistent with an aboriginal occupation in the area of Caddoan origin.

2. European Contact with the Caddo Nation

1. There has been considerable research activity of late in tracing the de Soto route through the Caddoan Area. For instance, the Trammell's Trace route for the Moscoso *entrada* in northeast Texas, proposed by Kenmotsu, Bruseth, and Corbin (1992), is a very detailed examination of the route, the location of Caddoan groups, and "provinces" along the route. Similarly, many of the papers in Young and Hoffman (in press) provide detailed treatment of other aspects and portions of the route after the *entrada* crossed the Mississippi River.

Interest in the de Soto route has never been higher, and its investigation has attracted scholars across the country. Preeminent among them is Dr. Charles Hudson of the University of Georgia who has published a series of provocative papers on the subject (see Hudson 1987a, 1987b, 1989, 1990; Hudson, DePratter, and Smith, 1989). Few de Soto period or Spanish sixteenth-century artifacts have been found at native American archaeological sites along the route, particularly west of the Mississippi River, and only the Martin site, in downtown Tallahassee, represents conclusive archaeological evidence of the de Soto *entrada* (Ewen 1988).

2. When the Spanish returned to East Texas in 1691, Fray Mazanet traveled with Domingo Terán de los Ríos from Coahuila recording native names for the creeks

and rivers that the expedition crossed. Most of the creeks and rivers east of the San Antonio area were recorded by Mazanet as having southern Caddoan names (Johnson 1991). The Caddoan peoples of East Texas were quite familiar with the area west of the Trinity River in Texas through seasonal deer- and bison-hunting trips.

3. Few of the East Texas and western Louisiana Spanish missions and presidios have been identified archaeologically, and only Mission Nuestra Señora Dolores de Ais (Corbin, Alex, and Karlina 1980; Corbin et al. 1990) and Mission San Miguel de los Linares de los Adaes (Gregory 1973, 1983) have been excavated to any extent. These sites are difficult to find: the wood ruins have deteriorated leaving only traces, few artifacts of the missionaries and converts remained to be found 200–250 years later, and most of the direct evidence for them must be adduced through intensive excavations and exhaustive survey reconnaissance efforts in the thickly wooded areas of the region.

With the recent rediscovery of an 1806 map drawn by Juan Pedro Walker (see John [1988] for more information about Walker the mapmaker) of the route of El Camino de los Tejas from the Trinity River to Nacogdoches, complete with notations on the locations of several mission ruins, Corbin (1991) has significantly narrowed down their possible locations. He is initiating a program of mission and presidio site identification in the Neches and Angelina River basins of East Texas.

4. Although not the subject of this study, archaeological sites associated with the influx of immigrant Indian groups into the Caddoan Area have recently been identified along the Red River in Northwest Louisiana and Southwest Arkansas. These include both Cherokee and Coushatta villages occupied between ca. 1780 and 1840 (McCrocklin 1990a, 1990b); the site of the U.S. Sulphur Fork factory; and associated Coushatta, Choctaw, or Delaware homesteads (Jeter et al. 1989, 266).

3. Archaeology and the Contact Era: Theory and Methodology

1. Vehik (1989, 115–125) has compiled a separate list of New World disease events in an attempt to identify which epidemics may have had an impact on southern plains aboriginal groups between ca. 1535 and 1850. Definite epidemics (i.e., those documented as occurring on the southern plains) identified by Vehik (1989, 116) include smallpox diseases in 1687–1691, 1737–1739, 1750, 1762–1766, 1780–1781, 1800–1802, 1815–1816, 1831–1832, and 1848–1850; plague, typhoid, and typhus 1777–1778; and cholera 1848–1850. Many of these occurrences have been documented among the Caddoan Indians in Northeast Texas, as well as in Florida and the lower Mississippi Valley (see Tables 4 and 5). The mortality rates for the epidemics were estimated to have been very high in 1687–1691, 1737–1739, 1777–1778, and 1800–1802. Probable epidemics (i.e., those documented in areas immediately adjacent to the southern plains but not directly documented among southern plains aboriginal groups) identified by Vehik (1989, Table 11) include an unspecified disease (possibly smallpox) in 1671, smallpox 1755–1760, possibly measles 1755–1760, and a cholera epidemic between 1830 and 1834.

2. All radiocarbon dates in the text are calibrated according to the dendrochro-

nology calibration curves presented by Stuiver and Becker (1986, 863–910) for A.D. 1950 to 2500 B.C. As pointed out by Bowman (1990, 45–46), these calibration curves do not take a monotonic form (i.e., increases in true age do not necessarily mean that radiocarbon ages increase), but "wiggle" back and forth through time over different periods.

In certain cases, a single radiocarbon date can correspond to more than one true date because these "wiggles" cause the calibration curves to overlap. Calibrated dates are thus not presented as central dates with an error term or standard deviation, but as a range of dates. When there are overlapping dates, the calibrated date and the series of date ranges are also presented in the discussion.

4. The Archaeological Record in the Caddoan Area, 1520–1685

1. In the absence of any viable taxonomic alternatives, we retain the use of the Angelina focus in this discussion. As presently defined, the Angelina focus encompasses the whole Caddoan archaeological sequence in the Angelina River drainage/Lake Sam Rayburn area of Northeast Texas (Story 1990, 169) and as such is in need of redefinition and reevaluation. The term *late Angelina focus* as used in this study refers to those sites in these localities that date after ca. 1400.

2. The Galt biface is a long (mean length, 23.9 centimeters), well-made two-sided, single-edged tool manufactured from exotic raw chert (Thurmond 1990a, 35). These bifaces occur as grave goods in Belcher and Titus phase contexts, either from Titus phase community cemeteries or with Belcher phase mound structures or burials. The Galt bifaces are associated with high-status Caddoes in the Cypress Creek basin and portions of the Red River Valley, and Thurmond (1990a, 35) interprets them as possible "badges of rank or office."

3. Information from collectors and from Robert Scott, M.A., an archaeologist with the U.S. Army Corps of Engineers, Fort Worth District, Permits Section (personal communication by phone, 10 July 1988), indicates that other deep shaft tombs of Titus phase age are known in the Cypress Creek basin. They appear to belong to the Big Cypress Creek subcluster (see Fig. 14), but the grave good associations are too poorly known to assign them to a period or subphase designation at this time.

4. Recently Dr. James E. Bruseth and I obtained two radiocarbon dates from 41AN87, a Frankston phase site on Mound Prairie Creek in the Neches River basin. Dates of the decorated ceramics in the trash middens are consistent with those of a Frankston phase 1 subdivision (Kleinschmidt 1982, Table 19). The calibrated dates of the samples are 1406 (Beta-43538) and 1425 (Beta-43537), with calibrated date ranges of 1387–1426 and 1403–1442.

5. The Mound Prairie area was named as it was by early Anglo-American settlers of Northeast Texas because of the large number of mound sites around the community of Jonesborough (Strickland 1937). At least six Caddoan mound sites are known on Mound Prairie, three of which (Sam Kaufman–Bob Williams, Frank Norris [41RR2], and Roden) had mounds constructed during the McCurtain phase. The Mound Prairie is not a natural tall-grass prairie, and it is suspected that it may have

formed because of aboriginally induced modifications of the local environment that suppressed forest growth.

5. The Archaeological and Ethnohistorical Record in the Caddoan Area, 1685–1800

1. There is a scant post-1800 Caddoan archaeological record in either Louisiana or Texas. This is particularly the case for Caddoan archaeological sites that postdate 1840, by which time most of the Caddoan groups had moved into the upper Trinity and Brazos River valleys to distance themselves from the advancing Anglo-American frontier (Perttula 1991). The locations of many of these 1840s–1850s Caddoan settlements are known from historic sources such as maps, land survey records, and state and federal papers (Helen Tanner, Ph.D., personal communication, 5 April 1991). Neighbours (1975, 121), for example, reproduces a mid-1850s map of the Brazos Indian Reservation that shows specific locations of Caddo, Anadarko, Waco, Tawacano (i.e., Tawakoni), Shawnee, and Tonkawa villages. Yet for the most part, finding these sites on the ground has proven to be extremely difficult. Nevertheless, the archaeological documentation of these later Historic Caddoan settlements, particularly those on the upper Brazos River Valley on the Brazos Indian Reservation, as well as those Caddoan villages that were occupied immediately preceding the 1854 establishment of the reservation, is absolutely crucial to developing a comprehensive understanding of the effects of contact between Caddoan and Anglo-American populations.

2. A more detailed investigation of the archaeological site files and collections in the repositories in Texas, Oklahoma, Arkansas, and Louisiana would undoubtedly reveal the existence of a much larger set of known post-1685 Caddoan archaeological sites. Many of the sites will probably be little known, their exact location uncertain, and much of their information and assemblage content ambiguous, but nevertheless the effort is warranted if for no other reason than to compile a reliable archaeological data base that can be employed in the study of Caddoan archaeological and ethnological cultures.

3. As previously mentioned, the *caddi* was a hereditary headman within a Caddo village and functioned as that village's political leader. According to Casanas, one of the early Spanish missionaries among the Hasinai tribes (Hatcher 1927, 216–217), the caddi was a governor who ruled the people in his village. In a model of the material culture of the Hasinai social elite, Wyckoff and Baugh (1980, 247–248) postulate that the residence of the caddi would have been spatially distinct from the village itself, larger in floor space than the remainder of the village houses, complemented with a nearby plaza area, and located near the village's cemetery area. On the Terán 1691 map of the upper Nasoni community, the caddi's house is thought to be at the far eastern edge of the community (see Fig. 23) near the Eli Moore site (41BW2).

4. Like the term *Caddo, Wichita* has a number of meanings in ethnographic and archaeological discussions of the aboriginal inhabitants of the southern Great Plains (Bell, Jelks, and Newcomb 1967). Affiliated tribes of Caddoan-speakers, the Tao-

vayas, Iscani, Tawakoni, Waco, Wichita, and, possibly, Kichai groups, did not refer to themselves collectively by the term *Wichita* until after the Civil War and the establishment in Oklahoma of the Wichita reservation in Indian Territory.

5. Kidder (1990b) argues, reasonably so, that the Ouachita Caddo were not indigenous inhabitants of the Ouachita River, but lived instead on the Red River in the vicinity of Natchitoches. Their settlement of the Ouachita River in the late seventeenth century may have been related to their participation in overland trade ventures in salt and other commodities with the Taensa, Tunica, and Koroa groups living between the Ouachita River and the Mississippi River.

6. My examination of the records, collections, and site forms at the Texas Archeological Research Laboratory indicates that there are only a handful of poorly known Historic Indian sites in the upper Sulphur, Cypress Bayou, and upper Sabine River basins of Northeast Texas (Perttula 1991, Fig. 4 and Table 1). Most of the sites include only limited European trade goods, such as glass beads, metal arrow points, sheet copper, and similar items, in some degree of association with Caddoan ceramics, usually in a burial context. There is no evidence currently available that indicates the existence of Historic Caddoan *rancherías* in these areas of Northeast Texas.

7. The Woldert site was named for Albert Woldert, a historian who lived in Tyler, Texas. He had heard about the site and the finds there from his father, and over the years was able to locate the general area where many of the European trade materials had been discovered by local farmers as early as the 1870s (Woldert 1952; Perttula and Skiles 1989). Woldert (1952) interpreted the concentrations of European trade goods at the site (actually a series of sites along Mill Race Creek [Perttula and Gilmore 1988, 55–56]) as the result of a raging skirmish between native Americans and Spanish explorers.

8. The "Statement of the Indian Nations living within the Territory of Texas, in 1810" indicated that the Nabedache and Hainai (the Texas or Hasinai tribes) lived in villages on the Neches and Angelina Rivers six to ten miles above the Camino Real. The Nacogdoche Caddo lived on the Angelina River north of the Spanish town of Nacogdoches, and the Nadaco had a village five miles north of the Nacogdoche. These Hasinai villages were estimated to have had between sixty to one hundred men per village in 1810 (Buquor 1853).

6. Special Aspects of the Eighteenth-Century Caddoan Archaeological Record

1. Two other Caddoan cemeteries of similar type in the vicinity include the A. P. Fourche and R. A. Simpson farm sites on Black Bayou and Black Cypress Bayou. These cemeteries included burials accompanied by glass trade beads, Jowell knives (large well-made chert bifaces), and numerous aboriginal ceramic vessels (Perttula 1991, Table 1).

2. The ethnic affiliation of the Womack, Gilbert, and Pearson sites is a matter of some discussion. The archival records suggest that these sites may have been occupied in Historic times by Nortenos—Yscani, Kichai, and/or Tawakoni groups—who

moved into the area in the early eighteenth century from the Arkansas and Canadian river basins to the north of Texas (Harris et al. 1965; Jelks 1967; Duffield and Jelks 1961; Story 1985b, 1990). I previously had argued that the Womack and Gilbert sites were southern Caddoan occupations of groups heavily involved in the fur trade (Perttula 1989a, 246–251), basing my reasoning at least in part on the close similarity of the native-manufactured ceramics between these Norteno sites and the ceramic wares found along the Red River and in Northeast Texas. Although I am unprepared to concede that these sites are Nortenos in ethnic affiliation (see chapter 5), I think it is appropriate to point out that at least based on the archaeological evidence (*a*) the Norteno sites were partially contemporaneous with late Titus phase Cypress cluster occupations; (*b*) the sites are a distinct phenomenon archaeologically from Northeast Texas Caddoan sites; and (*c*) that these groups apparently maintained some form of trade and interaction at the time. The overall relationship between the Norteno sites and southern-Caddoan speakers in the region remains to be unraveled.

3. The Taovayas and Wichita villages on the Red River in Montague County, Texas, and Jefferson County, Oklahoma (Bell et al. 1967), are not included here because investigations at these settlements have been less thorough than those at sites included in Table 20. Nevertheless, in the collections of European trade goods in private hands, and in the Benton-Whiteside Museum in Nocona, Texas, there is a staggering amount of gun parts and hardware (both French and English), lead balls and sprue, and native and European-made gunflints. The amounts recovered from the "Spanish fort" sites on the Texas side alone that I have seen total more than all together from the sites listed in Table 20.

4. The Pascagoula-Biloxi groups settled on the Red River in the Rapides District of Louisiana after ca. 1765 (Sibley 1832, 724). The particular village and cemetery, near the mouth of Rigolet de Bon Dieu, just south of where the Red River splits into Cane River and Rigolet de Bon Dieu, was shown on both the Nicholas King map of 1806 and the Darby 1816 map (Tanner 1974, 53).

5. Few of the young Caddo adults living in Oklahoma today speak any of the Caddoan dialects, and it is feared by the tribal leaders and elders that the Caddo language will no longer be spoken and be lost. The preservation and continued use of the Caddo language is of foremost concern to them, and they supported a 1991 language preservation study conducted by the University of Texas at Austin.

References

A voluminous literature records the archaeology and ethnohistory of the Caddoan peoples and the history of contact between Europeans and the native Americans of the southeastern United States. The references cited herein are just a small sampling. For those who wish to read and learn more about these topics, the excellent bibliographies prepared by Ewen (1990), Prucha (1977, 1982), Tate (1986), and Limp, Zahn, and Harcourt (1989) introduce the reader to the technical and general archaeological, ethnohistorical, and historical literature.

The thirty-volume sourcebook edited by David Hurst Thomas (1990b) on the Spanish Borderlands is particularly recommended as useful, as are the three volumes edited by Thomas (1989, 1990a, 1991), *Columbian Consequences,* published by Smithsonian Institution Press. For a current and detailed overview of the archaeology of the Caddoan Area and that of adjacent regions whose relevance to Caddoan archaeology has been discussed in this book, the reader should consult the excellent volumes prepared by Story et al. (1990), Jeter et al. (1989), Hofman et al. (1989), and Sabo et al. (1988) for the Southwestern Division of the U.S. Army Corps of Engineers. Finally, as a source of topical research articles, news, and commentary on Caddoan archaeology, the Oklahoma Archeological Survey has begun issuing the *Caddoan Archeology Newsletter*.

ALBERT, L. E.

1984 Survey of archaeological activity in Oklahoma. In *Prehistory of Oklahoma,* ed. R. E. Bell, 45–63. New York: Academic Press.

AMERICAN STATE PAPERS

1832–1834 *Documents Legislative and Executive, Class II, Indian Affairs.* Washington, D.C.: Gales & Seaton.

ANDERSON, H. A.

1990 The Delaware and Shawnee Indians and the Republic of Texas, 1820–1845. *Southwestern Historical Quarterly* 94:231–260.

ARCHIVES NATIONALES, ARCHIVES DES COLONIES, PARIS.

1679–1763 Serie C, Correspondence Generale, vols. 1–45.

ARCHIVO GENERAL DE INDIAS, SEVILLE

1492–1856 Audiencias e Indiferente, Legajos.

ARNOLD, J. B., AND R. WEDDLE

1978 *The nautical archeology of Padre Island: The Spanish shipwrecks of 1554*. New York: Academic Press.

ATEN, L. E.

1984 Woodland cultures of the Texas coast. In *Perspectives on Gulf Coast prehistory,* ed. D. D. Davis, 72–93. Ripley P. Bullen Monographs in Anthropology and History, no. 5, The Florida State Museum. Gainesville: University Presses of Florida.

AXTELL, J.

1985 *The invasion within: The contest of cultures in colonial North America.* New York: Oxford University Press.

1988 *After Columbus: Essays in the ethnohistory of colonial North America.* New York: Oxford University Press.

BAERREIS, D. A.

1983 A quantitative approach to culture change: The Delaware Indians as an ethnohistoric case study. In *Lulu Linear Punctated: Essays in honor of George Irving Quimby,* ed. R. C. Dunnell and D. K. Grayson, 185–207. Anthropological Papers, no. 72. Ann Arbor: University of Michigan Museum of Anthropology.

BAILEY, G. A.

1973 *Changes in Osage social organization 1673–1906*. Anthropological Papers, no. 5. Eugene: University of Oregon.

BANDELIER, F. (TRANSLATOR)

1964 [1904] *The journey of Alvar Núñez Cabeza de Vaca and his companions from Florida to the Pacific, 1528–1536*. Reprint. New York: Allerton Press.

BARKER, E. C.

1925 *The life of Stephen F. Austin, founder of Texas 1793–1836: A chapter in the westward movement of the Anglo-American people*. Austin: University of Texas Press.

BARNARD, H. D.

1939 Early history of research in Texas archeology by the Department of Anthropology, and the history of the Anthropology Museum of the University of Texas. M.A. thesis, The University of Texas at Austin.

BARNES, T. C., T. H. NAYLOR, AND C. W. POLZER

1981 *Northern New Spain: A research guide*. Tucson: University of Arizona Press.

BAUGH, T. G.

1982 *Edwards I (34BK2): Southern plains adaptations in the Protohistoric period*. Studies in Oklahoma's Past, no. 8. Norman: Oklahoma Archeological Survey.

1986 Cultural history and Protohistoric societies in the Southern Plains. In *Current trends in Southern Plains archaeology,* ed. T. G. Baugh, 167–187. Memoir 21, *Plains Anthropologist* (special issue) 31 (114).

BAUGH, T. G., AND F. E. SWENSON

1980 Comparative trade ceramics: Evidence for the southern plains macroeconomy. *Bulletin of the Oklahoma Anthropological Society* 29:83–102.

BEERS, H. P.

1979 *Spanish and Mexican records of the American Southwest: A bibliographical guide to archives and manuscript sources.* Tucson: University of Arizona Press.

BELL, M.

1981 *The Alex Justiss site: A Caddoan cemetery in Titus County, Texas.* Texas Department of Highways and Public Transportation, Highway Design Division, Publications in Archaeology, Report no. 21. Austin: Texas Department of Highways and Public Transportation.

BELL, R. E.

1981 Wichita Indians and the French trade on the Oklahoma frontier. *Bulletin of the Oklahoma Anthropological Society* 30:11–18.

1984a Arkansas Valley Caddoan: The Harlan phase. In *Prehistory of Oklahoma,* ed. R. E. Bell, 221–240. New York: Academic Press.

1984b Protohistoric Wichita. In *Prehistory of Oklahoma,* ed. R. E. Bell, 363–378. New York: Academic Press.

BELL, R. E., AND D. A. BAERREIS

1951 A survey of Oklahoma archaeology. *Bulletin of the Texas Archeological and Paleontological Society* 22:7–100.

BELL, R. E., E. B. JELKS, AND W. W. NEWCOMB (EDITORS)

1967 A pilot study of Wichita Indian archeology and ethnohistory. Final report submitted to the National Science Foundation on Grant GS-964. Dallas and Norman.

BELMONT, J. S.

1985 A reconnaissance of the Boeuf Basin, Louisiana. *Louisiana Archaeology* 10:271–284.

BENAVIDES, A.

1989 *The Béxar Archives (1717–1836): A name guide.* Austin: University of Texas Press.

BERLANDIER, J. L.

1969 *The Indians of Texas in 1830,* ed. J. C. Ewers. Washington, D.C.: Smithsonian Institution Press.

BERRY, J. M.

1917 The Indian policy of Spain in the Southwest, 1783–1795. *Mississippi Valley Historical Review* 3:462–477.

BINFORD, L. R.

1962 Archaeology as anthropology. *American Antiquity* 28:217–225.

1983 *Working at archaeology.* New York: Academic Press.

BLAKE, L. W.

1981 Early acceptance of watermelon by Indians of the United States. *Journal of Ethnobiology* 1:192–199.

BLAKELY, R. L. (EDITOR)

1988 *The King site: Continuity and contact in sixteenth-century Georgia.* Athens: University of Georgia Press.

BLAKELY, R. L., AND B. DETWEILER-BLAKELY

1989 The impact of European diseases in the sixteenth-century Southeast. *Midcontinental Journal of Archaeology* 14:62–89.

BLAKELY, R. L., AND D. S. MATHEWS

1990 Bioarchaeological evidence for a Spanish–native American conflict in the sixteenth-century Southeast. *American Antiquity* 55:718–743.

BOHANNON, C. F.

1973 *Excavations at the Mineral Springs site, Howard County, Arkansas.* Research series, no. 5. Fayetteville: Arkansas Archeological Survey.

BOLTON, H. E.

1908 The native tribes about the East Texas missions. *Texas State Historical Association Quarterly* 11:249–276.

1912 The Spanish occupation of Texas, 1519–1690. *Southwestern Historical Quarterly* 16:1–26.

1914 *Athanase de Mézières and the Louisiana-Texas Frontier, 1768–1780.* Vols. 1 and 2. Cleveland: Clark Publishing.

1915 *Texas in the middle eighteenth century: Studies in Spanish colonial history and administration.* Berkeley: University of California Press.

1917 The mission as a frontier institution in the Spanish-American colonies. *American Historical Review* 23:42–61.

1920 *The Spanish Borderlands: A chronicle of Old Florida and the Southwest.* New Haven: Yale University Press.

1987 *The Hasinais: Southern Caddoans as seen by the earliest Europeans.* Norman: University of Oklahoma Press.

BORAH, W. W.

1964 Americanas model: The demographic impact of European expansion upon the non-European world. In *Actas y Memorias, XXXV Congreso Internacional de Americanistas, México, 1962.* México D.F.: Editorial Libros de México.

1976 The historical demography of aboriginal and colonial America: An attempt at perspective. In *The native population of the Americas in 1492,* ed. W. M. Denevan, 13–34. Madison: University of Wisconsin Press.

BOURNE, E. G. (TRANSLATOR)

1904 *Narratives of the career of Hernando de Soto.* New York: Allerton.

BOWMAN, S.

1990 *Radiocarbon dating.* Berkeley and London: University of California Press.

BRACKENRIDGE, H. M.

1814 *Views of Louisiana; together with a journal of a voyage up the Missouri River in 1811*. Pittsburgh: Cramer, Spear, and Eichbaum.

BRADLEY, J. W.

1987 *Evolution of the Onondaga Iroquois: Accommodating change, 1500–1655*. Syracuse: Syracuse University Press.

BRADTMILLER, B.

1983 The biological effects of European contact among the Arikara. *American Journal of Physical Anthropology* 60:176.

BRAIN, J. P.

1975a *The archaeology of the Tunica: Trial on the Yazoo*. Lower Mississippi Survey, Preliminary Report. Cambridge: Peabody Museum.

1975b Artifacts of the Adelantado. *Conference on Historic Site Archaeology Papers* 8:129–138.

1978a The archaeological phase: Ethnographic fact or fancy. In *Archaeological essays in honor of Irving Rouse,* ed. R. C. Dunnell and E. S. Hall. The Hague: Mouton Publishers.

1978b Late Prehistoric settlement patterning in Yazoo Basin and Natchez Bluff regions. In *Mississippian Settlement Patterns,* ed. B. D. Smith, 331–368. New York: Academic Press.

1979 *Tunica treasure*. Papers of the Peabody Museum of Archaeology and Ethnology, Harvard University, vol. 71. Cambridge: Peabody Museum.

1983 Tunica triumph. *Geoscience and Man* 23:45–51.

1985a The archaeology of the Hernando de Soto expedition. In *Alabama and the Borderlands: From prehistory to statehood,* ed. R. R. Badger and L. A. Clayton, 96–107. University: University of Alabama Press.

1985b Introduction: Update of De Soto studies since the United States De Soto Expedition Commission report. In *Final Report of the United States De Soto Expedition Commission,* by J. R. Swanton, xi–lxxii. Classics in Anthropology Series. Washington, D.C.: Smithsonian Institution Press.

1989 *Tunica archaeology*. Papers of the Peabody Museum of Archaeology and Ethnology, Harvard University, vol. 78. Cambridge: Peabody Museum.

BRAIN, J. P., A. TOTH, AND A. RODRIQUEZ-BUCKINGHAM

1974 Ethnohistoric archaeology and the De Soto entrada into the lower Mississippi Valley. *Conference on Historic Site Archaeology Papers* 7:232–289.

BRAUDEL, F.

1984 *Civilization and capitalism: Fifteenth to eighteenth century*. Vol. 3, *The perspective of the world*. New York: Harper & Row.

BRAUN, D. D.

1985 Absolute seriation: A time-series approach. In *For concordance in archaeological analysis: Bridging data structure, quantitative technique, and theory,* ed. C. Carr, 509–539. Kansas City: Westport Publishers.

BRAY, R. T.

1978 European trade goods from the Utz site and the search for Fort Orleans. *The Missouri Archaeologist* 39:1–75.

BRENNER, E. M.

1988 Sociopolitical implications of mortuary ritual remains in seventeenth-century native southern New England. In *The recovery of meaning,* ed. M. P. Leone and P. B. Potter, 147–181. Washington, D.C.: Smithsonian Institution Press.

BROWMAN, D. L.

1981 Isotopic discrimination and correction factors in radiocarbon dating. In *Advances in archaeological method and theory,* vol. 4, ed. M. B. Schiffer, 241–295. New York: Academic Press.

BROWN, I. W.

1979a Bells. In *Tunica treasure,* by J. P. Brain, 197–205. Papers of the Peabody Museum of Archaeology and Ethnology, Harvard University, vol. 71. Cambridge: Peabody Museum.

1979b Functional group changes and acculturation: A case study of the French and the Indian in the lower Mississippi Valley. *Midcontinental Journal of Archaeology* 4:147–165.

1979c Historic artifacts and sociocultural change: Some warnings from the lower Mississippi Valley. *Conference on Historic Site Archaeology Papers* 13:109–121.

1980 Early eighteenth-century French-Indian culture contact in the Yazoo Bluffs region of the lower Mississippi Valley. Ph.D. diss., Brown University, Providence, R.I.

1982 An archaeological study of culture contact and change in the Natchez Bluffs region. In *La Salle and his legacy,* ed. P. K. Galloway, 176–193. Jackson: University Press of Mississippi.

1983 Historic aboriginal pottery from the Yazoo Bluffs region, Mississippi. *Southeastern Archaeological Conference Bulletin* 21:1–17.

1985 *Natchez Indian archaeology: Culture change and stability in the lower Mississippi Valley.* Archaeological report no. 15. Jackson: Mississippi Department of Archives and History.

BROWN, J. A.

1971 *Spiro Studies.* Vol. 3, *Pottery vessels.* First Part of the Third Annual Report of Caddoan Archaeology–Spiro Focus Research. Norman: University of Oklahoma Research Institute.

1975 The impact of the European presence on Indian culture. In *Contest for empire, 1500–1775,* ed. J. B. Elliott. Indianapolis: Indiana Historical Society.

1976 *Spiro Studies.* Vol. 4, *The artifacts.* Norman: University of Oklahoma Research Institute.

1981 The search for rank in Prehistoric burials. In *The archaeology of death,* ed. R. Chapman, I. Kinnes, and K. Randsborg, 25–37. Cambridge: Cambridge University Press.

1983 Spiro exchange connections revealed by sources of imported raw materials. In *Southeastern natives and their pasts,* ed. D. G. Wyckoff and J. L.

Hofman, 129–162. Studies in Oklahoma's Past, no. 11. Norman: Oklahoma Archeological Survey.

1984a Arkansas Valley Caddoan: The Spiro phase. In *Prehistory of Oklahoma,* ed. R. E. Bell, 241–263. New York: Academic Press.

1984b Observations of Caddoan settlement patterns. Paper presented at the Twenty-sixth Annual Caddo Conference, 23–24 March, at Stephen F. Austin State University, Nacogdoches, Tex.

1984c *Prehistoric southern Ozark marginality: A myth exposed.* Special Publications, no. 6. Columbia: Missouri Archaeological Society.

1990 Archaeology confronts history at the Natchez Temple. *Southeastern Archaeology* 9:1–10.

1991 Position Paper for "What is Caddo" Symposium. Paper presented at the Thirty-third Annual Caddo Conference, 22–24 March, Stephen F. Austin State University, Nacogdoches, Tex.

BROWN, J. A., R. E. BELL, AND D. G. WYCKOFF

1978 Caddoan settlement patterns in the Arkansas River drainage. In *Mississippian settlement patterns,* ed. B. D. Smith, 169–200. New York: Academic Press.

BRUSETH, J. E.

1987 Late Holocene environmental change and human adaptive strategies in Northeast Texas. Ph.D. diss., Department of Anthropology, Southern Methodist University, Dallas.

BRUSETH, J. E., AND T. K. PERTTULA

1981 *Prehistoric settlement patterns at Lake Fork Reservoir.* Texas Antiquities Committee, Texas Antiquities Permit Series, Report no. 2. Austin: Texas Historical Commission.

1991 1991 TAS Field School, The Sam Kaufman site (41RR16), Red River County, Texas. *Texas Archeology* 35(2):3, 13–14, 19.

BUCKLEY, E. C.

1911 The Aguayo expedition into Texas and Louisiana, 1719–1722. *Texas State Historical Association Quarterly* 15:1–65.

BUIKSTRA, J. E., AND J. H. MIELKE

1985 Demography, diet, and health. In *The analysis of Prehistoric diets,* ed. R. I. Gilbert, Jr., and J. H. Mielke, 360–422. Orlando: Academic Press.

BUQUOR, P. L. (TRANSLATOR)

1853 Translations of historical documents found in the archives of Bexar County at San Antonio in Texas. Commissioned as translator of certain Spanish records amongst the archives of Bexar County on February 12, 1853, by his excellency P. Hansborough Bell. Extracts, Department of Archives, University of Texas, 15 May 1935. Barker Texas History Center, The University of Texas at Austin.

BURNET, M., AND D. O. WHITE

1972 *Natural history of infectious disease.* 4th ed. Cambridge: Cambridge University Press.

BURNETT, B. A.

1986 A possibility of smallpox in the late Ouachita Caddo. Paper presented at the Twenty-eighth Annual Caddo Conference, 13–15 March, University of Arkansas, Little Rock.

1988 The bioarchaeological synthesis. In *Human adaptation in the Ozark and Ouachita mountains,* by G. Sabo III, A. M. Early, B. A. Burnett, J. C. Rose, J. P. Harcourt, and L. Vogele, Jr., 193–220. Final report submitted by the Arkansas Archeological Survey to the U.S. Army Corps of Engineers, Southwestern Division. Study Unit 1, Southwestern Division Archeological Overview. Research series, no. 31. Fayetteville: Arkansas Archeological Survey.

1990a The bioarchaeological synthesis of the eastern portion of the Gulf Coastal Plain. In *The Archeology and Bioarcheology of the Gulf Coastal Plain,* by D. A. Story, J. A. Guy, B. A. Burnett, M. D. Freeman, J. C. Rose, D. G. Steele, B. W. Olive, and K. J. Reinhard, 385–418. Research series, no. 38. Fayetteville: Arkansas Archeological Survey.

1990b The bioarcheology of the Hardman site (3CL418): Prehistoric and Protohistoric Caddoan samples. In *Hardman (3CL418): A Prehistoric salt processing site,* by I. Williams and A. M. Early, 11-1 to 11-147. Sponsored research program, Project report no. 642. Fayetteville: Arkansas Archeological Survey.

1990c The bioarcheology of Goldsmith Oliver 2 (3PU306). In *Goldsmith Oliver 2(3PU306): A Protohistoric archeological site near Little Rock, Arkansas,* by M. D. Jeter, K. H. Cande, and J. J. Mintz. Final report submitted to the Federal Aviation Administration, Southwest region, Fort Worth. Sponsored research program. Fayetteville: Arkansas Archeological Survey.

BURNETT, B. A., AND K. MURRAY

In press Biological effects of the entrada of the de Soto expedition in Arkansas. In *The expedition of Hernando de Soto in the West, 1541–1543,* ed. G. A. Young and M. P. Hoffman. Fayetteville: University of Arkansas Press.

CALAHORRA, FRAY JESUS DE

1760 Diario del Viage, October 24, 1760. Archivo General de Indias, Audiencia de México 92–6–22. Barker Texas History Center, The University of Texas Archives. Austin.

CAMPBELL, T. N.

1976 Articles on Indians in Texas. In *The handbook of Texas: A supplement,* vol. 3, ed. E. S. Branda. Austin: Texas State Historical Association.

CASTAÑEDA, C. E.

1936 *Our Catholic heritage in Texas.* 6 vols. Austin: V. Von Boeckmann–Jones Co.

CHAFE, W.

1983 The Caddo language, its relatives, and its neighbors. In *North American Indians: Humanistic perspectives,* ed. J. S. Thayer, 243–250. Papers in

Anthropology 24(2), Department of Anthropology. Norman: University of Oklahoma.

In press Caddo names in the de Soto documents. In *The expedition of Hernando de Soto in the West, 1541–1543,* ed. G. A. Young and M. P. Hoffman. Fayetteville: University of Arkansas Press.

CHAPMAN, C. H.

1974 *The origin of the Osage Indian tribe: An ethnographical, historical and archaeological study.* New York: Garland Press.

1980 *The archaeology of Missouri, II.* Columbia: University of Missouri Press.

1982 Osage Indians in Missouri and Oklahoma, A.D. 1796–1825. In *Pathways to Plains prehistory,* ed. D. G. Wyckoff and J. L. Hofman, 19–28. Memoir no. 3. Oklahoma City: Oklahoma Anthropological Society.

CLARK, G. A., M. A. KELLY, J. M. GRANGE, AND M. C. HILL

1987 The evolution of mycobacterial disease in human populations. *Current Anthropology* 28:45–62.

CLARK, J. G.

1970 *New Orleans, 1718–1812: An economic history.* Baton Rouge: Louisiana State University Press.

CLARK, J. W., AND J. E. IVEY

1974 *Archaeological and historical investigations at Martin Lake, Rusk and Panola Counties, Texas.* Research report 32. Austin: Texas Archeological Survey.

CLARK, R. C.

1902 Louis Juchereau de Saint-Denis and the re-establishment of the Tejas missions. *Texas State Historical Association Quarterly* 6:1–26.

CLAYTON, J. L.

1967 The growth and economic significance of the American fur trade, 1790–1890. In *Aspects of the fur trade: Selected papers of the 1965 North American Fur Trade Conference,* ed. R. W. Fridley and J. D. Holmquist, 62–72. St. Paul: Minnesota Historical Society.

COBB, J. E.

1976 The functional analysis of late Prehistoric remains from Bontke Shelter. M.A. thesis, University of Arkansas, Fayetteville.

COKER, W. S., AND T. D. WATSON

1986 *Indian traders and the Southeast Spanish Borderlands: Panton, Leslie and Co. and John Forbes and Co.* Gainesville: University Presses of Florida.

COLE, N. M.

1975 Early historic Caddoan mortuary practices in the Upper Neches drainage. Master's thesis, The University of Texas at Austin.

COOK, N. D.

1981 *Demographic collapse: Indian Peru, 1520–1620.* Cambridge: Cambridge University Press.

COOK, S. F.

1937 *The extent and significance of disease among the Indians of Baja Cali-*

fornia, 1697–1773. Ibero-Americana, no. 12. Berkeley: University of California.

1973 The significance of disease in the extinction of the New England Indians. *Human Biology* 45:485–508.

1976 *The conflict between the California Indian and white civilization.* Berkeley: University of California Press.

COOK, S. F., AND W. BORAH

1971–1974 *Essays in population history.* 2 vols. Berkeley: University of California Press.

CORBIN, J. E.

1989 Spanish-Indian interaction on the eastern frontier of Texas. In *Columbian consequences.* Vol. 1, *Archaeological and historical perspectives on the Spanish Borderlands West,* ed. D. H. Thomas, 269–276. Washington, D.C.: Smithsonian Institution Press.

1991 Retracing the *Camino de los Tejas* from the Trinity to Los Adaes: New insights into East Texas history. In *A Texas Legacy: The Old San Antonio Road and the Caminos Reales. A tricentennial history, 1691–1991,* ed. A. J. McGraw and J. W. Clark, Jr., pp. 191–219. Austin: Texas State Department of Highways and Public Transportation, Highway Design Division.

CORBIN, J. E., T. C. ALEX, AND A. KARLINA

1980 *Mission Dolores de los Ais: Archaeological investigations of an early Spanish colonial mission, San Augustine County, Texas.* Papers in Anthropology, no. 2, and Texas Antiquities Permit Series, Report no. 3. Nacogdoches: Stephen F. Austin State University.

CORBIN, J. E., H. A. BROWN, M. G. CANAVAN, AND S. TOUPS

1990 *Mission Dolores de los Ais (41SA25): San Augustine County, Texas. Archaeological Investigations, 1984.* Papers in Anthropology, no. 5. Nacogdoches: Stephen F. Austin State University.

CORBIN, J. E., J. M. STUDER, AND L. NUMMI

1978 *The Chayah site.* Papers in Anthropology, no. 1. Nacogdoches: Stephen F. Austin State University.

COX, I. J.

1906 *The early exploration of Louisiana.* University Studies, Series 2, vol. 11, no. 1. Cincinnati: University of Cincinnati.

1909 The significance of the Texas-Louisiana frontier. *Mississippi Valley Historical Association Proceedings* 3:198–213.

1922 *The journeys of René Robert Cavelier, Sieur de La Salle.* New York: Allerton Book Co.

CRANE, V. W.

1929 *The southern frontier, 1670–1732.* Ann Arbor: University of Michigan Press.

CREEL, D. G.

1982a Artifacts of non-native manufacture. In *The Deshazo site, Nacogdoches County, Texas,* ed. D. A. Story, 113–130. Texas Antiquities Committee,

Texas Antiquities Permit Series, Report no. 7. Austin: Texas Historical Commission.

1982b Site description and investigation. In *The Deshazo site, Nacogdoches County, Texas,* ed. D. A. Story, 35–50. Texas Antiquities Committee, Texas Antiquities Permit Series, Report no. 7. Austin: Texas Historical Commission.

1982c Transcribed interview with William C. Beatty on WPA archaeology at the Hatchel and Mitchell sites, Bowie County, Texas. Manuscript on file at the Texas Archeological Research Laboratory.

1991a Bison hides in late Prehistoric exchange in the southern plains. *American Antiquity* 56:40–49.

1991b Burial seriation and occupational history at the Hatchell-Mitchell-Moore Complex, Bowie County, Texas. Paper presented at the Thirty-third Annual Caddo Conference, 22–24 March, Stephen F. Austin State University, Nacogdoches, Tex.

CRONON, W.

1983 *Changes in the land: Indians, colonists, and the ecology of New England.* New York: Hill and Wang.

CROSBY, A. W.

1967 *Conquistador y pestilencia:* The first New World pandemic and the fall of the great Indian empires. *Hispanic American Historical Review* 47: 321–337.

1972 *The Columbian exchange: Biological and cultural consequences of 1492.* Westport, Conn.: Greenwood Press.

1976 Virgin soil epidemic as a factor in aboriginal population decline. *The William and Mary Quarterly* 33:289–299.

1986 *Ecological imperialism: The biological expansion of Europe, 900–1900.* Cambridge: Cambridge University Press.

1987 *The Columbian voyages, the Columbian exchange, and their historians.* Washington, D.C.: American Historical Association.

CROSBY, C. A.

1988 From myth to history, or why King Philip's ghost walks abroad. In *The recovery of meaning,* ed. M. P. Leone and P. B. Parker, 183–209. Washington, D.C.: Smithsonian Institution Press.

CURREN, C.

1984 *The Protohistoric period in Central Alabama.* Camden: Alabama Tombigbee Regional Commission.

DAVIS, D. D.

1984 Protohistoric cultural interaction on the northern Gulf Coast. In *Perspectives on Gulf Coast prehistory,* ed. D. D. Davis, 216–231. Ripley F. Bullen Monographs in Anthropology and History, no. 5, Florida State Museum. Gainesville: University Presses of Florida.

DAVIS, E. M.

1961 Proceedings of the Fifth Conference on Caddoan Archaeology. *Bulletin of the Texas Archeological Society* 31:77–150.

1970 Archaeological and historical assessment of the Red River basin in Texas. In *Archaeological and historical resources of the Red River basin,* ed. H. A. Davis, 25–65. Research Series, no. 1. Fayetteville: Arkansas Archeological Survey.

1979 The first quarter century of the Texas Archeological Society. *Bulletin of the Texas Archeological Society* 50:159–194.

DAVIS, H. A.

1967 The puzzle of Point Remove. *Field Notes* 33:2–7.

DAVIS, H. A. (EDITOR)

1983 *A state plan for the conservation of archaeological resources in Arkansas.* Research Series, no. 21. Fayetteville: Arkansas Archeological Survey.

DEAGAN, K.

1983 *Spanish St. Augustine: The archaeology of a colonial creole community.* New York: Academic Press.

1984 Reconstructing aboriginal population dynamics through Euro-American archaeological contexts. Paper presented at the Forty-ninth Annual Meeting of the Society for American Archaeology, 12–14 April, Portland, Ore.

1985 Spanish-Indian interaction in sixteenth-century Florida and Hispaniola. In *Cultures in contact,* ed. W. W. Fitzhugh, 281–318. Washington, D.C.: Smithsonian Institution Press.

1987 *Artifacts of the Spanish colonies of Florida and the Caribbean, 1500–1800.* Vol. 1, *Ceramics, glassware, and beads.* Washington, D.C.: Smithsonian Institution Press.

DEBO, A.

1942 *And still the waters run: The betrayal of the five civilized tribes.* Norman: University of Oklahoma Press.

DELANGEZ, J.

1938 *The journal of Jean Cavelier: The account of a survivor of La Salle's Texas expedition, 1684–1688.* Chicago: Institute of Jesuit History.

1944 The voyages of Tonti in North America. *Mid-America* 26:255–297.

1946 The "Récit des voyages et des découvertes du Père Jacques Marquette." *Mid-America* 28:173–194, 211–258.

DICKENS, R. S., H. T. WARD, AND R. P. STEPHEN DAVIS

1987 *The Siouan project: Seasons I and II.* Research Laboratories of Anthropology, Monograph Series, no. 1, Chapel Hill: University of North Carolina.

DICKINSON, S. D.

1936 Ceramic relationship of the pre-Caddo pottery from the Crenshaw site. *Bulletin of the Texas Archeological and Paleontological Society* 8:56–70.

1941 Certain vessels from the Clements Place, an historic Caddo site. *Bulletin of the Texas Archeological and Paleontological Society* 13:117–132.

1980 Historic tribes of the Ouachita drainage system in Arkansas. *The Arkansas Archeologist* 21:1–11.

1987 Arkansas's Spanish halberds. *The Arkansas Archeologist* 25/26:53–62.

DICKINSON, S. D., AND S. C. DELLINGER

1940 A survey of the historic earthenware of the Lower Arkansas River Valley. *Bulletin of the Texas Archeological and Paleontological Society* 12: 76–96.

DICKINSON, S. D., AND H. J. LEMLEY

1939 Evidence of the Marksville and Coles Creek complexes at the Kirkham Place, Clark County, Arkansas. *Bulletin of the Texas Archeological and Paleontological Society* 11:139–189.

DIN, G. C.

1973 Spain's immigration policy in Louisiana and the American penetration, 1792–1803. *Southwestern Historical Quarterly* 76:255–276.

DIXON, R. B.

1913 Some aspects of North American archaeology. *American Anthropologist* 15:549–565.

DOBYNS, H. F.

1966 An appraisal of techniques for estimating aboriginal American population with a new hemispheric estimate. *Current Anthropology* 7:395–441.

1980 The study of Spanish colonial frontier institutions. In *Spanish colonial frontier research,* ed. H. F. Dobyns, 5–25. Spanish Borderlands Research, no. 1. Albuquerque: Center for Anthropological Studies.

1983 *Their number become thinned: Native American population dynamics in eastern North America.* Knoxville: University of Tennessee Press.

1984 Native American population collapse and recovery. In *Scholars and the Indian experience,* ed. W. R. Swagerty, 17–35. Bloomington: Indiana University Press.

DOBYNS, H. F. (EDITOR)

1976 Brief perspective on a scholarly transformation: Widowing the "virgin land." *Ethnohistory* 23:95–197.

DORSEY, G. A.

1905a Caddo customs of childhood. *Journal of American Folk-Lore* 18:226–228.

1905b *Traditions of the Caddo.* Publication 41. Washington, D.C.: Carnegie Institution of Washington.

DOUGHTY, R. W.

1987 *At home in Texas: Early views of the land.* College Station: Texas A&M University Press.

DOWNER, A. S.

1990 Tribal sovereignty and historic preservation: Native American participation in cultural resource management on Indian lands. In *Preservation on the reservation: Native Americans, Native American lands, and archaeology,* ed. A. L. Klesert and A. S. Downer, 67–100. Navajo Nation Papers in Anthropology, no. 26. Window Rock, Az.: Navajo Nation Archaeology Department, Navajo Nation Historic Preservation Department.

DUFFIELD, L. F., AND E. B. JELKS

1961 *The Pearson site: A historic Indian site in Iron Bridge Reservoir, Rains County, Texas.* Archaeology Series, no. 4. Austin: Department of Anthropology, The University of Texas.

DUFFY, J.

1953 *Epidemics in colonial America.* Baton Rouge: Louisiana State University Press.

DUNNELL, R. C.

1970 Seriation method and its evaluation. *American Antiquity* 35:305–319.

1971 *Systematics in prehistory.* New York: The Free Press.

1978 Style and function: A fundamental dichotomy. *American Antiquity* 43:192–202.

1986 Five decades of American archaeology. In *American Archaeology past and future,* ed. D. J. Meltzer, D. D. Fowler, and J. A. Sabloff, 23–49. Washington, D.C.: Smithsonian Institution Press.

1991 Methodological impacts of catastrophic depopulation on American archaeology and ethnology. In *Columbian consequences.* Vol. 3, *The Spanish Borderlands in Pan-American perspective,* ed. D. H. Thomas, 561–580. Washington, D.C.: Smithsonian Institution Press.

DYE, D. H.

1986 Introduction. In *The Protohistoric period in the Mid-South: 1500–1700,* ed. D. H. Dye and R. C. Brister, xi–xiv. Archaeological Reports, no. 18. Jackson: Mississippi Department of Archives and History.

DYE, D. H., AND R. C. BRISTER (EDITORS)

1986 *The Protohistoric period in the Mid-South, 1500–1700: Proceedings of the 1983 Mid-South Archaeological Conference.* Archaeological Reports, no. 18. Jackson: Mississippi Department of Archives and History.

EARLY, A. M.

1978 Turquoise beads from the Standridge site, 3MN53. *The Arkansas Archeologist* 19:25–30.

1982a Caddoan settlement systems in the Ouachita River basin. In *Arkansas archeology in review,* ed. N. L. Trubowitz and M. D. Jeter, 198–232. Research Series, no. 15. Fayetteville: Arkansas Archeological Survey.

1982b An outline of the culture history of the eastern Ouachitas. In *Fancy Hill: Archeological studies in the southern Ouachita Mountains,* ed. A. M. Early and W. F. Limp, 33–46. Research Series, no. 16. Fayetteville: Arkansas Archeological Survey.

1983 Summary. *The Arkansas Archeologist* 22:51–60.

1985 A brief history of archeological work in the Ouachita River Valley, Arkansas. *Louisiana Archaeology* 10:1–24.

1986 Dr. Thomas L. Hodges and his contributions to Arkansas archeology. *The Arkansas Archeologist* 23/24:1–11.

1988 *Standridge: Caddoan settlement in a mountain environment.* Research Series, no. 29. Fayetteville: Arkansas Archeological Survey.

1990 Hardman and salt making. In *Hardman (3CL418): A Prehistoric salt processing site,* by I. Williams and A. M. Early, 13-1 to 13-31. Sponsored Research Program, Project Report no. 642. Fayetteville: Arkansas Archeological Survey.

ECCLES, W. J.

1973 French aims and means in colonial North America. In *France and North America: Over 300 years of dialogue,* ed. M. Allain and G. Conrad, 57–70. Lafayette: University of Southwest Louisiana Press.

ERICSON, J. E., AND E. A. COUGHLIN

1984 Pigments analysis of painted ceramics and within grave offerings on a late Caddo site at Cedar Grove, Arkansas. In *Cedar Grove: An interdisciplinary investigation of a Late Caddo farmstead in the Red River Valley,* ed. N. L. Trubowitz, 171–173. Research Series, no. 23. Fayetteville: Arkansas Archeological Survey.

ESPEY, HUSTON, AND ASSOCIATES, INC.

1983 The archaeological investigation of the Louis Procello site, 16DS212, De Soto Parish, Louisiana. Document No. 82360. Austin.

ESPINOSA, I. F.

1716 Diario Derrotero de la Nueva España a la Provincia de los Tejas, año de 1716. Archivos General de Naciones, Provincias Internas, vol. 181. University of Texas Archives, Barker Texas History Center, Austin.

EVERETT, D.

1990 *The Texas Cherokee: A people between two fires 1819–1840.* Norman: University of Oklahoma Press.

EWEN, C. R.

1988 *The discovery and excavation of Hernando de Soto's first winter encampment.* De Soto Working Paper no. 7. Tuscaloosa: University of Alabama and State Museum of Natural History.

1990 *The archaeology of Spanish colonialism in the southeastern United States and the Caribbean.* Columbian Quincentenary Series, Guides to the Archaeological Literature of the Immigrant Experience in America, no. 1. Ann Arbor: Society for Historical Archaeology.

EWERS, J. C.

1955 *The horse in Blackfoot Indian culture, with comparative material from other western tribes.* Bulletin 159. Washington, D.C.: Bureau of American Ethnology.

1973 The influence of epidemics on the Indian populations and cultures of Texas. *Plains Anthropologist* 18:104–115.

1974 Symbols of chiefly authority in Spanish Louisiana. In *The Spanish in the Mississippi Valley,* ed. J. McDermott, 272–286. Urbana: University of Illinois Press.

FAIRBANKS, C. H.

1985 From exploration to settlement: Spanish strategies for colonization. In *Alabama and the Borderlands: From prehistory to statehood,* ed. R. R.

Badger and L. A. Clayton, 128–139. University: University of Alabama Press.

FIELDHOUSE, D. K.

1966 *The colonial empires: A comparative survey from the eighteenth century.* London: G. Weidenfeld and Nicolson.

FIELDS, R. C.

1981 Analysis of the native ceramics from the Deshazo site. Master's thesis, The University of Texas at Austin.

FISH, S. K., AND P. R. FISH

1979 Historic demography and ethnographic analogy. *Early Georgia* 6:29–43.

FISH, S. K., AND S. A. KOWALEWSKI (EDITORS)

1990 *The archaeology of regions: A case for full-coverage survey.* Washington, D.C.: Smithsonian Institution Press.

FITZHUGH, W. W.

1985 The South—Labor, tribute and social policy: The Spanish legacy. Commentary on Part 4. In *Cultures in contact: The impact of European contacts on native American cultural institutions,* A.D. *1000–1800,* ed. W. W. Fitzhugh, 269–279. Washington, D.C.: Smithsonian Institution Press.

FLORES, D. L.

1984 *Jefferson and southwestern exploration: The Freeman and Custis accounts of the Red River expedition of 1806.* Norman: University of Oklahoma Press.

1985 *Journal of an Indian trader: Anthony Glass and the Texas frontier, 1790–1810.* College Station: Texas A&M University Press.

FORD, J. A.

1936 *An analysis of Indian village site collections from Louisiana and Mississippi.* Anthropological Study 2. Baton Rouge: Department of Conservation, Louisiana Geological Survey.

1951 *Greenhouse: A Troyville–Coles Creek period site in Avoyelles Parish, Louisiana.* Anthropological Papers 44(1). New York: American Museum of Natural History.

1961 *Menard site: The Quapaw village of Osotouy on the Arkansas River.* Anthropological Papers 48(2). New York: American Museum of Natural History.

FORD, J. A., AND G. R. WILLEY

1941 An interpretation of the prehistory of the eastern United States. *American Anthropologist* 43:325–363.

FREEMAN, J. E.

1962 The Neosho focus: A late prehistoric culture in Northeastern Oklahoma. *Bulletin of the Oklahoma Anthropological Society* 10:1–25.

FRITZ, G. J.

1986a Dessicated botanical remains from three Bluff Shelter sites in the Pine Mountains project area, Crawford County, Arkansas. In *Contributions to Ozark prehistory,* ed. G. Sabo III, 86–97. Research Series, no. 26. Fayetteville: Arkansas Archeological Survey.

1986b Prehistoric Ozark Agriculture, the University of Arkansas Rockshelter Collections. Ph.D. diss., University of North Carolina—Chapel Hill.

1989 Evidence of plant use from Copple Mound at the Spiro site. In *Contributions to Spiro archeology: Mound excavations and regional perspectives,* ed. J. D. Rogers, D. G. Wyckoff, and D. A. Peterson, 65–87. Studies in Oklahoma's Past, no. 16. Norman: Oklahoma Archeological Survey.

FRITZ, G. J., AND R. H. RAY

1982 Rock art sites in the southern Arkansas Ozarks and Arkansas River Valley. In *Arkansas Archeology in Review,* ed. N. L. Trubowitz and M. D. Jeter, 240–276. Research Series, no. 15. Fayetteville: Arkansas Archeological Survey.

GALLOWAY, P. K. (EDITOR)

1982 *La Salle and his legacy: Frenchmen and Indians in the Lower Mississippi Valley.* Jackson: University Press of Mississippi.

GARRETT, J. K.

1944 Letters and documents: Dr. John Sibley and the Louisiana-Texas frontier, 1803–1814. *Southwestern Historical Quarterly* 47(4):388–391.

1946a Notes and documents: Dr. John Sibley and the Louisiana-Texas frontier, 1803–1814. *Southwestern Historical Quarterly* 49(3):399–431.

1946b Notes and documents: Dr. John Sibley and the Louisiana-Texas Frontier, 1803–1814. *Southwestern Historical Quarterly* 49(4):599–614.

GIBSON, C.

1989 Spanish Indian policies. In *Handbook of North American Indians.* Vol. 4, *History of Indian-white relations,* ed. W. E. Washburn, 96–102. Washington, D.C.: Smithsonian Institution Press.

GIBSON, J. L.

1985a An evaluatory history of archaeology in the Ouachita Valley of Louisiana. *Louisiana Archaeology* 10:25–101.

1985b Ouachita prehistory. *Louisiana Archaeology* 10:319–335.

GILMORE, K.

1978 Spanish colonial settlements in Texas. In *Texas Archeology: Essays honoring R. King Harris,* ed. K. D. House, 132–145. Dallas: Southern Methodist University Press.

1983 *Caddoan interaction in the Neches Valley, Texas.* Reprints in Anthropology, vol. 27. Lincoln: J&L Reprints.

1986a *French-Indian interaction at an early eighteenth-century post: The Roseborough Lake Site, Bowie County, Texas.* Contributions in Archaeology, No. 3. Denton: Institute of Applied Sciences, North Texas State University.

1986b La Salle's Fort St. Louis in Texas. *Bulletin of the Texas Archeological Society* 55:61–72.

GILMORE, K. K., AND M. FORET

1988 Ethnohistoric investigations. In *Archaeological survey along Mill Race*

Creek and tributaries, Wood County, Texas: 1987–1988, ed. T. K. Perttula and K. K. Gilmore, 91–99. Contributions in Archaeology, no. 6. Denton: Institute of Applied Sciences, University of North Texas.

GIRAUD, M.

1957 *Histoire de la Louisiane Française.* Vol. 2, *Années de transition, 1715–1717.* Paris: Presses Universitaires de France.

1963 *Histoire de la Louisiane Française.* Vol. 3, *Le Système de law, 1717–1720.* Paris: Presses Universitaires de France.

1974a *Histoire de la Louisiane Française.* Vol. 4, *La Louisiane après le système de law, 1721–1723.* Paris: Presses Universitaires de France.

1974b *A history of French Louisiana.* Vol. 1, *The reign of Louis XIV, 1698–1715.* Baton Rouge: Louisiana State University Press.

GOOD, C. E.

1982 Analysis of structures, burials, and other cultural features. In *The Deshazo site, Nacogdoches County, Texas,* ed. D. A. Story, 51–112. Texas Antiquities Committee, Texas Antiquities Permit Series, no. 7. Austin: Texas Historical Commission.

GREGORY, H. F.

1973 Eighteenth-Century Caddoan archaeology: A study in models and interpretation. Ph.D. diss., Southern Methodist University, Dallas.

1978 A historic Tunica burial at the Coulee des Grues site in Avoyelles Parish, Louisiana. In *Texas archeology: Essays in honor of R. King Harris,* ed. K. D. House, 146–164. Dallas: Southern Methodist University Press.

1980 A continuity model for Caddoan adaptation on the Red River in Louisiana. *Louisiana Archaeology* 5:347–360.

1981 Another response to Perttula. *Louisiana Archaeology* 7:126–131.

1983 Los Adaes: The archaeology of an ethnic enclave. *Geoscience and Man* 23:53–57.

1986 Introduction. In *The southern Caddo: An anthology,* ed. H. F. Gregory, xiii–xx. New York: Garland Publishing.

GREGORY, H. F., AND C. H. WEBB

1965 European trade beads from six sites in Natchitoches Parish, Louisiana. *The Florida Anthropologist* 18:15–44.

GRIFFIN, J. B.

1967 Eastern North American archaeology: A summary. *Science* 156:175–191.

1985 Changing concepts of the Prehistoric Mississippian cultures of the eastern United States. In *Alabama and the Borderlands: From prehistory to statehood,* ed. R. R. Badger and L. A. Clayton, 40–63. University: University of Alabama Press.

GRIFFITH, W. J.

1954 *The Hasinai Indians of East Texas as seen by Europeans, 1687–1772.* Middle American Research Institute, Philological and Documentary Studies, volume 2, no. 3. New Orleans: Tulane University.

GUY, J. A.

1988 A history of archeological research within the West Gulf Coastal Plain. Master's thesis, The University of Texas at Austin.

1990 Previous archeological investigations. In *The archeology and bioarcheology of the Gulf Coastal Plain,* by D. A. Story, J. A. Guy, B. A. Burnett, M. D. Freeman, J. C. Rose, D. G. Steele, B. W. Olive, and K. J. Reinhard, 27–130. Research Series, no. 38. Fayetteville: Arkansas Archeological Survey.

HABIG, M.

1984 *Spanish Texas pilgrimage: The old Franciscan missions and other Spanish settlements of Texas, 1632–1821.* Chicago: Franciscan Herald Press.

HACKETT, C. W. (EDITOR AND TRANSLATOR)

1931–1946 *Pichardo's treatise on the limits of Louisiana and Texas.* 4 vols. Austin: University of Texas Press.

HAGGARD, J. V.

1945 The neutral ground between Louisiana and Texas, 1806–1821. *Louisiana Historical Quarterly* 28:1001–1128.

HAHN, J. H.

1986 Demographic patterns and changes in mid–seventeenth-century Timucua and Apalachee. *Florida Historical Quarterly* 64:371–392.

HALLY, D. J.

1972 The Plaquemine and Mississippian Occupations of the Upper Tensas Basin, Louisiana. Ph.D. diss., Harvard University, Cambridge.

HAMELL, G. R.

1983 Trading in metaphors: The magic of beads. Another perspective on Indian-European contact in northeastern North America. In *Proceedings of the 1982 Glass Trade Bead Conference,* ed. C. F. Hayes, 5–28. Rochester: Rochester State Museum.

HAMILTON, T. M.

1960a The gunsmith's cache discovered at Malta Bend, Missouri. In *Indian trade guns,* compiled by T. M. Hamilton, 150–171. *The Missouri Archaeologist,* vol. 22.

1960b Some gun parts from eighteenth-century Osage sites. In *Indian trade guns,* compiled by T. M. Hamilton, 120–149. *The Missouri Archaeologist,* vol. 22.

1980 *Colonial frontier guns.* Chadron, Nebr.: Fur Trade Press.

HANSON, J. R.

1987 *Hidatsa culture change, 1780–1845: A cultural ecological approach.* Reprints in Anthropology, vol. 34. Lincoln: J&L Reprints.

HARMON, A. M., AND J. C. ROSE

1989 Bioarcheology of the Louisiana and Arkansas study area. In *Archeology and bioarcheology of the lower Mississippi Valley and Trans-Mississippi South in Arkansas and Louisiana,* by M. D. Jeter, J. C. Rose, G. I. Williams, Jr., and A. M. Harmon, 323–354. Research Series, no. 37. Fayetteville: Arkansas Archeological Survey.

HARRINGTON, M. R.

1920 *Certain Caddo sites in Arkansas.* Indian Notes and Monographs, Miscellaneous Series, vol. 10. New York: Museum of the American Indian, Heye Foundation.

1924 The Ozark Bluff–Dwellers. *American Anthropologist* 26:1–21.

1960 *The Ozark Bluff–Dwellers.* Indian Notes and Monographs, volume 12. New York: Museum of the American Indian, Heye Foundation.

HARRIS, R. K.

1953 The Sam Kaufman site, Red River County, Texas. *Bulletin of the Texas Archeological Society* 24:43–68.

HARRIS, R. K., AND I. M. HARRIS

1980 Distribution of Natchitoches Engraved ceramics. *Louisiana Archaeology* 6:223–230.

HARRIS, R. K., I. M. HARRIS, J. C. BLAINE, AND J. BLAINE

1965 A preliminary archeological and documentary study of the Womack site, Lamar County, Texas. *Bulletin of the Texas Archeological Society* 36: 287–365.

HARRIS, R. K., I. M. HARRIS, AND M. P. MIROIR

1980 The Atlanta State Park site in Northeastern Texas. *Louisiana Archaeology* 6:231–239.

HARTLEY, J. D., AND A. F. MILLER

1977 *Archaeological investigations at the Bryson-Paddock site: An early Contact period site on the southern plains.* Archaeological Site Report, no. 32. Norman: Oklahoma River Basin Survey, University of Oklahoma.

HATCHER, M. A.

1921 The Louisiana background of the colonization of Texas, 1763–1803. *Southwestern Historical Quarterly* 24:169–194.

1927 Descriptions of the Tejas or Asinai Indians, 1691–1722. *Southwestern Historical Quarterly* 30:206–218, 283–304; 31:50–62, 150–180.

1932 The expedition of Don Domingo Terán de los Ríos into Texas. *Preliminary Studies of the Texas Catholic Historical Society* 2:3–62.

HAVEN, S. F.

1856 *Archaeology in the United States.* Smithsonian Contributions to Knowledge, vol. 8. Washington, D.C.: Government Printing Office.

HEMMINGS, E. T.

1982 *Human adaptations in the Grand Marais Lowland.* Research Series, no. 17. Fayetteville: Arkansas Archeological Survey.

1983 Spirit Lake (3LA83): Test excavations in a late Caddo site on the Red River, Southwest Arkansas. In *Contributions to the archeology of the Great Bend region in Southwest Arkansas,* ed. F. F. Schambach and F. Rackerby, 55–89. Research Series, no. 22. Fayetteville: Arkansas Archeological Survey.

HEMMINGS, J.

1978 *Red gold: The conquest of the Brazilian Indians, 1500–1760.* Cambridge: Harvard University Press.

HENIGE, D.

1986 Primary source by primary source? On the role of epidemics in New World depopulation. *Ethnohistory* 33:293–312.

HERRINGTON, L.

1979 Lake Bob Sandlin: A case study of the mitigation process in a reservoir area. Texas Antiquities Committee, Technical Report no. 32. Austin: Texas Historical Commission.

HESTER, T. R.

1989a Perspectives on the material culture of the mission Indians of the Texas–northeastern Mexico Borderlands. In *Columbian consequences.* Vol. 1, *Archaeological and historical perspectives on the Spanish Borderlands West,* ed. D. H. Thomas, 213–229. Washington, D.C.: Smithsonian Institution Press.

1989b Texas and northeastern Mexico: An overview. In *Columbian consequences.* Vol. 1, *Archaeological and historical perspectives on the Spanish Borderlands West,* ed. D. H. Thomas, 191–211. Washington, D.C.: Smithsonian Institution Press.

HILL, E. E. (COMPILER)

1965 *Records of the Bureau of Indian Affairs.* 2 vols. Preliminary Inventories of the National Archives, National Archives and Records Service, General Services Administration, no. 163. Washington, D.C.: Government Printing Office.

HODDER, I.

1982 *Symbols in action: Ethnoarchaeological studies of material culture.* Cambridge: Cambridge University Press.

HODGES, MRS. T. L.

1957 The Cahinnio Caddo: A contact unit in the eastern margin of the "Caddo Area." *Bulletin of the Texas Archeological Society* 28:190–197.

HODGES, T. L., AND MRS. T. L. HODGES

1943 The Watermelon Island site in Arkansas. *Bulletin of the Texas Archeological and Paleontological Society* 15:66–79.

1945 Suggestions for the identification of certain Mid-Ouachita pottery as Cahinnio Caddo. *Bulletin of the Texas Archeological and Paleontological Society* 16:98–116.

HOFFMAN, M. P.

1970 Archeological and historical assessment of the Red River basin in Arkansas. In *Archeological and historical resources of the Red River basin,* ed. H. A. Davis, 135–194. Research Series, no. 1. Fayetteville: Arkansas Archeological Survey.

1971 A partial archaeological sequence for the Little River Region, Arkansas. Ph.D. diss., Harvard University, Cambridge.

1977a The Kinkead-Mainard site, 3PU2: A late Prehistoric Quapaw phase site near Little Rock, Arkansas. *The Arkansas Archeologist* 16–18:1–41.

1977b *Ozark reservoir papers: Archeology in West-Central Arkansas 1965–*

1970. Research Series, no. 10. Fayetteville: Arkansas Archeological Survey.

1983 Changing mortuary patterns in the Little River Region, Arkansas. In *Southeastern natives and their pasts,* ed. D. G. Wyckoff and J. L. Hofman, 163–182. Studies in Oklahoma's Past, no. 11. Norman: Oklahoma Archeological Survey.

1986 Protohistory of the Lower and Central Arkansas River Valley in Arkansas. In *The Protohistoric period in the Mid-South: 1500–1700: Proceedings of the 1983 Mid-South Archaeological Conference,* ed. D. H. Dye and R. C. Brister, 24–37. Archaeological Report no. 18. Jackson: Mississippi Department of Archives and History.

1987 Who's wearing the white hats? The Arkansas act to prohibit burial desecration and its implications for Caddoan archaeology. *Newsletter of the Southeastern Archaeological Conference* 29(2): 22–28.

HOFMAN, J. L., R. L. BROOKS, J. S. HAYS, D. W. OWSLEY, R. L. JANTZ, M. K. MARKS, AND M. H. MANHEIN

1989 *From Clovis to Comanchero: Archeological overview of the southern Great Plains*. Research Series, no. 35. Fayetteville: Arkansas Archeological Survey.

HOLMES, J. D. L.

1975 Spanish policy toward the southern Indians in the 1790s. In *Four centuries of southern Indians,* ed. C. M. Hudson, 65–82. Athens: University of Georgia Press.

HOLMES, W. H.

1903 Aboriginal pottery of the eastern United States. In *Bureau of American ethnology, Twentieth Annual Report*. Washington, D.C.: Smithsonian Institution.

1914 Areas of American culture characterization tentatively outlined as an aid in the study of the antiquities. *American Anthropologist* 16: 413–446.

HOUSE, J. H.

1991 The Mississippian sequence in the Menard locality, eastern Arkansas. In *Arkansas before the Americans,* ed. H. A. Davis, 6–39. Research Series, no. 40. Fayetteville: Arkansas Archeological Survey.

HOUSE, J. H., AND H. MCKELWAY

1983 Mississippian and Quapaw on the Lower Arkansas. In *A state plan for the conservation of archeological resources in Arkansas,* ed. H. A. Davis, SE41–47. Research Series, no. 21. Fayetteville: Arkansas Archeological Survey.

HUDSON, C. M.

1981 Why the southeastern Indians slaughtered deer. In *Indians, animals, and the fur trade,* ed. S. Krech III, 155–176. Athens: University of Georgia Press.

1985 De Soto in Arkansas: A brief synopsis. *Field Notes* 205: 3–12.

1986 Hernando De Soto in the Caddo area. Paper presented at the Twenty-eighth Annual Caddo conference, 13–15 March, University of Arkansas, Little Rock.

1987a An unknown South: Spanish explorers and southeastern chiefdoms. In *Visions and revisions: Ethnohistoric perspectives on southern cultures,* ed. G. Sabo III and W. M. Schneider, 6–24. Southern Anthropological Society Proceedings, vol. 20. Athens: University of Georgia Press.

1987b *The uses of evidence in reconstructing the route of the Hernando de Soto expedition.* De Soto Working Paper 1. Tuscaloosa: Alabama De Soto Commission.

1989 Tracking the elusive de Soto. *Archaeology* 42(3):32–35.

1990 A synopsis of the Hernando De Soto expedition, 1539–1543. In *De Soto Trail: De Soto National Historic Trail Study,* by the National Park Service, Southeastern Regional Office, 75–126. Washington, D.C.: National Park Service.

HUDSON, C. M., AND D. MORSE

In press History of the case for a new route of the de Soto expedition. In *The expedition of Hernando de Soto in the West, 1541–1543,* ed. G. A. Young and M. P. Hoffman. Fayetteville: University of Arkansas Press.

HUDSON, C. M., C. B. DEPRATTER, AND M. T. SMITH

1989 Hernando de Soto's expedition through the southern United States. In *First encounters: Spanish explorations in the Caribbean and the United States, 1492–1570,* ed. J. T. Milanich and S. Milbreath, 77–98. Ripley F. Bullen Monographs in Anthropology and History, no. 9. Gainesville: University of Florida Press.

HUDSON, C. M., M. T. SMITH, AND C. B. DEPRATTER

1984 The Hernando De Soto expedition: From Apalachee to Chiaha. *Southeastern Archaeology* 3:65–77.

HUDSON, C. M., M. T. SMITH, D. HALLY, R. POLHEMUS, AND C. B. DEPRATTER

1985 Coosa: A chiefdom in the sixteenth-century southeastern United States. *American Antiquity* 50:723–737.

HUMPHREY, W.

1986 *The collected stories of William Humphrey.* New York: Dell Publishing Co., Laurel Books.

HUTCHINSON, D. L., AND C. S. LARSEN

1988 Determination of stress episode duration from linear enamel hypoplasias: A case study from St. Catherines Island, Georgia. *Human Biology* 60(1):93–110.

JACKSON, A. T.

n.d.a Exploration of a burial site on Clements Bros. farm in Cass County, Texas. Manuscript on file, Texas Archeological Research Laboratory, The University of Texas at Austin.

n.d.b Exploration of a burial site on Goode Hunt farm in Cass County, Texas. Manuscript on file, Texas Archeological Research Laboratory, The University of Texas at Austin.

1932 Exploration of a burial site on E. H. Moore's plantation in Bowie County, Texas. Manuscript on file, Texas Archeological Research Laboratory, The University of Texas at Austin.

1934 Types of East Texas pottery. *Bulletin of the Texas Archeological and Paleontological Society* 6:38–57.

1935 Ornaments of East Texas Indians. *Bulletin of the Texas Archeological and Paleontological Society* 7:11–28.

JACKSON, J.

1986 *Los Mesteños: Spanish ranching in Texas, 1721–1821.* College Station: Texas A&M University Press.

JACKSON, J., R. S. WEDDLE, AND W. DEVILLE

1990 *Mapping Texas and the Gulf Coast: The contributions of Saint-Denis, Olivan, and Le Maire.* College Station: Texas A&M University Press.

JACKSON, R. H.

1985 Demographic change in northwestern New Spain. *The Americas* 41(4): 462–479.

1986 Indian demographic patterns in colonial New Spain: The case of Baja California missions. *Proceedings of the Pacific Coast Council on Latin American Studies* 12:37–46.

JACOBS, W. R.

1971 The fatal confrontation: Early native-white relations on the frontiers of Australia, New Guinea, and America—A comparative study. *Pacific Historical Review* 60:293–309.

1974 The tip of the iceberg: Pre-Columbian Indian demography and some implications for revisionism. *William and Mary Quarterly* 31:123–132.

JELKS, E. B.

1961 *Excavations at Texarkana Reservoir, Sulphur River, northeastern Texas.* Bulletin 179, River Basin Survey Papers, no. 21. Washington, D.C.: Bureau of American Ethnology, Smithsonian Institution.

1965 The archeology of McGee Bend Reservoir, Texas. Ph.D. diss., The University of Texas—Austin.

1970 Documentary evidence of Indian occupation at the Stansbury site (41-39B1-1). *Bulletin of the Texas Archeological Society* 41:277–286.

JELKS, E. B. (EDITOR)

1967 The Gilbert site: A Norteno focus site in Northeastern Texas. *Bulletin of the Texas Archeological Society* 37:1–248.

JENSEN, H. P.

1968 Coral Snake Mound, X16SA48. *Bulletin of the Texas Archeological Society* 39:9–44.

JETER, M. D.

1986 Tunicans west of the Mississippi: A summary of early historic and archaeological evidence. In *The Protohistoric period in the Mid-South, 1500–1700: Proceedings of the 1983 Mid-South Archaeological Conference,* ed. D. H. Dye and R. C. Brister, 38–63. Archaeological Reports, no. 18. Jackson: Mississippi Department of Archives and History.

1990 *Edward Palmer's Arkansaw Mounds.* Fayetteville: University of Arkansas Press.

JETER, M. D., K. H. CANDE, AND J. J. MINTZ

1990 Goldsmith Oliver 2 (3PU306): A protohistoric archeological site near Little Rock, Arkansas. Final report submitted to Federal Aviation Administration, Southwest Region, Fort Worth, Texas. Sponsored research program. Fayetteville: Arkansas Archeological Survey.

JETER, M. D., D. B. KELLEY, AND G. P. KELLEY

1979 The Kelley-Grimes site: A Mississippi period burial mound, Southeast Arkansas, excavated in 1936. *The Arkansas Archeologist* 20:1–51.

JETER, M. D., J. C. ROSE, G. I. WILLIAMS, JR., AND A. M. HARMON

1989 *Archeology and Bioarcheology of the lower Mississippi Valley and Trans-Mississippi South in Arkansas and Louisiana.* Research Series, no. 37. Fayetteville: Arkansas Archeological Survey.

JOHANSSON, S. R.

1982 The demographic history of the native peoples of North America: A selective bibliography. *Yearbook of Physical Anthropology* 25:133–152.

JOHN, E. A. H.

1975 *Storms brewed in other men's worlds.* College Station: Texas A&M University Press.

1985 La situación y visión de los indios de la frontera norte de Nueva España (siglos XVI–XVIII). *América Indigena* 45(3):465–483.

1988 The riddle of mapmaker Juan Pedro Walker. In *Essays on the history of North American discovery and exploration,* ed. S. H. Palmer and D. Reinhartz, 102–132. College Station: Texas A&M University Press.

JOHNSON, L., JR.

1987 A plague of phases. *Bulletin of the Texas Archeological Society* 57: 1–26.

1991 Notes on Mazanet's stream names, with comments on their linguistic and ethnohistorical value. In *A Texas legacy: The Old San Antonio Road and the Camino Reales. A tricentennial history, 1691–1991,* ed. A. J. McGraw and J. W. Clark, 121–128. Austin: Texas State Department of Highways and Public Transportation, Highway Design Division.

JOHNSON, L., JR., AND E. B. JELKS

1958 The Tawakoni-Yscani village, 1760: A study in archeological site identification. *Texas Journal of Science* 10:405–422.

JONES, B. C.

1968 The Kinsloe focus: A study of seven historic Caddoan sites in Northeast Texas. Master's thesis, University of Oklahoma, Norman.

JONES, R. B.

1985 Archaeological investigations in the Ouachita River Valley, Bayou Bartholomew to Riverton, Louisiana. *Louisiana Archaeology* 10:103–169.

JORALEMON, D.

1982 New World depopulation and the case of disease. *Journal of Anthropological Research* 38:108–127.

JOUTEL, H.

1906 [1713]. *An historical journal of the late Monsieur de LaSalle's last voyage into North America to discover the River Mississippi,* ed. H. R. Stiles. Reprint. New York: Joseph McDonough.

KARKLINS, K.

1985 *Glass beads: The nineteenth century Levin catalogue and Venetian bead book and guide to description of glass beads.* Studies in Archaeology, Architecture and History, National Historic Parks and Sites Branch. Ottowa: Parks Canada.

KAY, J.

1984 The fur trade and native American population growth. *Ethnohistory* 31: 265–287.

KAY, M.

1984 Late Caddo subtractive technology in the Red River basin. In *Cedar Grove: An interdisciplinary investigation of a late Caddo farmstead in the Red River Valley,* ed. N. L. Trubowitz, 174–206. Research Series, no. 23. Fayetteville: Arkansas Archeological Survey.

KELLEY, D. B.

1978 Summary of regional archeological knowledge. In New Hope: An archeological assessment of a proposed surface mining operation in the Gulf Coastal Plain of Southwest Arkansas, assembled by T. C. Klinger. Manuscript on file. Fayetteville: Arkansas Archeological Survey.

KELLEY, J. C.

1955 Juan Sabeata and diffusion in aboriginal Texas. *American Anthropologist* 57:981–995.

KENMOTSU, N.

1987a The Mayhew site, 41NA21, a possible Hasinai Caddo farmstead in Bayou Loco, Nacogdoches County, Texas. Manuscript on file, Texas Archeological Research Laboratory, Austin.

1987b A study of Texas gunflints. Paper presented at the Annual Meeting of the Texas Archeological Society, 30 October–1 November, Waco, Tex.

1990 Gunflints: A study. *Historical Archaeology* 24(2):92–124.

KENMOTSU, N., J. E. BRUSETH, AND J. E. CORBIN

1992 Moscoso and the expedition in Texas. In *The expedition of Hernando De Soto in the West, 1541–1543,* ed. G. A. Young and M. P. Hoffman. Fayetteville: University of Arkansas Press.

KIDDER, T. R.

1986 Protohistoric and Early Historic culture dynamics in Southeast Arkansas and Northeast Louisiana, A.D. 1500–1700. Paper presented at the Southeastern Archaeological Conference, 5–8 November, Nashville.

1987 Prehistory and early history of the lower Ouachita River basin. *Southeastern Archaeological Conference Bulletin* 30:41.

1988 Protohistoric and Early Historic culture dynamics in Southeast Arkansas and Northeast Louisiana, A.D. 1500–1700. Ph.D. diss., Harvard University, Cambridge.

1990a Ceramic chronology and culture history of the southern Ouachita River basin: Coles Creek to the Early Historic period. *Midcontinental Journal of Archaeology* 15:51–99.

1990b The Ouachita Indians of Louisiana: An ethnohistorical and archaeological investigation. *Louisiana Archaeology* 12:179–201.

KIELMAN, C. V.

1967 *The University of Texas archives: A guide to the historical manuscript collections of the University of Texas.* Austin: University of Texas Press.

KINNAIRD, L.

1932 American penetration into Spanish Louisiana. In *New Spain and the Anglo-American West: Historical contributions submitted to Herbert Eugene Bolton,* 1:211–237. Lancaster: Lancaster Press.

1949 *Spain in the Mississippi Valley, 1765–1794.* 2 vols. Annual Report for the Year 1945. Washington, D.C.: American Historical Association.

KINNAIRD, L., AND L. B. KINNAIRD

1980 Choctaws west of the Mississippi, 1766–1800. *Southwestern Historical Quarterly* 83(4):349–370.

KLEINSCHMIDT, U. K.

1982 Review and analysis of the A. C. Saunders site, 41AN19, Anderson County, Texas. M.A. thesis, The University of Texas at Austin.

1984 The A. C. Saunders site, Anderson County, Texas. Paper presented at the Twenty-sixth Annual Caddo Conference, 23–24 March, Stephen F. Austin State University, Nacogdoches, Tex.

KNIFFEN, F. B., H. F. GREGORY, AND G. A. STOKES

1987 *The historic Indian tribes of Louisiana: From 1542 to the present.* Baton Rouge: Louisiana State University Press.

KNIGHT, V. J.

1986 The institutional organization of Mississippian religion. *American Antiquity* 51:675–687.

KRECH, S.

1983 The influence of disease and the fur trade on Arctic drainage lowlands Dene, 1800–1850. *Journal of Anthropological Research* 39:123–146.

KRESS, M. K., AND M. A. HATCHER

1932 Diary of a visit of inspection of the Texas missions made by Fray Gaspar José de Solis in the Year 1767–1768. *Southwestern Historical Quarterly* 35:28–76.

KRIEGER, A. D.

1944 Archaeological horizons in the Caddo Area. In *El Norte de México y el Sur de los Estados Unidos,* 154–156. Mexico, D.F.: Sociedad Mexicana de Antropología.

1946 *Culture complexes and chronology in northern Texas.* Publication 4640. Austin: University of Texas.

1947 The first symposium on the Caddoan archaeological area. *American Antiquity* 12:198–207.

1953 New World culture history: Anglo-America. In *Anthropology Today,* ed. A. L. Kroeber, 238–264. Chicago: University of Chicago Press.

KROEBER, A. L.

1939 *Cultural and natural areas of native North America.* University of California Publications in American Archaeology and Ethnology, no. 38. Berkeley: University of California.

LARSEN, C. S.

1987a Bioarchaeological interpretation and early contact populations on St. Catherines Island, Georgia. Paper presented at the Annual Meeting of the American Association of Physical Anthropologists, New York.

1987b Stress and adaptation at Santa Catalina de Guale: Analysis of human remains. Paper presented at the Society for Historical Archaeology symposium, Missions of Spanish Florida: New perspectives from Guale, Timucua, and Apalachee, 8–9 January, Savannah, Ga.

LEHMER, D. J.

1977 The other side of the fur trade. In *Selected writings of Donald J. Lehmer,* ed. W. R. Wood, 91–104. Reprints in Anthropology, vol. 8. Lincoln: J&L Reprints.

LEMLEY, H. J.

1936 Discoveries indicating a pre-Caddo culture on Red River in Arkansas. *Bulletin of the Texas Archeological and Paleontological Society* 8: 25–55.

LEMONNIER, P.

1986 The study of material culture today: Toward an anthropology of technical systems. *Journal of Anthropological Archaeology* 5:147–186.

LESSER, A., AND G. WELTFISH

1932 *Composition of the Caddoan linguistic stock.* Smithsonian Miscellaneous Collections, vol. 87(6). Washington, D.C.

LEUTENEGGER, FR. B. (TRANSLATOR)

1973 Excerpts from the *Libros de los decretos* of the Missionary College of Zacatecas, 1707–1828. In *The Zacatecan missionaries in Texas, 1716–1834,* 1–104. Texas Historical Survey Committee, Office of the State Archeologist, Report no. 23. Austin.

1979 *The Texas missions of the College of Zacatecas in 1749–1750.* Documentary Series, no. 5. San Antonio: Old Spanish Missions Historical Research Library at San Jose Mission.

LEWIS, G. A.

1987 The Clements Brothers' farm site 41CS25. Master's thesis, Department of Anthropology, The University of Texas at Austin.

LIMP, W. F., E. ZAHN, AND J. P. HARCOURT (EDITORS)

1989 *The archeological literature of the South-Central United States.* 4 vols. Research Series, no. 36. Fayetteville: Arkansas Archeological Survey.

LONG, A., AND B. RIPPETEAU

1974 Testing contemporaneity and averaging radiocarbon dates. *American Antiquity* 39:205–215.

LOTTINVILLE, S. (EDITOR)
1980 *A journal of travels into the Arkansas territory during the year 1819*, by Thomas Nuttall. Norman: University of Oklahoma Press.

LOVELAND, C. J.
1987 Human skeletal remains from the Clark and Holdeman sites, Red River County, Texas. *Bulletin of the Texas Archeological Society* 57:165–181.

LYON, E. A.
1982 New Deal archaeology in the southeast: WPA, TVA, NPS, 1934–1942. Ph.D. diss., Louisiana State University, Baton Rouge.

MCCROCKLIN, C.
1990a The Lost Prairie Cherokee Indian sites of Miller County, Arkansas. *Field Notes* 226:3–5.
1990b The Red River Coushatta Indian villages of Northwest Louisiana 1790–1835. *Louisiana Archaeology* 12:129–178.

MCEWAN, B. G., AND J. M. MITCHEM
1984 Indian and European acculturation in the eastern United States as a result of trade. *North American Archaeologist* 5:271–285.

MCKERN, W. C.
1939 The Midwestern Taxonomic Method as an aid to archaeological study. *American Antiquity* 4:301–313.

MCLEAN, M. D. (COMPILER AND EDITOR)
1988 *Papers concerning Robertson's colony in Texas.* Vol. 14, *March 18 through July 22, 1836: The Battle of San Jacinto and the fall of Fort Parker.* Arlington: University of Texas at Arlington Press.
1989 *Papers concerning Robertson's colony in Texas.* Vol. 15, *July 23, 1836 through August 9, 1837: The gentleman from Milam.* Arlington: University of Texas at Arlington Press.

MCVAUGH, R.
1956 *Edward Palmer: Plant explorer of the American West.* Norman: University of Oklahoma Press.

MCWILLIAMS, R. G. (EDITOR AND TRANSLATOR)
1981 *Iberville's Gulf journals.* University: University of Alabama Press.

MCW. QUICK, P.
1986 *Proceedings: Conference on reburial issues.* Chicago: Society for American Archaeology and Society of Professional Archeologists.

MAGNAGHI, R. M.
1978 Sulphur Fork factory, 1817–1822. *Arkansas Historical Quarterly* 37:168–183.

MAINFORT, R. C.
1985 Wealth, space, and status in a historic Indian cemetery. *American Antiquity* 50:555–579.

MARGRY, P.
1877–1886 *Découvertes et établissements des Français dans l'ouest et dans le sud de l'Amérique Septentrionale (1614–1754).* 6 vols. Paris.

MARTIN, C.

1974 The European impact on the culture of a northeastern Algonquian tribe: An ecological interpretation. *William and Mary Quarterly* 31:3–26.

1978 *Keepers of the game: Indian-animal relationships and the fur trade.* Berkeley: University of California Press.

MASON, C. I.

1976 Historic identification and Lake Winnebago focus Oneota. In *Cultural change and continuity,* ed. C. E. Cleland. New York: Academic Press.

MELTZER, D. J.

1979 Paradigms and the nature of change in American archaeology. *American Antiquity* 44:644–657.

MELTZER, D. J., D. D. FOWLER, AND J. A. SABLOFF (EDITORS)

1986 *American archaeology past and future: A celebration of the Society for American Archaeology 1935–1985.* Washington, D.C.: Smithsonian Institution Press.

MERBS, C. F.

1989 Effects of European contact on patterns of health and disease in southwestern Indians. In *Columbian Consequences,* vol. 1, ed. D. H. Thomas. Washington, D.C.: Smithsonian Institution Press.

MERRELL, J. H.

1984 The Indians' New World: The Catawba experience. *William and Mary Quarterly* 41:537–565.

MILANICH, J. T.

1987a Corn and Calusa: De Soto and demography. In *Coasts, plains and deserts: Essays in honor of Reynold J. Ruppe,* ed. S. W. Gaines, 173–184. Anthropological Research Papers, no. 38. Tempe: Arizona State University.

1987b Hernando de Soto and the expedition in *La Florida.* Miscellaneous Project Report no. 32. Gainesville: Florida State Museum.

1988 The impact of exploration: Examining depopulation and settlement shifts among the sixteenth-century Florida aborigines. Paper presented at the 1988 Society for Historical Archaeology Conference, 15–16 January, Reno, Nev.

MILANICH, J. T., AND S. MILBRATH

1989a Another world. In *First encounters: Spanish explorations in the Caribbean and the United States, 1492–1570,* ed. J. T. Milanich and S. Milbrath, 1–26. Ripley F. Bullen Monographs in Anthropology and History, no. 9. Gainesville: University of Florida Press.

MILANICH, J. T., AND S. MILBRATH (EDITORS)

1989b *First encounters: Spanish explorations in the Caribbean and the United States, 1492–1570.* Ripley F. Bullen Monographs in Anthropology and History, no. 9. Gainesville: University of Florida Press.

MILLER, C. L., AND G. R. HAMELL

1986 A new perspective on Indian-White contact: Cultural symbols and colonial trade. *Journal of American History* 73:311–328.

MILLER, E.

1988 Health and disease among contact populations in Texas. Paper presented at the Fifty-Ninth Annual Texas Archeological Society Meeting, 28–30 October, Houston.

MILLS, L.

1968 Mississippian head vases of Arkansas and Missouri. *The Missouri Archaeologist* 30:1–83.

MILNER, G. R.

1980 Epidemic disease in the post contact Southeast: A reappraisal. *Midcontinental Journal of Archaeology* 5:39–56.

MIROIR, M. P., R. K. HARRIS, J. C. BLAINE, AND J. MCVAY

1973 Benard de la Harpe and the Nassonite post. *Bulletin of the Texas Archeological Society* 44:113–168.

MITCHEM, J. M.

1989 Artifacts of exploration: Archaeological evidence from Florida. In *First encounters: Spanish explorations in the Caribbean and the United States, 1492–1570,* ed. J. T. Milanich and S. Milbrath, 99–109. Ripley F. Bullen Monographs in Anthropology and History, no. 9. Gainesville: University of Florida Press.

MITCHEM, J. M., AND D. L. HUTCHINSON

1986 Interim report on excavations at the Tatham Mound, Citrus County, Florida: Season II. Miscellaneous Project Report, Series no. 28. Department of Anthropology, Florida State Museum, Gainesville.

1987 Interim report on archaeological research at the Tatham Mound, Citrus County, Florida: Season III. Miscellaneous Project Report, Series no. 30. Department of Anthropology, Florida State Museum, Gainesville.

MITCHEM, J. M., AND B. G. MCEWAN

1988 New data on early bells from Florida. *Southeastern Archaeology* 7: 39–49.

MITCHEM, J. M., M. T. SMITH, A. C. GOODYEAR, AND R. R. ALLEN

1985 Early Spanish contact on the Florida Gulf Coast: The Weeki Wachee and Ruth Smith Mounds. In *Indians, colonists, and slaves: Essays in memory of Charles H. Fairbanks,* ed. K. W. Johnson, J. M. Leader, and R. C. Wilson, 179–219. Special Publication no. 4. Gainesville: Florida Journal of Anthropology.

MOONEY, J.

1896 *The Ghost-Dance religion, and the Sioux outbreak of 1890.* Fourteenth Annual Report of the Bureau of Ethnology, 1892–1893, pt. 2. Washington, D.C.: Bureau of Ethnology, Smithsonian Institution.

1928 *The aboriginal population of America north of Mexico,* ed. J. R. Swanton. Smithsonian Miscellaneous Collections, vol. 80(7). Washington, D.C.

MOORE, C. B.

1908 Certain mounds of Arkansas and of Mississippi. *Academy of Natural Sciences of Philadelphia Journal* 13 (pts. 1–4).

1909 Antiquities of the Ouachita Valley. *Academy of Natural Sciences of Philadelphia Journal* 14 (pt. 1).

1912 Some aboriginal sites on Red River. *Academy of Natural Sciences of Philadelphia Journal* 14 (pt. 4).

1913 Some aboriginal sites in Louisiana and in Arkansas. *Academy of Natural Sciences of Philadelphia Journal* 16 (pt. 1).

MOREY, N. C., AND R. V. MOREY

1973 Foragers and farmers: Differential consequences of Spanish contact. *Ethnohistory* 20:229–246.

MORFI, FR. J. A. DE

1935 *History of Texas, 1663–1779*. Quivira Society Publications, no. 6, ed. C. E. Castañeda. Santa Fe: Quivira Society.

MORSE, D. F., AND P. A. MORSE

1983 *Archaeology of the Central Mississippi Valley*. New York: Academic Press.

MULLER, J. D.

1978 The Southeast. In *Ancient native Americans,* ed. J. D. Jennings, 281–325. San Francisco: W. H. Freeman.

1986 *Archaeology of the lower Ohio River Valley*. Orlando: Academic Press.

MURPHY, R.

1937 The journey of Pedro de Rivera, 1724–1728. *Southwestern Historical Quarterly* 41:125–141.

MURPHY, R. F., AND J. H. STEWARD

1956 Trappers and tappers: Parallel processes in acculturation. *Economic Development and Culture Change* 4:335–355.

NASATIR, A. P., AND N. M. LOOMIS

1967 *Pedro Vial and the roads to Santa Fe*. Norman: University of Oklahoma Press.

NASH, G. B.

1972 The image of the Indian in the southern colonial mind. *William and Mary Quarterly* 29:197–230.

NATIONAL ARCHIVES

1809–1821 Natchitoches–Sulphur Fork Agency Ledgers. Record Group T1029. Washington, D.C.

1825–1848 Office of Indian Affairs (War Department), Reports and Special Files. Washington, D.C.

1849–1939 Reports of the Commissioner of Indian Affairs (Department of the Interior). Washington, D.C.

NEIGHBOURS, K. F.

1957 Chapters from the history of the Texas Indian reservation. *West Texas Historical Association Year Book* 33:3–16.

1973 *Indian exodus: Texas Indian affairs, 1835–1859*. Quannah: Nortex Offset Publications.

1975 *Robert Simpson Neighbors and the Texas frontier, 1836–1859*. Waco: Texian Press.

NEITZEL, R. S.

1965 *Archeology of the Fatherland site: The grand village of the Natchez.* Anthropological Papers 51(1). New York: American Museum of Natural History.

1983 *The grand village of the Natchez revisited.* Archaeological Report no. 12. Jackson: Mississippi Department of Archives and History.

NEUMAN, R. W.

1984 *An introduction to Louisiana archaeology.* Baton Rouge: Louisiana State University Press.

NEWELL, H. P., AND A. D. KRIEGER

1949 *The George C. Davis site, Cherokee County, Texas.* Society for American Archaeology, Memoirs, no. 5.

NEWKUMET, V. B., AND H. L. MEREDITH

1988 *Hasinai: A traditional history of the Caddo confederacy.* College Station: Texas A&M University Press.

NEWMAN, M. T.

1976 Aboriginal New World epidemiology and medical care, and the impact of the Old World disease imports. *American Journal of Physical Anthropology* 45:667–672.

ORR, K. G.

1946 The archaeological situation at Spiro, Oklahoma: A preliminary report. *American Antiquity* 11:228–256.

1952 Survey of Caddoan Area archaeology. In *Archaeology of the eastern United States,* ed. J. B. Griffin. Chicago: University of Chicago Press.

ORSER, C. E., JR.

1984 Trade good flow in Arikara villages: Expanding Ray's "Middleman Hypothesis." *Plains Anthropologist* 29:1–12.

ORSER, C. E., AND L. J. ZIMMERMAN

1984 A computer simulation of Euro-American trade good flow to the Arikara. *Plains Anthropologist* 29:199–210.

OSBORN, A. J.

1983 Ecological aspects of equestrian adaptations in aboriginal North America. *American Anthropologist* 85:563–591.

O'SHEA, J. M.

1981 Social configurations and the archaeological study of mortuary practices: A case study. In *The archaeology of death,* ed. R. Chapman, I. Kinnes, and K. Randsborg, 39–52. Cambridge: Cambridge University Press.

1984 *Mortuary variability: An archaeological investigation.* New York: Academic Press.

PADILLA, J. A.

1919 [1820]. Texas in 1820: Report on the barbarous Indians of the Province of Texas. Translated by M. A. Hatcher. *Southwestern Historical Quarterly* 23:47–68.

PALKOVICH, A. M.

1981 Demography and disease patterns in a Protohistoric Plains group: A study of the Mobridge Site (39WW1). *Plains Anthropologist* 17:71–84.

PARKER, P.

1990 Keepers of the treasures: Protecting historic properties and cultural traditions on Indian Lands. A report on tribal preservation funding needs submitted to Congress. U.S. Department of the Interior, National Park Service, Interagency Resources Division. Washington, D.C.

PARSONS, E. C.

1941 Notes on the Caddo. *Memoirs of the American Anthropological Association* 57:1–76.

PEABODY, C., AND W. K. MOOREHEAD

1904 *The exploration of Jacobs Cavern, McDonald County, Missouri.* Department of Archaeology, Bulletin 1. Andover, Mass.: Phillips Academy.

PEAKE, O. B.

1954 *A history of the United States Indian factory system, 1795–1822.* Denver: Sage Books.

PEARCE, J. E.

1919 Indian mounds and other relics of Indian life in Texas. *American Anthropologist* 21:223–234.

1932a The archaeology of East Texas. *American Anthropologist* 34:670–687.

1932b The present status of Texas archeology. *Bulletin of the Texas Archeological and Paleontological Society* 4:44–54.

1932c The significance of the East Texas archaeological field. In *Conference on southern pre-history,* 53–58. Washington, D.C.: National Research Council.

PERINO, G.

1978 Four McCurtain focus Caddoan vessels. *Central States Archaeological Journal* 25:74–76.

1979 The identification of three Early Historic Caddoan vessels. *Central States Archaeological Journal* 26:24–26.

1981 *Archaeological investigations at the Roden site, McCurtain County, Oklahoma.* Idabel: Museum of the Red River.

1983 *Archaeological research at the Bob Williams site, Red River County, Texas.* Idabel: Museum of the Red River.

1985 *Selected preforms, points and knives of the North American Indians,* vol. 1. Idabel: Museum of the Red River.

PERTTULA, T. K.

1980 Comments on G. Perino's "The identification of three Early Historic Caddoan vessels." *Central States Archaeological Journal* 27:23–24.

1982 Review of "Archaeological investigations at the Roden site, McCurtain County, Oklahoma" by G. Perino. *Plains Anthropologist* 27:182–184.

1984 The Loftin site and phase in western Ozark prehistory. In *The Loftin Component,* assembled by W. R. Wood, 40–62. *The Missouri Archaeologist,* vol. 44.

1987 Excavations at the Quince site (34AT134), Atoka County, Oklahoma.

Vol. 5, pt. 2, of the McGee Creek Archaeological Project reports. Institute of Applied Sciences, North Texas State University, Denton.

1989a Contact and interaction between Caddoan and European peoples: The Historic archaeological and ethnohistorical records. Ph.D. diss., University of Washington, Seattle.

1989b The looting and vandalism of archaeological sites in East Texas: A status report. Final report on a project conducted for the Archeological Planning and Review and Office of the State Archeologist, Texas Historical Commission, Austin.

1989c A study of mound sites in the Sabine River basin, Northeast Texas and Northwest Louisiana. Final report submitted to the Texas Historical Commission by the University of North Texas, Institute of Applied Sciences, Denton.

1990 The development of agricultural subsistence, regional and diachronic variability in Caddoan subsistence, and implications for the Caddoan archaeological record. Part I in Historic context: The evolution of agricultural societies in Northeast Texas before A.D. 1600. Manuscript on file, Department of Archeological Planning and Review, Texas Historical Commission, Austin.

1991 Effect of European contact on native and immigrant Indians in Northeast Texas. Manuscript on file, Department of Archeological Planning and Review, Texas Historical Commission, Austin.

In press Caddoan archeology and issues of reburial and repatriation. In *Archaeological ethics and treatment of the dead,* ed. L. Zimmerman. Southhampton, England: World Archaeological Congress.

PERTTULA, T. K., C. J. CRANE, AND J. E. BRUSETH

1983 A consideration of Caddoan subsistence. *Southeastern Archaeology* 1: 89–102.

PERTTULA, T. K., AND K. K. GILMORE

1988 *Archaeological survey along Mill Race Creek and tributaries, Wood County, Texas: 1987–1988.* Contributions in Archaeology, no. 6. Denton: Institute of Applied Sciences, University of North Texas.

PERTTULA, T. K., K. GILMORE, P. MCGUFF, AND B. D. SKILES

1988 Archaeological survey and testing along Mill Race Creek and tributaries, Wood County, Texas: In search of the French trading post Le Dout. *Texas Archeology* 32(1):7–8.

PERTTULA, T. K., AND P. MCGUFF

1985 Woodland and Caddoan settlement in the McGee Creek drainage, Southeast Oklahoma. *Plains Anthropologist* 30:219–235.

PERTTULA, T. K., AND A. F. RAMENOFSKY

1982 An archaeological model of Caddoan culture change: The Historic period. *Southeastern Archaeological Conference Bulletin* 24:13–15.

PERTTULA, T. K., AND B. D. SKILES

1989 Another look at an eighteenth-century archaeological site in Wood County, Texas. *Southwestern Historical Quarterly* 92(3):417–435.

PERTTULA, T. K., B. D. SKILES, M. B. COLLINS, M. C. TRACHTE, AND F. VALDEZ, JR.

1986 *"This everlasting sand bed": Cultural resources investigations at the Texas Big Sandy Project, Wood and Upshur Counties, Texas.* Reports of Investigations, no. 52. Austin: Prewitt and Associates, Inc.

PERTTULA, T. K., B. D. SKILES, AND B. C. YATES

1992 The Goldsmith site (41WD208): Investigations of the Titus phase in the upper Sabine River basin, Northeast Texas. *Bulletin of the Texas Archeological Society* 61.

PERTTULA, T. K., R. R. TURBEVILLE, AND B. D. SKILES

1987 New thermoluminescence and radiocarbon dates from the upper Sabine River basin, East Texas. *Texas Archeology* 31(2):7–9.

PETERSON, D. A.

1989 A history of excavations and interpretations of artifacts from the Spiro Mounds site. In *The southeastern ceremonial complex: Artifacts and analysis,* ed. P. Galloway, 114–121. Lincoln: University of Nebraska Press.

PETERSON, J.

1978 Hunter-gatherer/farmer exchange. *American Anthropologist* 80:335–351.

PHILLIPS, P.

1970 *Archaeological survey in the lower Yazoo basin, Mississippi, 1949–1955.* Papers, vol. 60. Cambridge: Peabody Museum of American Archaeology and Ethnology, Harvard University.

PHILLIPS, P., AND J. A. BROWN

1984 *Pre-Columbian shell engravings from the Craig Mound at Spiro.* Vols. 4–6. Cambridge: Peabody Museum Press.

PIPER, H. M., K. W. HARDIN, AND J. G. PIPER

1983 Cultural responses to stress: Patterns observed in American Indian burials of the Second Seminole War. *Southeastern Archaeology* 1:122–137.

PLOG, S.

1980 *Stylistic variation in Prehistoric ceramics.* Cambridge: Cambridge University Press.

POYO, G. E., AND G. M. HINOJOSA

1988 Spanish Texas and Borderlands historiography in transition: Implications for United States history. *Journal of American History* 75(2):393–416.

PREWITT, E. R.

1981 Cultural chronology in Central Texas. *Bulletin of the Texas Archeological Society* 52:65–89.

PREWITT, T. J.

1969 Stylistic variation in a Caddoan ceramic type. *Bulletin of the Oklahoma Anthropological Society* 17:59–74.

1974 Regional interaction networks and the Caddoan Area. *Papers in Anthropology* 15(2):73–101.

PRIKRYL, D. J.

1987 A synthesis of the prehistory of the Lower Elm Fork of the Trinity River. Master's thesis, The University of Texas at Austin.

1990 *Lower Elm Fork prehistory: A redefinition of cultural concepts and chronologies along the Trinity River, North Central Texas.* Office of the State Archeologist, Report no. 37. Austin: Texas Historical Commission.

PRUCHA, F. P.

1962 *American Indian policy in the formative years: The Indian Trade and Intercourse acts, 1790–1834.* Lincoln: University of Nebraska Press.

1977 *A bibliographic guide to the history of Indian-white relations in the United States.* Chicago: University of Chicago Press.

1982 *Indian-white relations in the United States: A bibliography of works published 1975–1980.* Lincoln: University of Nebraska Press.

1984 *The great father: The United States government and the American Indians.* 2 vols. Lincoln: University of Nebraska Press.

PURSER, J.

1964 The administration of Indian affairs in Louisiana, 1803–1820. *Louisiana History* 5:401–419.

QUINN, D. B. (EDITOR)

1979 *New American world: A documentary history of North America to 1612.* Vol. 2, *Major Spanish searches in eastern North America: Franco-Spanish clash in Florida. The beginnings of Spanish Florida,* and vol. 5, *The extension of settlement in Florida, Virginia, and the Spanish Southwest.* New York: Arno Press.

RAMENOFSKY, A. F.

1982 The archaeology of population collapse: Native American response to the introduction of infectious disease. Ph.D. diss., University of Washington, Seattle.

1984 Population estimates and time: Methodological issues in the archaeology of European contact. Paper presented at the Forty-ninth Annual Meeting of the Society for American Archaeology, 12–14 April, Portland.

1985a The introduction of European disease and the aboriginal population collapse. *Mississippi Archaeologist* 20:2–18.

1985b Review of "Their Number Become Thinned: Native American population dynamics in eastern North America" by H. F. Dobyns. *American Antiquity* 50:198–199.

1986 A consideration of stability or change in the sixteenth-century southeast. Paper presented at the Southeastern Archaeological Conference, 5–8 November, Nashville.

1987a Diffusion of disease at European contact. Paper presented at the Fifty-second Annual Meeting of the Society for American Archaeology, 6–10 May, Toronto.

1987b *Vectors of death: The archaeology of European contact.* Albuquerque: University of New Mexico Press.

1990 Loss of innocence: Explanations of differential persistence in the sixteenth-century southeast. In *Columbian consequences*. Vol. 2, *Archaeological and historical perspectives on the Spanish Borderlands East,* ed. D. H. Thomas, 27–43. Washington, D.C.: Smithsonian Institution Press.

RAY, A. J.

1974 *Indians on the fur trade: Their role as hunters, trappers and middlemen in the lands southwest of Hudson Bay 1660–1870*. Toronto: University of Toronto Press.

1978 History and archaeology of the fur trade. *American Antiquity* 43:26–34.

RECORDS OF THE SUPERIOR COUNCIL (CABILDO), 1763 – 1803. LOUISIANA HISTORICAL CENTER, NEW ORLEANS.

REFF, D. T.

1985 The demographic and cultural consequences of Old World diseases in the Greater Southwest, 1520–1660. Ph.D. diss., The University of Oklahoma, Norman.

1987a Contact shock and the routes of contagion during the early Historic period in the Greater Southwest. Paper presented at the Annual Meeting of the Society for American Archaeology, 6–10 May, Toronto.

1987b The introduction of smallpox in the Greater Southwest. *American Anthropologist* 89:704–708.

REITZ, E. J., AND C. M. SCARRY

1985 *Reconstructing historic subsistence with an example from sixteenth-century Spanish Florida*. Special Publication, no. 3. Albuquerque: Society for Historical Archaeology.

RENFREW, C., AND P. BAHN

1991 *Archaeology: Theories, methods, and practice*. New York: Thames and Hudson.

RICKEY, H. W. (TRANSLATOR)

1937 Description of the Ouachita in 1786 by Jean Filhoil. *Louisiana Historical Quarterly* 20:476–485.

RILEY, C. L.

1986 An overview of the Greater Southwest in the Protohistoric period. In *Ripples in the Chichimec Sea: New considerations of Southwestern-Mesoamerican interaction,* ed. F. J. Mathien and R. H. McGuire, 45–54. Carbondale: Southern Illinois University Press.

ROBERTSON, J. A. (TRANSLATOR AND EDITOR)

1933 *True relation of the hardships suffered by Governor Fernando de Soto and certain Portuguese gentlemen during the discovery of the province of Florida now newly set forth by a gentleman of Elvas*. Publications of the Florida Historical Society, no. 11. De Land, Fla.: Florida Historical Society.

ROBINSON, P. A., M. A. KELLEY, AND P. E. RUBERTONE

1985 Preliminary biocultural interpretations from a seventeenth-century Narragansett Indian cemetery in Rhode Island. In *Cultures in contact: The impact of European contacts on native American cultural institutions*

A.D. *1000–1800,* ed. W.W. Fitzhugh, 107–130. Washington, D.C.: Smithsonian Institution Press.

ROGERS, J. D.

1982 Specialized buildings in northern Caddo prehistory. In *Southern Plains Archaeology,* ed. S.C. Vehik, 105–117. Papers in Anthropology 23(1). Norman: Department of Anthropology, University of Oklahoma.

1983 Social ranking and change in the Harlan and Spiro phases of eastern Oklahoma. In *Southeastern natives and their pasts,* ed. D.G. Wyckoff and J.L. Hofman, 17–128. Studies in Oklahoma's Past, no. 11. Norman: Oklahoma Archeological Survey.

1987 Patterns of change on the western margins of the Southeast, A.D. 600–900. Manuscript on file, Department of Anthropology, University of California, Los Angeles.

1991 A perspective on Arkansas basin and Ozark highland prehistory. *Caddoan Archeology* 2(1):9–16.

In press The Caddos. Manuscript to appear in *Handbook of the North American Indians* (Southeast volume). Washington, D.C.: Smithsonian Institution Press.

ROGERS, J. D., D. G. WYCKOFF, AND D. A. PETERSON (EDITORS)

1989 *Contributions to Spiro archeology: Mound excavations and regional perspectives.* Studies in Oklahoma's Past, no. 16. Norman: Oklahoma Archeological Survey.

ROHRBAUGH, C. L.

1973 *Hugo Reservoir III: A report on the early formative cultural manifestations in Hugo Reservoir, and in the Caddoan Area.* Archaeological Site Report no. 24. Norman: Oklahoma River Basin Survey.

1982 An hypothesis for the origin of the Kichai. In *Pathways to Plains prehistory,* ed. D.G. Wyckoff and J.L. Hofman, 51–63. Memoir No. 3. Norman: Oklahoma Anthropological Society.

1984 Arkansas Valley Caddoan: Fort Coffee focus and Neosho focus. In *Prehistory of Oklahoma,* ed. R.E. Bell, 265–285. New York: Academic Press.

ROLINGSON, M. A., AND F. F. SCHAMBACH

1981 *The Shallow Lake site (3UN9/52) and its place in regional prehistory.* Research Series, no. 12. Fayetteville: Arkansas Archeological Survey.

ROSE, J. C.

1984 Bioarchaeology of the Cedar Grove site. In *Cedar Grove: An interdisciplinary investigation of a late Caddo farmstead in the Red River Valley,* ed. N.L. Trubowitz, 227–256. Research Series, no. 23. Fayetteville: Arkansas Archeological Survey.

ROSE, J. C., J. P. HARCOURT, AND B. A. BURNETT

1988 Bioarcheology of the OAO study area. In *Human adaptation in the Ozark and Ouachita mountains,* by G. Sabo III, A. M. Early, J. C. Rose, B. A. Burnett, J. P. Harcourt, and L. Vogele, Jr., 171–192. Final report submitted by the Arkansas Archeological Survey to the U.S. Army Corps of Engineers, Southwestern Division. Study Unit 1 of the Southwestern Division Archeological Overview. Research Series, no. 31, Fayetteville.

ROWLAND, D., A. G. SANDERS, AND P. K. GALLOWAY (EDITORS)

1984 *Mississippi provincial archives: French dominion 1729–1763.* Vols. 4 and 5. Baton Rouge: Louisiana State University Press.

SABO, G., III

1982 The Huntsville site (3MA22): A Caddoan civic-ceremonial center in the Arkansas Ozarks. Paper presented at the Forty-seventh Annual Meeting of the Society for American Archaeology, Minneapolis.

1987 Reordering their world: A Caddoan ethnohistory. In *Visions and revisions: Ethnohistoric perspectives on southern cultures,* ed. G. Sabo III and W. M. Schneider, 25–47. Athens: University of Georgia Press.

1988 In service of kings and gods: Medal chiefs and eighteenth-century Caddoan interaction with Europeans. Paper presented at the Forty-first Plains Conference, 2–5 November, Wichita State University, Wichita.

1989 Acculturation revisited: Interpreting Spanish-Caddoan contact. Paper presented at the Annual Meeting of the American Society for Ethnohistory, 2–5 November, D'Arcy McNickle Center for the History of the American Indian, The Newberry Library, Chicago.

In press Caddos and Europeans: Encounters and images. Historical Reflection.

SABO, G., III (EDITOR)

1986 *Contributions to Ozark prehistory.* Research Series, no. 26. Fayetteville: Arkansas Archeological Survey.

SABO, G., III, A. M. EARLY, J. C. ROSE, B. A. BURNETT, L. VOGELE, AND J. P. HARCOURT

1988 *Human adaptation in the Ozark-Ouachita mountains.* Final report submitted by the Arkansas Archeological Survey to the U.S. Army Corps of Engineers, Southwestern Division. Study Unit 1 of the Southwestern Division Archeological Overview. Research Series, no. 31. Fayetteville: Arkansas Archeological Survey.

SABO, G., III, D. B. WADDELL, AND J. H. HOUSE

1982 *A cultural resource overview of the Ozark–St. Francis national forests.* Atlanta: U.S. Department of Agriculture, U.S. Forest Service, Southern Region.

SAYLES, E. B.

1935 *An archaeological survey of Texas.* Medallion Papers, no. 17. Globe, Ariz.: Lancaster Press.

SCHAMBACH, F. F.

1970 Pre-Caddoan cultures in the Trans-Mississippi South: A beginning sequence. Ph.D. diss., Harvard University, Cambridge.

1982 An outline of Fourche Maline culture in Southwest Arkansas. In *Arkansas archeology in review,* ed. N. L. Trubowitz and M. D. Jeter, 132–197. Research Series, no. 15. Fayetteville: Arkansas Archeological Survey.

1983 The archeology of the Great Bend region in Arkansas. In *Contributions to the archeology of the Great Bend region,* ed. F. F. Schambach and

F. Rackerby, 1–11. Research Series, no. 22. Fayetteville: Arkansas Archeological Survey.

1988 The archaeology of Oklahoma. *Quarterly Review of Archaeology* 9:5–9.

1989 The end of the trail: The route of Hernando De Soto's army through Southwest Arkansas and East Texas. *Arkansas Archeologist Bulletin* 27/28:9–33.

1990a Mounds, embankments and ceremonialism in the Trans-Mississippi South. Proceedings of the Eleventh Annual Mid-South Archeological Conference.

1990b The "Northern Caddoan Area" was not Caddoan. *Caddoan Archeology* 1(4):4–9.

SCHAMBACH, F. F. (EDITOR)

1991 *Coles Creek and Mississippi period foragers in the Felsenthal region of the lower Mississippi Valley: Evidence from the Bangs Slough site, Southeast Arkansas.* Research Series, no. 40. Fayetteville: Arkansas Archeological Survey.

SCHAMBACH, F. F., AND A. M. EARLY

1983 Southwest Arkansas. In *A state plan for the conservation of archeological resources in Arkansas,* ed. H. A. Davis. Research Series, no. 21. Fayetteville: Arkansas Archeological Survey.

SCHAMBACH, F. F., AND J. E. MILLER

1984 A description and analysis of the ceramics. In *Cedar Grove: An interdisciplinary investigation of a late Caddo farmstead in the Red River Valley,* ed. N. L. Trubowitz, 109–170. Research Series, no. 23. Fayetteville: Arkansas Archeological Survey.

SCHAMBACH, F. F., N. L. TRUBOWITZ, F. RACKERBY, E. T. HEMMINGS, W. F. LIMP, AND J. E. MILLER

1983 Test excavations at the Cedar Grove site (3LA97): A late Caddo farmstead in the Great Bend region, Southwest Arkansas. In *Contributions to the archeology of the Great Bend region,* ed. F. F. Schambach and F. Rackerby, 90–129. Research Series, no. 22. Fayetteville: Arkansas Archeological Survey.

SCHILZ, T. F., AND D. E. WORCESTER

1987 The spread of firearms among the Indian tribes on the northern frontier of New Spain. *American Indian Quarterly* 11(1):1–10.

SCHOENINGER, M. J., K. M. HIEBERT, AND N. VAN DER MERWE

1987 Decrease in diet quality between the Prehistoric and the Contact period on St. Catherines Island. Paper presented at the American Association of Physical Anthropologists Conference, New York.

SCURLOCK, J. D.

1962 The Culpepper site, A late Fulton aspect site in Northeast Texas. *Bulletin of the Texas Archeological Society* 32:285–316.

SENEX, JOHN

1717 A map of Louisiana and the Mississippi River. Louisiana Room, map no. 1134, Northwestern State University, Natchitoches, Louisiana.

SHAFER, H. J.

1981 Archeological investigations at the Attaway site, Henderson County, Texas. *Bulletin of the Texas Archeological Society* 52:147–179.

SIBLEY, J.

1832 Historical sketches of several Indian tribes in Louisiana, south of the Arkansas River, and between the Mississippi and River Grande. In *American state papers* (Class II, Indian Affairs), vol. 1, 721–725. Washington, D.C.: Gales & Seaton.

1922 *A report from Natchitoches in 1807,* ed. A. H. Abel. Indian notes and monographs. New York: Museum of the American Indian and the Heye Foundation.

SILVERBERG, R.

1968 *Mound builders of ancient America: The archaeology of a myth.* New York: Graphic Society.

SKILES, B. D., J. E. BRUSETH, AND T. K. PERTTULA

1980 A synthesis of the upper Sabine River basin culture history. *The Record* 36:1–12.

SKINNER, S. A., R. K. HARRIS, AND K. M. ANDERSON (EDITORS)

1969 *Archaeological investigations at the Sam Kaufman site, Red River County, Texas.* Contributions in Anthropology, no. 5. Dallas: Southern Methodist University.

SMITH, B. D.

1982 The division of mound exploration of the Bureau of (American) Ethnology and the birth of American archaeology. *Bulletin of the Southeastern Archaeological Conference* 24:51–54.

1985 Introduction. In *Report on the mound explorations of the Bureau of Ethnology,* by C. Thomas, 1–17. Classics in Anthropology Series. Washington, D.C.: Smithsonian Institution Press.

1986 The archaeology of the southeastern United States: From Dalton to De Soto, 10,500 B.P.–500 B.P. In *Advances in world archaeology,* ed. F. Wendorf and A. E. Close, 1–92. New York: Academic Press.

SMITH, B. D. (EDITOR)

1990 *The Mississippian emergence.* Washington, D.C.: Smithsonian Institution Press.

SMITH, M. T.

1984 Depopulation and culture change in the early Historic period interior Southeast. Ph.D. diss., University of Florida, Gainesville.

1987 *Archaeology of aboriginal culture change in the interior Southeast: Depopulation during the Early Historic period.* Gainesville: University of Florida Press.

1989 Indian responses to European contact: The Coosa example. In *First encounters: Spanish exploration in the Caribbean and the United States, 1492–1570,* ed. J. T. Milanich and S. Milbrath, 135–149. Ripley F. Bullen Monographs in Anthropology and History, no. 9. Gainesville: University of Florida Press.

SNOW, D. R., AND K. M. LANPHEAR

1988 European contact and Indian depopulation in the Northeast: The timing of the first epidemics. *Ethnohistory* 35:15–33.

SNOW, D. R., AND W. A. STARNA

1984 Sixteenth-century depopulation: A preliminary view from the Mohawk Valley. Paper presented at the Forty-ninth Annual Meeting of the Society for American Archaeology, Portland.

SOCIAL SCIENCE RESEARCH COUNCIL

1954 Acculturation: An exploratory formulation. *American Anthropologist* 56 (3):973–1002.

SPAULDING, A. C.

1983 Archaeological theory: 1936. In *Lulu Linear Punctated: Essays in honor of George Irving Quimby,* ed. R. C. Dunnell and D. K. Grayson, 19–25. Anthropological Papers, no. 72. Ann Arbor: Museum of Anthropology, University of Michigan.

SPICER, E. H.

1962 *Cycles of conquest: The impact of Spain, Mexico, and the United States on the Indians of the Southwest, 1533–1960.* Tucson: University of Arizona Press.

SPIELMANN, K. A.

1983 Late Prehistoric exchange between the Southwest and southern plains. *Plains Anthropologist* 28:257–272.

1989 Colonists, hunters, and farmers: Plains-pueblo interaction in the seventeenth century. In *Columbian consequences.* Vol. 1, *Archaeological and historical perspectives on the Spanish Borderlands West,* ed. D. H. Thomas, 101–113. Washington, D.C.: Smithsonian Institution Press.

SPIESS, A. E., AND B. D. SPIESS

1987 New England pandemic of 1616–1622: Cause and archaeological implications. *Man in the Northeast* 34:71–83.

STEELY, S.

1986 *Six months from Tennessee.* Wolfe City, Texas: Hennington Publishing Co.

STEPONAITIS, V. P.

1986 Prehistoric archaeology in the southeastern United States, 1970–1985. *Annual Reviews in Anthropology* 15:363–404.

STEVENS, W. E.

1916 The organization of the British fur trade, 1760–1800. *Mississippi Valley Historical Review* 3:172–202.

STEWARD, J. H.

1942 The direct historical approach to archaeology. *American Antiquity* 7: 337–343.

1954 Theory and application in a social science. *Ethnohistory* 1:292–302.

STODDARD, A.

1812 *Sketches, historical and descriptive, of Louisiana.* Philadelphia: William Carey.

STODDER, A. L. W.

1986 Pueblo health in the Protohistoric: Paleopathology and other lines of evidence. Paper presented at the Second Annual Conference on Health and Disease in the Prehistoric Southwest, 22 November, University of New Mexico, Albuquerque.

STORY, D. A.

1967 Pottery vessels from the Gilbert site. In *The Gilbert site: A Norteno focus site in Northeastern Texas,* ed. E. B. Jelks, 37–112. *Bulletin of the Texas Archeological Society,* vol. 37.

1978 Some comments on anthropological studies concerning the Caddo. In *Texas Archeology,* ed. K. D. House, 46–68. Dallas: Southern Methodist University Press.

1981 An overview of the archaeology of East Texas. *Plains Anthropologist* 26:139–156.

1984 A review of the investigations at Cedar Grove. In *Cedar Grove: An interdisciplinary investigation of a late Caddo farmstead in the Red River Valley,* ed. N. L. Trubowitz, 278–280. Research Series, no. 23. Fayetteville: Arkansas Archeological Survey.

1985a Adaptive strategies of archaic cultures of the West Gulf Coastal Plain. In *Prehistoric food production in North America,* ed. R. I. Ford. Anthropological Papers, no. 75. Ann Arbor: Museum of Anthropology, University of Michigan.

1985b The Walton site: An historic burial in McLennan County, Texas. *Central Texas Archaeologist* 10:66–96.

1990 Cultural history of the native Americans. In *The archeology and bioarcheology of the Gulf Coastal Plain,* by D. A. Story, J. A. Guy, B. A. Burnett, M. D. Freeman, J. C. Rose, D. G. Steele, B. W. Olive, and K. J. Reinhard, 163–366. Research Series, no. 38. Fayetteville: Arkansas Archeological Survey.

STORY, D. A. (EDITOR)

1982 *The Deshazo site, Nacogdoches County, Texas.* Vol. 1. Texas Antiquities Committee, Texas Antiquities Permit Series, no. 7. Austin: Texas Historical Commission.

n.d. *The Deshazo site, Nacogdoches County, Texas.* Vol. 2, The native-made artifacts and synthesis. Manuscript on file, Texas Archeological Research Laboratory, The University of Texas at Austin.

STORY, D. A., AND D. G. CREEL

1982 The cultural setting. In *The Deshazo site, Nacogdoches County, Texas,* ed. D. A. Story, 20–34. Texas Antiquities Committee, Texas Antiquities Permit Series, no. 7. Austin: Texas Historical Commission.

STORY, D. A., AND E. M. DAVIS

1983 Woodland and Caddoan cultural units in the Trans-Mississippi South. Manuscript on file, Department of Anthropology, The University of Texas at Austin.

STORY, D. A., J. GUY, B. A. BURNETT, M. D. FREEMAN, J. C. ROSE, D. G. STEELE, B. W. OLIVE, AND K. J. REINHARD

1990 *Archeology and bioarcheology of the Gulf Coastal Plain.* 2 vols. Research Series, no. 38. Fayetteville: Arkansas Archeological Survey.

STRICKLAND, R. W.

1937 Anglo-American activities in northeastern Texas 1803–1845. Ph.D. diss., The University of Texas at Austin.

1942 Moscoso's journey through Texas. *Southwestern Historical Quarterly* 46:109–137.

STUBBS, J. R.

1982 The Chickasaw contact with the La Salle expedition in 1682. In *La Salle and his Legacy: Frenchmen and Indians in the lower Mississippi Valley,* ed. P. K. Galloway, 41–47. Jackson: University Press of Mississippi.

STUIVER, M., AND B. BECKER

1986 High-precision decadal calibration of the radiocarbon time scale, A.D. 1950–2500 B.C. *Radiocarbon* 28(2B):863–910.

STYLES, B. W., AND J. R. PURDUE

1984 Faunal exploitation at the Cedar Grove site. In *Cedar Grove: An interdisciplinary investigation of a late Caddo farmstead in the Red River Valley,* ed. N. L. Trubowitz, 211–226. Research Series, no. 23. Fayetteville: Arkansas Archeological Survey.

SUHM, D. A., AND E. B. JELKS

1962 *Handbook of Texas archeology: Type descriptions.* Texas Archeological Society Special Bulletin 1 and Texas Memorial Museum Bulletin 4. Austin: Texas Archeological Society and Texas Memorial Museum.

SUHM, D. A., A. D. KRIEGER, AND E. B. JELKS

1954 *An introductory handbook of Texas archeology. Bulletin of the Texas Archeological Society,* vol. 25.

SURREY, N. M. M.

1916 *The commerce of Louisiana during the French regime, 1699–1763.* Columbia University Studies in History, Economics, and Public Law, vol. 71. New York: Columbia University.

SWAGERTY, W. R.

1984 Spanish-Indian relations, 1513–1821. In *Scholars and the Indian experience: Critical review of recent writings in the social sciences,* ed. W. R. Swagerty, 36–78. Bloomington: Indiana University Press for the D'Arcy McNickle Center for the History of the American Indian.

1989 Indian trade in the Trans-Mississippi West to 1870. In *Handbook of North American Indians.* Vol. 4, *History of Indian-white relations,* ed. W. E. Washburn, 351–374. Washington, D.C.: Smithsonian Institution Press.

SWANTON, J. R.

1911 *Indian tribes of the Lower Mississippi Valley and adjacent coast of the Gulf of Mexico.* Bulletin 43. Washington, D.C.: Bureau of American Ethnology, Smithsonian Institution.

1939 *Final report of the United States De Soto Expedition Commission.* Report prepared for the U.S. House of Representatives, 76th Cong., 1st sess. H. Doc. 71.

1942 *Source material on the history and ethnology of the Caddo Indians.* Bulletin 132. Washington, D.C.: Bureau of American Ethnology, Smithsonian Institution.

1946 *The Indians of the Southeastern United States.* Bulletin 137. Washington, D.C.: Bureau of American Ethnology, Smithsonian Institution.

SWANTON, J. R., AND R. B. DIXON

1914 Primitive American history. *American Anthropologist* 16:376–412.

TANNER, H. H.

1974 The territory of the Caddo tribe of Oklahoma. In *Caddoan Indians,* vol. 4, 9–144. New York: Garland Publishings.

TATE, M. L.

1986 *The Indians of Texas: An annotated research bibliography.* Native American Bibliography Series, no. 9. Metuchen, N.J.: Scarecrow Press.

TERÁN, DON MANUEL DE MIER Y

1870 Noticia de las tribus de salvajes conocidos que habitan el Departamento de Tejas, y del número de familias de que consta cada tribu, puntos en que habitan y terrenos en que acampan. *Sociedad de Geografía y Estadística de La República Méxicana Boletín* (n.s.) 2:264–269.

THOMAS, A. B. (EDITOR AND TRANSLATOR)

1935 *After Coronado: Spanish exploration northeast of New Mexico, 1696–1727: Documents from the archives of Spain, Mexico, and New Mexico.* Norman: University of Oklahoma Press.

THOMAS, C.

1894 *Report of the mound explorations of the Bureau of Ethnology.* Twelfth Annual Report of the Bureau of Ethnology. Washington, D.C.: Bureau of Ethnology, Smithsonian Institution.

THOMAS, D. H.

1987 The archaeology of Mission Santa Catalina de Guale: 1. Search and discovery. *Anthropological Papers of the American Museum of Natural History* 63 (pt. 2):47–161.

1988 Saints and soldiers at Santa Catalina: Hispanic designs for colonial America. In *The recovery of meaning,* ed. M. P. Leone and P. B. Potter, 73–140. Washington, D.C.: Smithsonian Institution Press.

THOMAS, D. H. (EDITOR)

1989 *Columbian consequences.* Vol. 1, *Archaeological and historical perspectives on the Spanish Borderlands West.* Washington, D.C.: Smithsonian Institution Press.

1990a *Columbian consequences.* Vol. 2, *Archaeological and historical perspectives on the Spanish Borderlands East.* Washington, D.C.: Smithsonian Institution Press.

1990b *The Spanish Borderlands sourcebooks.* 30 vols. New York: Garland Publishing.

1991 *Columbian consequences.* Vol. 3, *The Spanish Borderlands in Pan-American perspective.* Washington, D.C.: Smithsonian Institution Press.

THORNTON, R.

1986 *We shall live again: The 1870 and 1890 Ghost Dance movements as demographic revitalization.* New York: Cambridge University Press.

1987 *American Indian holocaust and survival: A population history since 1492.* Norman: University of Oklahoma Press.

THORNTON, R., AND J. M. THORNTON

1981 Estimating prehistoric Indian population size for United States area: Implications of the nineteenth-century population decline and nadir. *American Journal of Physical Anthropology* 55:47–53.

THURMOND, J. P.

1981 Archeology of the Cypress Creek drainage basin, Northeastern Texas and Northwestern Louisiana. Master's thesis, The University of Texas at Austin.

1985 Late Caddoan social group identifications and sociopolitical organization in the upper Cypress Basin and its vicinity, Northeastern Texas. *Bulletin of the Texas Archeological Society* 54:185–200.

1990a *Archeology of the Cypress Creek drainage basin, Northeastern Texas and Northwestern Louisiana.* Studies in Archeology, no. 5. Austin: Texas Archeological Research Laboratory, The University of Texas at Austin.

1990b Was the Cypress Cluster one of the (many) victims of the 1539–1543 De Soto expedition? *Caddoan Archeology Newsletter* 1(3):5–11.

TRIGGER, B. G.

1975 Brecht and ethnohistory. *Ethnohistory* 22:51–56.

1980 Archaeology and the image of the American Indian. *American Antiquity* 45:662–676.

1981a Archaeology and the ethnographic present. *Anthropologica* 23:1–17.

1981b Ontario native people and the epidemics of 1634–1640. In *Indians, animals, and the fur trade,* ed. S. Krech III, 19–38. Athens: University of Georgia Press.

1982 Ethnohistory: Problems and prospects. *Ethnohistory* 29:1–19.

1983 American archaeology as native history: A review essay. *William and Mary Quarterly* 40:413–452.

1985 *Natives and newcomers: Canada's 'Heroic Age' reconsidered.* Montreal: McGill-Queen's University Press.

1986a Ethnohistory: The unfinished edifice. *Ethnohistory* 33:253–267.

1986b Prehistoric archaeology and American society. In *American archaeology past and future: A celebration of the Society for American Archaeology 1935–1985,* ed. D. J. Meltzer, D. D. Fowler, and J. A. Sabloff, 187–215. Washington, D.C.: Smithsonian Institution Press.

1990 North American archaeology in the 1990s. *Antiquity* 64:778–787.

TRIMBLE, M. K.

1985 Epidemiology on the northern plains: A cultural perspective. Ph.D. diss., University of Missouri–Columbia.

1986 *An ethnohistorical interpretation of the spread of smallpox in the northern plains utilizing concepts of disease ecology.* Reprints in Anthropology, no. 33. Lincoln: J&L Reprints.

1988 Cycles of infectious disease on the upper Missouri. Paper presented at the Forty-first Plains Conference, 2–5 November, Wichita State University, Wichita.

TRUBOWITZ, N. L.

1984 *Cedar Grove: An interdisciplinary investigation of a late Caddo farmstead in the Red River Valley.* Research Series, no. 23. Fayetteville: Arkansas Archeological Survey.

1987 New goods on old routes: Exchange in the Contact era in eastern North America. Paper presented at the Fifty-second Annual Meeting of the Society for American Archaeology, 6–10 May, Toronto.

TURNER, F. J.

1977 [1891]. *The character and influence of the Indian trade in Wisconsin: A study of the trading post as an institution.* Ed. D. H. Miller and W. W. Savage, Jr. Norman: University of Oklahoma Press.

TURNER, R. L.

1978 The Tuck Carpenter site and its relation to other sites within the Titus focus. *Bulletin of the Texas Archeological Society* 49:1–110.

TYSON, C. N.

1981 *The Red River in southwestern history.* Norman: University of Oklahoma Press.

UBELAKER, D. H.

1976 The sources and methodology for Mooney's estimates of North American Indian populations. In *The native populations of the Americas in 1492*, ed. W. M. Denevan, 243–288. Madison: University of Wisconsin Press.

UBELAKER, D. H., AND R. L. JANTZ

1986 Biological history of the aboriginal population of North America. *Rassengeschichte der Menschheit* 2:7–79.

UPHAM, S.

1986 Smallpox and climate in the American Southwest. *American Anthropologist* 88:115–128.

1987 Understanding the disease history of the Southwest: A reply to Reff. *American Anthropologist* 89:708–710.

U.S. CONGRESS. HOUSE.

1847 *Report on the Texas Indians—Report of Mssrs. Butler and Lewis.* 29th Cong., 2d sess. H. Doc. 76.

U.S. CONGRESS. SENATE.

1989 A Report of the Special Committee on Investigations of the Select Committee on Indian Affairs. Final report and legislative recommendations. 101st Cong., 1st sess. Report 101-216.

U.S. TREASURY DEPARTMENT

1790–1884 *Annual reports.* 48th Cong., 1st sess. H. Misc. Doc. 49, pt. 2, 32,130. Serial 2236.

USNER, D. H.

1981 Frontier exchange in the lower Mississippi Valley: Race relations and economic life in Colonial Louisiana, 1699–1763. Ph.D. diss., Duke University, Durham, N.C.

1985 The deerskin trade in French Louisiana. In *Proceedings of the Tenth Meeting of the French Colonial Historical Society,* ed. P. B. Boucher, 75–93. Boston: University Press of America.

1987 The frontier exchange economy of the lower Mississippi Valley in the eighteenth century. *William and Mary Quarterly* 44:165–192.

1989 Economic relations in the Southeast until 1783. In *Handbook of North American Indians.* Vol. 4, *History of Indian-white relations,* ed. W. E. Washburn, 391–395. Washington, D.C.: Smithsonian Institution Press.

In press Indians, settlers, and slaves in a frontier exchange economy: The lower Mississippi Valley before 1783. *William and Mary Quarterly.*

VARNER, J. G., AND J. J. VARNER (EDITORS AND TRANSLATORS)

1951 *The Florida of the Inca.* Austin: University of Texas Press.

VEGA, G. DE LA

1951 *The Florida of the Inca,* ed. and trans. J. G. Varner and J. J. Varner. Austin: University of Texas Press.

VEHIK, S. C.

1986 Onate's expedition to the southern plains: Routes, destinations, and implications for late Prehistoric cultural adaptations. *Plains Anthropologist* 31:13–33.

1988 Late Prehistoric exchange on the southern plains and its periphery. *Midcontinental Journal of Archaeology* 13:41–68.

1989 Problems and potential in Plains Indian demography. In *Plains Indian historical demography and health: Perspectives, interpretations, and critiques,* ed. G. R. Campbell, 115–125. *Plains Anthropologist* 34(124), pt. 2, Memoir 23.

1990 Late Prehistoric Plains trade and economic specialization. *Plains Anthropologist* 35(128):125–145.

VERLEY, M.

1964 The Camden ceramic complex within Ouachita County, Arkansas. Master's thesis, University of Illinois, Urbana.

VOORRIPS, A., AND J. M. O'SHEA

1987 Conditional spatial patterning: Beyond the nearest neighbor. *American Antiquity* 52:500–521.

WADE, M.

1989 French Indian Policies. In *Handbook of North American Indians.* Vol. 4, *History of Indian-white relations,* ed. W. E. Washburn, 20–28. Washington, D.C.: Smithsonian Institution Press.

WALKER, P. L., P. LAMBERT, AND M. J. DENIRO

1989 The effects of European contact on the health of Alta California Indians. In *Columbian consequences.* Vol. 1, *Archaeological and historical per-*

spectives on the Spanish Borderlands West, ed. D. H. Thomas, 349–364. Washington, D.C.: Smithsonian Institution Press.

WALKER, W. M.

1932 Prehistoric cultures of Louisiana. In *Conferences of southern pre-history.* Division of Anthropology and Psychology, Committee on State Archaeological Surveys, Birmingham, Ala. Washington, D.C.: National Research Council.

1935 *A Caddo burial site at Natchitoches, Louisiana.* Smithsonian Miscellaneous Collections, vol. 94(14). Washington, D.C.: Smithsonian Institution.

1936 *The Troyville mounds, Catahoula Parish, Louisiana.* Bulletin 113. Washington, D.C.: Bureau of American Ethnology, Smithsonian Institution.

WALLERSTEIN, I.

1974–1980 *The modern world-system.* 2 vols. New York: Academic Press.

WASELKOV, G. A.

1989 Seventeenth-century trade in the colonial southeast. *Southeastern Archaeology* 8:117–133.

WASHBURN, W. E. (EDITOR)

1989 *Handbook of North American Indians.* Vol. 4, *History of Indian-white relations.* Washington, D.C.: Smithsonian Institution Press.

WATKINS, B.

1984 Historical background. In *Cedar Grove: An interdisciplinary investigation of a late Caddo farmstead in the Red River Valley,* ed. N. L. Trubowitz, 44–55. Research Series, no. 23. Fayetteville: Arkansas Archeological Survey.

WEBB, C. H.

1945 Second Historic Caddo site at Natchitoches. *Bulletin of the Texas Archeological and Paleontological Society* 16:52–83.

1959 *The Belcher mound, a stratified Caddoan site in Caddo Parish, Louisiana.* Memoirs, no. 16. Kenosha, Wis.: Society for American Archaeology.

1983 The Bossier focus revisited: Montgomery I, Werner, and other unicomponent sites. In *Southeastern natives and their pasts,* ed. D. G. Wyckoff and J. L. Hofman, 183–240. Studies in Oklahoma's Past, no. 11. Norman: Oklahoma Archeological Survey.

1984 Ceremonial materials in Caddoan burial assemblages on the Red River in Northwestern Louisiana. Paper presented at the Southern Ceremonial Complex Conference, 27–29 September, Cottonlandia Museum, Greenwood, Miss.

WEBB, C. H., AND M. DODD

1939 Further excavations at the Gahagan Mound: Connections with a Florida culture. *Bulletin of the Texas Archeological and Paleontological Society* 11:92–128.

1941 Pottery types from the Belcher Mound site. *Bulletin of the Texas Archeological and Paleontological Society* 13:88–116.

WEBB, C. H., AND H. F. GREGORY

1978 *The Caddo Indians of Louisiana.* Louisiana Archaeological Survey and Antiquities Commission, Anthropological Study no. 2. Baton Rouge: Louisiana Department of Culture, Recreation and Tourism.

WEBB, C. H., AND R. R. MCKINNEY

1975 Mounds Plantation (16CD12), Caddo Parish, Louisiana. *Louisiana Archaeology* 2:39–128.

WEBB, C. H., F. MURPHEY, W. G. ELLIS, AND H. R. GREEN

1969 The Resch site, 41HS16, Harrison County, Texas. *Bulletin of the Texas Archeological Society* 40:3–106.

WEDDLE, R. S.

1973 *Wilderness manhunt: The Spanish search for La Salle.* Austin: University of Texas Press.

1985 *Spanish sea: Discovery on the Gulf of Mexico, 1500–1685.* College Station: Texas A&M University Press.

WEDEL, M. M.

1971 J. B. Bénard de La Harpe: Visitor to the Wichitas in 1719. *Great Plains Journal* 10(2):37–70.

1972 Claude-Charles Dutisné: A review of his 1719 journeys, part I. *Great Plains Journal* 12(1):5–25.

1973 Claude-Charles Dutisné: A review of his 1719 journeys, part II. *Great Plains Journal* 12(2):147–173.

1974 The Bénard de La Harpe historiography on French colonial Louisiana. *Louisiana Studies* 13(1).

1978 *La Harpe's 1719 post on Red River and nearby Caddo settlements.* Bulletin 30. Austin: The Texas Memorial Museum.

1979 The ethnohistoric approach to Plains Caddoan origins. *Nebraska History* 60:183–196.

1981 *The Deer Creek site, Oklahoma: A Wichita village sometimes called Ferdinandiana, an ethnohistorian's view.* Series in Anthropology, no. 5. Oklahoma City: Oklahoma Historical Society.

1982 The Wichita Indians in the Arkansas River basin. In *Plains Indian studies: A collection of essays in honor of John C. Ewers and Waldo R. Wedel,* ed. D. H. Ubelaker and H. J. Viola, 118–133. Smithsonian Contributions to Anthropology, no. 30. Washington, D.C.: Smithsonian Institution Press.

1988 *The Wichita Indians 1541–1750: Ethnohistorical essays.* Reprints in Anthropology, vol. 38. Lincoln: J&L Reprint Co.

WEINSTEIN, R. A., AND D. B. KELLEY

1984 *Archaeology and paleogeography of the upper Felsenthal region: Cultural resources investigations in the Calion Navigation Pool, South-Central Arkansas.* Baton Rouge: Coastal Environments.

WHITAKER, A. P.

1928 The commerce of Louisiana and the Floridas at the end of the eighteenth century. *Hispanic American Historical Review* 8:190–203.

WHITE, D.

1970 Investigations of the cemetery at the Gee's landing site, 3DR17. *The Arkansas Archeologist* 11:1–20.

WHITE, R.

1983 *The roots of dependency: Subsistence, environment, and social change among the Choctaws, Pawnees, and Navajos*. Lincoln: University of Nebraska Press.

WHITE, R., AND W. CRONON

1989 Ecological change and Indian-white relations. In *Handbook of North American Indians*. Vol. 4, *History of Indian-white relations,* ed. W. E. Washburn, 417–429. Washington, D.C.: Smithsonian Institution Press.

WIEGERS, R. P.

1988 A proposal for Indian slave trading in the Mississippi Valley and its impact on the Osage. *Plains Anthropologist* 33(120):187–202.

WILLEY, G. R., AND P. PHILLIPS

1958 *Method and theory in American archaeology.* Chicago: University of Chicago Press.

WILLEY, G. R., AND J. A. SABLOFF

1974 *A history of American archaeology*. San Francisco: W. H. Freeman.

WILLIAMS, I., AND A. M. EARLY

1990 Hardman (3CL418): A prehistoric salt processing site. Sponsored Research Program, Arkansas Archeological Survey. Final report, Project no. 642, Fayetteville.

WILLIAMS, J. W.

1942 Moscoso's trail in Texas. *Southwestern Historical Quarterly* 46:138–157.

1979 *Old Texas trails*. Austin: Eakin Press.

WILLIAMS, S.

1964 The aboriginal locations of the Kadohadacho and related tribes. In *Exploration in cultural anthropology,* ed. W. Goodenough, 545–570. New Haven: Yale University Press.

1980 The Armorel phase: A very late complex in the lower Mississippi Valley. *Bulletin of the Southeastern Archaeological Conference* 22:105–110.

WILLIAMS, S., AND J. P. BRAIN

1983 *Excavations at the Lake George site, Yazoo County, Mississippi, 1958–1960*. Papers of the Peabody Museum of Archaeology and Ethnology, Harvard University, vol. 74. Cambridge: Peabody Museum.

WILSON, R.

1962 The A. W. Davis site, Mc-6, of McCurtain County, Oklahoma. *Bulletin of the Oklahoma Anthropological Society* 10:103–152.

WILSON, S. M., AND J. D. ROGERS

1992 Historical dynamics in the Contact era. In *Perspectives on change: Ethnohistorical and archaeological approaches to culture contact,* ed. J. D. Rogers and S. M. Wilson. New York: Plenum Press.

WINFREY, D. H., AND J. M. DAY (EDITORS)

1966 *The Indian papers of Texas and the Southwest, 1825–1916.* 5 vols. Austin: Pemberton Press.

WISSLER, C.

1914 Material cultures of the North American Indians. *American Anthropologist* 16:447–505.

WITTHOFT, J.

1967 Archaeology as a key to the colonial fur trade. In *Aspects of the fur trade: Selected papers of the 1965 North American fur trade conference,* ed. R. W. Fridley and J. D. Holmquist, 55–61. St. Paul: Minnesota Historical Society.

WITTY, T. A.

1983 An archaeological review of the Scott County Pueblo. *Bulletin of the Oklahoma Anthropological Society* 32:99–106.

WOLDERT, A.

1942 The expedition of Luis de Moscoso in Texas in 1542. *Southwestern Historical Quarterly* 46:158–166.

1952 Relics of possible Indian battle in Wood County, Texas. *Southwestern Historical Quarterly* 55:484–489.

WOLF, E. R.

1982 *Europe and the people without history.* Berkeley: University of California Press.

1984 Culture: Panacea or problem? *American Antiquity* 49:393–400.

WOLFE, R. J.

1982 Alaska's great sickness, 1900: An epidemic of measles and influenza in a virgin soil population. *Proceedings of the American Philosophical Society* 126:92–121.

WOLFMAN, D.

1982 Archeomagnetic dating in Arkansas and the border areas of adjacent states. In *Arkansas archeology in review,* ed. N. L. Trubowitz and M. D. Jeter, 277–300. Research Series, no. 15. Fayetteville: Arkansas Archeological Survey.

1984 Cedar Grove chronometrics. In *Cedar Grove: An interdisciplinary investigation of a late Caddo farmstead in the Red River Valley,* ed. N. L. Trubowitz, 257–262. Research Series, no. 23. Fayetteville: Arkansas Archeological Survey.

WOOD, P. H.

1989 The changing population of the colonial South: An overview by race and region, 1685–1790. In *Powhatan's mantle: Indians in the colonial Southeast,* ed. P. H. Wood, G. A. Waselkov, and M. T. Hatley, 35–103. Lincoln: University of Nebraska Press.

WOODALL, J. N.

1969 Cultural ecology of the Caddo. Ph.D. diss., Southern Methodist University, Dallas.

1980 The Caddoan confederacies—Some ecological considerations. *Louisiana Archaeology* 6:127–171.

WOODS, P. D.

1980 *French-Indian relations on the southern frontier, 1699–1762.* Studies in American History and Culture, no. 18. Ann Arbor: University of Michigan Research Press.

WORCESTER, D. E.

1944 The spread of Spanish horses in the Southwest. *New Mexico Historical Review* 19:225–232.

WYCKOFF, D. G.

1967 *The E. Johnson site and prehistory in southeast Oklahoma.* Oklahoma River Basin Survey, Archaeological Site Report no. 6. Norman: University of Oklahoma.

1970 Archaeological and historical assessment of the Red River basin in Oklahoma. In *Archaeological and historical assessment of the Red River basin,* ed. H. A. Davis, 67–134. Research Series, no. 1. Fayetteville: Arkansas Archeological Survey.

1974 *The Caddoan area: An archaeological perspective.* New York: Garland Press.

1980 Caddoan adaptive strategies in the Arkansas basin, eastern Oklahoma. Ph.D. diss., Washington State University, Pullman.

WYCKOFF, D. G., AND T. G. BAUGH

1980 Early historic Hasinai elites: A model for the material culture of governing elites. *Midcontinental Journal of Archaeology* 5:225–283.

WYCKOFF, D. G., AND L. R. FISHER

1985 *Preliminary testing and evaluation of the Grobin Davis archaeological site, 34Mc-253, McCurtain County, Oklahoma.* Archeological Resource Survey Report no. 22. Norman: Oklahoma Archeological Survey.

YATES, B. C.

1986 Vertebrate faunal remains. In *French-Indian interaction at an eighteenth-century frontier post: The Roseborough Lake site, Bowie County, Texas,* by K. Gilmore, 107–129. Contributions in Archaeology, no. 3. Denton: Institute of Applied Sciences, North Texas State University.

YELTON, J. K.

1985 The depopulation of the Osage and Missouri tribes. Osage and Missouri Indian life cultural change: 1675–1825, Part Four. Final Performance Report on National Endowment for the Humanities Research Grant RS-20296, University of Missouri, Columbia.

YOUNG, G. A., AND M. P. HOFFMAN (EDITORS)

In press *The Expedition of Hernando de Soto in the West, 1541–1543.* Proceedings of the de Soto Expedition Symposia, University Museum, University of Arkansas, October 1988 and March 1990. Fayetteville: University of Arkansas Press.

ZUBROW, E.

1990 The depopulation of native America. *Antiquity* 64:754–764.

Index